School Programs in
Speech-Language

School Programs in Speech-Language

Organization and Management

Third Edition

Elizabeth A. Neidecker, Associate Professor Emerita
Bowling Green State University

Jean L. Blosser, Professor
University of Akron

PRENTICE HALL
ENGLEWOOD CLIFFS, NEW JERSEY 07632

Library of Congress Cataloging-in-Publication Data

Neidecker, Elizabeth A.
    School programs in speech-language : organization and management /
Elizabeth A. Neidecker, Jean L. Blosser. — 3rd ed.
        p.   cm.
    Includes bibliographical references and index.
    ISBN 0-13-792268-X
    1. Speech therapy for children—United States—Curricula.
2. Speech therapy—Vocational guidance—United States. I. Blosser,
Jean. II. Title.
LB3454.N44   1991
371.91'42—dc20   92–18228
                                                                                    CIP

Acquisition Editor: Julie Berrisford
Production Editors: Fred Dahl and Rose Kernan
Copy Editor: Rose Kernan
Designers: Fred Dahl and Rose Kernan
Prepress Buyer: Kelly Behr
Manufacturing Buyer: Mary Ann Gloriande

© 1993 by Prentice Hall
A Simon & Schuster Company
Englewood Cliffs, New Jersey 07632

PRINTED IN THE UNITED STATES OF AMERICA

10 9 8 7 6 5

ISBN 0-13-792268-X

PRENTICE-HALL INTERNATIONAL (UK) LIMITED, *London*
PRENTICE-HALL OF AUSTRALIA PTY. LIMITED, *Sydney*
PRENTICE-HALL CANADA INC., *Toronto*
PRENTICE-HALL HISPANOAMERICANA, S.A., *Mexico*
PRENTICE-HALL OF INDIA PRIVATE LIMITED, *New Delhi*
PRENTICE-HALL OF JAPAN, INC., *Tokyo*
PRENTICE-HALL OF SOUTHEAST ASIA PTE. LTD., *Singapore*
EDITORA PRENTICE-HALL DO BRASIL, LTDA., *Rio de Janeiro*

This book is dedicated to our families:
Mary, Bill, Renick, Trevor and
in memory of
Fred, Alpha, John, and Nancy

Contents

CHAPTER 8

Intervention: Planning, Implementing, Evaluating, 206

CHAPTER 9

Working with Others: Collaboration and Consultation, 252

Preface

In this, the third edition of *School Programs in Speech-Language: Organization and Management,* you will see a new name: Jean Blosser, Ed.D., who is my co-author; I am happy to introduce her to you. Jean brings to the book her experience as a public school clinician, a university professor, an author and editor, a frequent participant in national and state professional programs and organizations, and a supervisor of students in the public schools and the university clinic. Dr. Blosser is Director of the Speech and Hearing Center, School of Communicative Disorders, The University of Akron.

In this new edition we have sought not only to bring the text up-to-date but also to re-write it to meet the needs of a new generation of students about to enter the profession in the schools. We have also geared this edition to the school speech-language pathologist already in the field who is facing a vast array of new information, research, roles, program options, government regulations, and the expanding scope and responsibilities inherent in the school system.

The major premise of this book, however, remains the same: the school speech-language pathologist is committed to the idea that communication skills are prerequisite to the acquisition of educational skills and knowledge of a subject. The role of the school clinician is to prevent, alleviate, and remove communication barriers that hinder the student from profiting from the instruction offered in the classroom. There is much talk today about improving schools in the United States. It seems to us that the school speech-language pathologist can have an important role in this endeavor by removing communication barriers thereby enhancing the child's access to a good education.

Chapter One traces the growth and development of the profession in the schools, including the philosophy that invited speech and hearing programs into the school system and the expansion of those programs, both geographically and professionally.

Chapter Two discusses professionalism, accreditation, certification, and licensure. Ethical considerations are examined as well as professional agencies and organizations. The current Code of Ethics of the American Speech-Language-Hearing Association is included in this chapter.

Chapter Three presents the foundations of school programs, including organizational structure of the school system, funding for speech, language, and hearing programs, as well as Public Laws 94-142, 99-457, and 101-476 and their impact on current practices. The prevalence and incidence of speech, language, and hearing problems among school children is also discussed. The role of parents as team members with speech-language pathologists and school personnel is explored.

Chapter Four is concerned with the management roles of the school speech-language clinician, including the management of time, resources, and personnel. Writing goals and objectives for the program is described as well as the application of management principles and strategies for long range planning.

Chapter Five is a comprehensive description of the "tools of the trade." These include physical facilities, space, materials, equipment, and technology (augmentative and alternative communication systems, assistive listening devices, computers, and software). A checklist for assessing the quality of physical facilities and equipment is included. Facility requirements for special populations are described. The process of assuring quality improvement in program implementation is explained and a quality improvement plan appropriate for the school setting is provided. The need to exercise caution in order to control the spread of infectious diseases is explained and includes a risk management plan. Record and report systems are also examined including the managing, storing, and retrieving of clinical records.

Chapter Six describes case finding and case selection—two of the most important functions of the school clinician. Traditional, as well as current, practices are discussed in detail with many helpful ideas included. Numerous suggestions and practical forms are provided for obtaining referrals from teachers and assessing students. The need to establish criteria for eligibility, severity, and priority in the case selection process is explained with several examples of criteria scales and charts. The importance of the school clinician's role on the placement team is examined.

Chapter Seven highlights models of service delivery and scheduling. It describes various service delivery options including traditional approaches, collaborative-consultative models, classroom-based intervention, community-based intervention, intervention assistance teams, and inservice models. Service delivery and scheduling considerations in a variety of school settings and with different populations are discussed. Guidelines for determining caseload size and composition with emphasis on infants, toddlers, and students with severe impairments. Several service delivery options are described.

Chapter Eight discusses planning intervention programs and treatment strategies including a sample Individualized Education Program and Individualized Family Service Plan. There is also a comprehensive lesson planning format. Particular emphasis is placed on making treatment relevant to students' academic needs and working with teachers to facilitate development of communication skills required for classroom success. Counseling, as one of the tasks of the speech-language pathologist, is also discussed.

Chapter Nine focuses on the school clinician's role as a collaborative-consultant with other professionals and the student's family. The importance of collaborating with others to develop creative solutions to students' communication problems is discussed. It explains the responsibilities and roles of various professionals and suggests practical methods for developing effective communication and interaction with educators, students, family members, administrators, and the community.

Chapter Ten is a sampling of programs. It contains questions to, and answers from, four experienced speech, language pathologists in school systems in Arizona, Illinois, Georgia, and Ohio.

Student teaching is the topic of Chapter Eleven. It describes the many aspects of the student teaching experience along with practical information and advice to the prospective student teacher.

Chapter Twelve discusses what goes on in the world of work after college. Topics examined include continuing education, research, collective bargaining, writing for publication, becoming involved in professional organizations, preparing for due process hearings, and maintaining a good public image. Information on getting your first job includes where to start, the credential file and portfolio, preparing a resume, and tips on putting your best foot forward in a job interview.

At the end of each chapter there are discussion questions and projects. They are included to help students make practical applications of theoretical knowledge and factual information and to stimulate dialogue with each other and with the instructor of the course.

The authors wish to thank the reviewers for their time and input. They are: Mary C. Twitchell, Ph.D. from Radford University; David L. Ratusnik, Ph.D. from the University of Central Florida; and Betsy Vinson from the University of Florida, Gainesville.

The writing of a textbook would not be possible without the encouragement and generous help of colleagues and students—both past and present. It would not be possible to name all of them but Dr. Blosser and I are especially indebted to Sally DeWitt Tippett, Jane Scaglione Frobose, Deborah Kendall, Lynne Coleman, John Butler, Colleen Conner, Roberta DePompei, Tammy Lastohkein, Collette Glay-Moon, Denise Vargas, and Rose Kernan.

Elizabeth A. Neidecker
Associate Professor Emerita
Bowling Green State University

School Programs in Speech-Language

The Growth and Development of the Profession in the Schools

Introduction

This chapter provides a historical background of the profession of speech, language, and hearing and the development of programs within the schools of the United States. The philosophy of education that invited speech, language, and hearing programs into the schools is described. Also discussed is the expansion of school programs, both professionally and geographically. The chapter points out the role of the school pathologists in the early days and changes in that role, as well as the factors that influenced those changes. It also considers the prevailing philosophy and legislation mandating equal educational opportunities for all children with disabilities and its implications for both the programs of the future and the roles and responsibilities of the school pathologist.

Early History

Although speech, language, and hearing problems have been with us since the early history of humankind, rehabilitative services for children with communication handicaps were not realized until the early part of the twentieth century. The growth of the profession and the establishment of the American Academy of Speech Correction in 1925 reflect the realization of the needs and special problems of the individuals with disabilities.

According to Moore and Kester (1953), the educational philosophy that invited speech correction into the schools was expressed in the preface to a teacher's manual published in 1897, which contained John Dewey's "My Ped-

2

**Chapter 1:
The Growth
and
Development
of the
Profession in
the Schools**

agogic Creed." The preface, written by Samuel T. Dutton, superintendent of schools, Brookline, Massachusetts, stated

> The isolation of the teacher is a thing of the past. The processes of education have come to be recognized as fundamental and vital in any attempt to improve human conditions and elevate society.
>
> The missionary and the social reformer have long been looking to education for counsel and aid in their most difficult undertakings. They have viewed with interest and pleasure the broadening of pedagogy so as to make it include not only experimental physiology and child study, but the problems of motor training, physical culture, hygiene, and the treatment of defectives and delinquents of every class.
>
> The schoolmaster, always conservative, has not found it easy to enter this large field; for he has often failed to realize how rich and fruitful the result of such researches are; but remarkable progress has been made, and a changed attitude on the part of the educators is the result.

Moore and Kester (1953) suggested that child labor laws influenced the growth of speech programs in the schools. Barring children from work forced both the atypical and the normal child to remain in school, and teachers soon asked for help with the exceptional children. A few got help, including assistance with children having speech defects.

According to Moore and Kester (p. 49), it was in 1910 that the Chicago public schools started a program of speech correction. Ella Flagg Young, the superintendent of schools, in her annual report in 1910 said

> Immediately after my entrance upon the duties of superintendent, letters began to arrive filled with complaints and petitions by parents of stammering children—complaints that the schools did nothing to help children handicapped by stammering to overcome their speech difficulty, but left them to lag behind and finally drop out of the schools; and petitions that something be done for those children. It was somewhat peculiar and also suggestive that these letters were followed by others from people who had given much attention to the study of stammering and wished to undertake the correction of that defect in stammerers attending the public schools. Soon after the schools were opened in the fall, I sent out a note, requesting each principal to report the number of stammerers in the school. It was surprising to find upon receiving the replies that there were recognized as stammerers 1,287 children. A recommendation was made to the committee on school management to the effect that the head of the department of oral expression in the Chicago Teachers' College be authorized to select ten of the members of the graduating class who showed special ability in the training given at the college in that particular subject and should be further empowered to give additional training of these students preparatory to their undertaking, under the direction of the department, the correction of the speech defects of these 1,287 children. The Board appropriated $3,000.00 toward the payment of these students who should begin their

work after graduation at the rate of $65 a month during a period extending from February 1 to June 30.

Instead of gathering the children into one building or into classes to be treated for their troubles, a plan was adopted of assigning to the young teacher a circuit and having her travel from school to school during the day. The object of this plan was to protect the young teacher from the depression of spirit and low physical condition that often ensue from continued confinement in one room for several successive hours at work upon abnormal conditions. It was soon found that the term "stammering" had been assumed to be very general in its application and many children who had been reported as stammerers had not the particular defect reported but some other form of speech defect.

The superintendent of schools in New York City in 1909 requested an investigation of the need for speech training in the schools, and two years later the following recommendations were presented to the board of education: First, the number of speech handicapped children was to be ascertained and case histories obtained; second, speech centers were to be established providing daily lessons of from 30 to 60 minutes; third, English teachers were to be given further training and utilized as instructors; and fourth, a department for training teachers was to be established. It was not until four years later, however, that a director of speech improvement was appointed to carry out the recommendations (Moore and Kester, 1953).

The Michigan Story

In their fascinating history of the early years of the Michigan Speech-Language-Hearing Association, Costello and Curtis (1989) described the beginnings of the Detroit public school speech correction program.

In 1909, Mrs. Frank Reed, of the Reed School of Stammering in Detroit, contacted the superintendent of the Detroit Public Schools and offered to train two teachers, free of charge, in the Reed Method of the Correction of Stammering, provided the program would be incorporated in the Detroit Schools. A survey was made of the need and 247 cases were found. In May 1910, Mrs. Reed's offer was accepted and during the summer two teachers trained. They were Miss Clara B. Stoddard and Miss Lillian Morley. In September 1910, two centers were opened in Detroit, one on the east side and one on the west side of the city. Wednesday was kept free from classes to call on parents, visit children in the regular classroom and for other activities associated with their work. In 1914, classes for children with other speech defects were begun.

In 1916, Miss Stoddard recommended the establishment of a special clinic at which a thorough physical examination and Binet test be given to children who seemed to have special problems. Regular monthly staff meetings were held and the latest literature on speech was reviewed. The

4

Chapter 1:
The Growth
and
Development
of the
Profession in
the Schools

cooperation of teachers and parents was enlisted in the correction of speech. The speech department personnel very early recognized the need for medical care for some of the children. A program for the mentally subnormal in special rooms was inaugerated in 1914. (Costello and Curtis, 1989.)

Early Growth

During this same decade there was an increasing number of public school systems employing speech clinicians. Among them were Detroit, Grand Rapids, Cleveland, Boston, Cincinnati, and San Francisco (Paden, 1970). In 1918, Dr. Walter B. Swift of Cleveland wrote an article entitled "How to Begin Speech Correction in the Public Schools" (reprinted in *Language, Speech and Hearing Services in Schools*, April 1972).

To the state of Wisconsin goes the credit for establishing at the University of Wisconsin the first training program for prospective specialists in the field and for granting the first doctor of philosophy degree in the area of speech disorders to Sara M. Stinchfield in 1921. Wisconsin was also the first state to enact enabling legislation for public school speech services and to appoint in 1923 a state supervisor of speech correction, Pauline Camp. Meanwhile, other universities throughout the United States were developing curricula in the area of speech disorders. Until 1940, however, only eight additional states added similar laws to their statute books (Irwin, 1959). By 1963, a study by Haines (1965) indicated that 45 of the states had passed legislation placing speech and hearing programs in the public schools. These laws provided for financial help to school districts maintaining approved programs, supervision by the state, responsibility for administering the law, and the establishment of standards. The laws described minimum standards, which the programs were expected to exceed (Haines, 1965).

The first state supervisors, in cooperation with the school clinicians in their respective states, did a remarkably far-sighted job in establishing statewide programs in regard to the organizational aspects. With no precedents to follow, they established standards that have retained merit through many years. The Vermont program (Dunn, 1949), providing speech and hearing services to children in rural areas, and the Ohio plan (Irwin, 1949) furnish two such examples. They addressed themselves to such topics as finding children who need the services, diagnostic services, caseload, the scheduling of group and individual therapy sessions, rooms for the therapist, equipment and supplies, coordination day, summer residence programs, in-service training of parents and teachers, and periodic rechecks of children.

A Period of Expansion

The decades of the 1940s and the 1950s were times of growth for all aspects of the profession. In 1943 the American Medical Association requested that a list of ethical speech correction schools and clinics be provided for distribution to physicians. During World War II the entire membership was listed in the National Roster of Scientific Personnel. The organization that started life in 1926 as The American Academy of Speech Correction with 25 dedicated and determined individuals changed its name in 1948 to The American Speech and Hearing Association and in 1979 to The American Speech-Language-Hearing Association. Its membership increased from the original 25 persons in 1926 to 330 in 1940, to 1,623 in 1950, and again to 6,249 in 1960. In 1964, the "associate" category was eliminated and there were 11,703 members. By 1975, the membership had climbed to 21,435 with a steady increase until the present time when the membership exceeds 65,000.

The official publication, *Journal of Speech Disorders,* was first published in 1936 at Ohio State University with G. Oscar Russell as editor. In 1957 the American Speech and Hearing Association established a permanent national office and appointed a professional executive secretary, Kenneth Johnson. In 1959 an employment bulletin, *Trends,* and a monthly professional magazine, *Asha,* were published.

Hearing Handicapped

Initially, programs for the children with hearing impairments in this country were designed for children who were deaf and the needs of those with mild-to-moderate hearing impairments were, for the most part, neglected. Educational programs for the deaf were first established in the United States in 1817 with the founding of the American School for the Deaf at Hartford, Connecticut (Bender, 1960). Deaf children were educated in residential schools or institutions until the establishment of classrooms in regular schools. The child in the regular classroom with a mild to moderate to possibly a severe hearing loss was dealt with by the classroom teacher. In his book, *Speech Correction Methods,* Ainsworth (1948) pointed out that "substitutions and omissions were frequently found in children with hearing loss and may be attacked with articulatory principles employing also visual and kinaesthetic avenues of approach." During this era, professionals in the schools were "speech correctionists" and dealt with most communication problems as articulatory problems.

Later the "speech correctionist" became a "speech and hearing therapist" and the public school therapists included hard-of-hearing children in their caseloads on the same basis as the speech handicapped child. There were also classroom teachers of the hard-of-hearing in the public schools.

Concern for the hearing handicapped child in the classroom was indicated by one of the sessions in the 33rd annual convention of the American Speech and Hearing Association held in 1957 in Cincinnati, Ohio. The title of the session was "The Hard of Hearing Child in the Public Schools" and covered such topics as "The Public School Program for the Hard of Hearing in a Large School System," "Types of Public School Programs Presently in Existence in Small School Systems," "the Preparation for Teachers of the Hard of Hearing in the Public Schools," and "The Use of Amplification in Public School Programs for the Hard of Hearing."

Speech Improvement Programs

School programs designed to help all children develop the ability to communicate effectively in acceptable speech, voice, and language patterns were first called *speech improvement* programs. Such programs were usually carried out by the classroom teacher, with the speech-language specialist serving as a consultant and doing demonstration teaching in the classroom. Many such programs were initiated in the 1920s, 1930s, and 1940s and were concentrated on the kindergarten and first-grade levels. One of the purposes was to reduce the number of minor speech problems.

The programs were not considered part of the school clinician's regular duties in many states. However, in some cities, speech improvement programs were carried out successfully despite lack of state support. According to Garrison and colleagues (1961), the communities of Arlington County, Virginia; Brea, California; Des Moines, Iowa; Hartford, Connecticut; Hingham, Massachusetts; New York City; Wauwatosa, Wisconsin; Wichita, Kansas; and Youngstown, Ohio, were recognized as having well-organized speech improvement programs.

It was also during these decades that the public school programs increased and expanded, both professionally and geographically. School clinicians found themselves wearing many hats. In addition to selling the idea of such a program to the school system and the community, the clinician had to

Devise a set of forms to be used for record keeping and reporting

Locate the children with speech and hearing handicaps

Schedule them for therapy after talking with their teachers for the most convenient time for all concerned

Provide the diagnosis and the therapy

Work with the school nurse on locating the children with hearing losses

Counsel the parents

Answer hundreds of questions from teachers who were often totally unfamiliar with such a program

Keep the school administration informed

Confer with persons in other professional disciplines

And, at the same time, remain healthy, well groomed, trustworthy, modest, friendly, cheerful, courteous, patient, enthusiastic, tolerant, cooperative, businesslike, dependable, prompt, creative, interesting, and unflappable

Furthermore, the clinician had to keep one eye on the clock and the calendar and the other eye on state standards.

Language and Speech

Speech-language pathologists have been dealing with children with language problems for many years. Before research and experience sharpened diagnostic tools and awareness, these children were referred to as having "severe articulation disorders," "delayed speech," or "immature language." During the 1940s, 1950, and early 1960s, there was considerable interest among professionals in articulation and speech sounds. The focus changed in the late 1960s and early 1970s to an interest in syntactic structures and sentence forms. The past several decades have increased both knowledge and awareness of language problems. Indeed, the title of the professional organization was changed, in recognition of this, from the "American Speech and Hearing Association" to the "American Speech-Language-Hearing Association."

Along with this growing awareness of language problems was the realization that the school clinician had a commitment to the student whose language is disordered or delayed; the language problem may be the underlying cause of a student's difficulty in mastering reading or arithmetic skills. In addition, language problems may be present in the child who is hearing impaired, mentally retarded, learning disabled, physically handicapped, emotionally disturbed or environmentally disadvantaged.

Improvement in Quality

The growth in numbers of clinicians serving the schools was steady during the 1950s and the 1960s. That era concentrated on the improvement of quality as well as quantity by emphasizing increased training for clinicians through advanced certification standards set by the American Speech and Hearing Association.

A major project geared toward improving speech and hearing services to children in the schools was undertaken by the U.S. Office of Education, Purdue University, and the Research Committee of the American Speech and Hearing Association (Steer et al., 1961). The major objectives were to provide authoritative information about current practices in the public schools and to identify unresolved problems. On the basis of these findings, priorities were established for identification of urgently needed research. With the cooperation of hundreds of clinicians, supervisors, classroom teachers, and training institution personnel, a list of topics for further study and research was distilled by the work groups. Given highest priority were the following topics: the collection of longitudinal data on speech; comparative studies of program organization (with special attention to the frequency, duration, and intensity of therapy); and comparative studies of the use of different remedial procedures with children of various ages presenting different speech, voice, and language problems.

Six additional topics were also identified and assigned a high priority: the development of standardized tests of speech, voice, and language; the development of criteria for selection of primary-grade children for inclusion in remedial programs; comparative studies of speech improvement and clinical programs; comparative studies of group, individual, and combined group and individual therapy programs; studies of the adjustment of children and their language usage in relation to changes in speech accomplished during participation in therapy programs; and comparative studies of different curricula and clinical training programs for prospective public school speech and hearing personnel.

The study also addressed itself to such topics as the professional roles and relationships of the school clinician, the supervision of programs, diagnosis and measurement, and the recruitment of professional personnel to meet the growing needs of children with communication handicaps in the schools.

The "Quiet Revolution"

Things were changing rapidly in the late 1960s and early 1970s for school programs, and the "quiet revolution" referred to by O'Toole and Zaslow (1969) became less quiet as the school speech-language specialists talked about breaking the cycle of mediocrity, lowering caseloads, giving highest priority to the most severe cases, scheduling on intensive cycles rather than intermittently, extending programs throughout the summer, utilizing diagnostic teams, and many other issues. The emphasis had shifted, slowly but surely, from quantity to quality.

The appointment in 1969 by the American Speech and Hearing Association of a full-time staff member to serve as Associate Secretary for School/Clinic Affairs; the publication in 1971 of *Language, Speech and Hearing Services in Schools;* and the appointment by ASHA of a standing committee on Language, Speech and Hearing Services in Schools all attest to the recognition of the public school speech-language specialist as a large and important part of the profession.

It was not the professional organization's thinking alone that brought about the many changes. Outside influences—mainly the changes in the philosophy and conditions surrounding the American education system—began to effect changes in the profession. Increased populations, tightened school budgets, focus on the lack of reading skills in the elementary school, more attention to special populations such as children who are mentally retarded and socially or economically disadvantaged—all had an impact.

Participant or Separatist?

It was during this period that Ainsworth (1965) examined two possible roles for the speech and hearing specialist in the public schools which he described as the "participant" and the "separatist" roles. The "separatist," according to Ainsworth, worked as an independent professional responsible for diagnosing and treating speech disorders of children in public schools and viewed his responsibilities fulfilled when he successfully carried out the clinical activities.

Regarding the "participant's" role, Ainsworth felt that the child receiving treatment as part of the school program would receive better quality care if therapy were integrated into the educational process. Indeed, he felt that an entirely new concept of funding speech therapy would need to be developed if the separatist role were to be the school pathologist's role.

Federal Legislation

In 1954, the U.S. Supreme Court's decision in the case of *Brown* vs. *Board of Education* set into motion a new era and struck down the doctrine of segregated education. This decision sparked such issues as women's rights; the right to education and treatment for the handicapped; and the intrinsic rights of individuals, including blacks and minority groups.

Parent organizations have long been a catalyst in bringing about change, and in the case of children with disabilities they were certainly no exception. According to Reynolds and Rosen (1976)

> Parents of handicapped children began to organize about thirty years ago to obtain educational facilities for their offspring and to act as watchdogs of the institutions serving them. At first, the organizations concentrated on political action; since 1970, however, they have turned to the courts. This fact may be more important than any other in accounting for the changes in special education that are occurring now and are likely to occur in the near future.

The PARC Case

An extension of the *Brown v. Board of Education* decision, according to Reynolds and Rosen, was the consent decree established in the case of the Pennsylvania Association for Retarded Children. This decree stated that no matter how serious the handicap, every child has the right to education. The PARC case established the right of parents to become involved in making decisions concerning their child and stipulated that education must be based on programs appropriate to the needs and capacities of each individual child.

Mainstreaming

One of the unexpected aftermaths of the PARC case was to place the stamp of judicial approval on *mainstreaming*. According to Reynolds and Rosen (p. 558)

> Mainstreaming is a set or general predisposition to arrange for the education of children with handicaps or learning problems within the environment provided for all other children—the regular school and normal home and community environment—whenever feasible.

The intent of mainstreaming is to provide handicapped children with an appropriate educational program in as "normal" or "regular" an environment as possible. Thus, depending on the nature and/or severity of the handicapping condition, the child may be in a self-contained classroom or a regular classroom for all or part of the educational program, in other words, in the "least restrictive environment."

Mainstreaming has special implications for the regular classroom teacher as well as other personnel involved in the education of children with handicaps. Reynolds and Rosen (pp. 557–58) say

> Obviously, mainstreaming makes new demands on both regular classroom and special education teachers. In the past, a regular education teacher was

10

Chapter 1:
The Growth
and
Development
of the
Profession in
the Schools

expected to know enough about handicapping conditions to be able to identify children with such problems for referral out of the classroom into special education settings. At the same time, special education teachers were trained to work directly with the children with certain specific handicaps (as in the days of residential schools) in separate special settings.

Under mainstreaming, different roles are demanded for both kinds of teachers. The trend for training special education teachers for indirect resource teacher roles rather than narrow specialists is well established in many preparation centers. Concurrently, programs are underway to provide regular education teachers with training in the identification of learning problems. At the local school level, regular and special education teachers in mainstreamed programs are no longer isolated in separate classrooms. They work together in teams to share knowledge, skills, observations, and experiences to enhance the programs for children with special problems, whether the children are permanently or temporarily handicapped. Thus, it has become essential for special teachers to learn the skills of consultation and for both teachers to learn techniques of observation as well as communication.

Bureau of Education for the Handicapped

In 1967 the Congress created the Bureau of Education for the Handicapped and began a program of grants to speed the development of educational programs.

In 1974, Edwin W. Martin, then director of the Bureau of Education for the Handicapped, in an address to the members of the American Speech and Hearing Association, stated that he did not feel we were successfully integrating our roles as speech and hearing specialists in the educational system. He urged that speech-language pathologists and audiologists in schools must be actively involved in interdisciplinary efforts with parents, learning disability specialists, administrators, guidance counselors, classroom teachers, and all educational colleagues.

Legislation: PL 94-142

The most sweeping and significant change concerning the education of children with disabilities took place on November 29, 1975, when President Gerald Ford signed into law The Education For All Handicapped Children Act (Public Law 94-142). According to Ratliff, PL 94-142 was "conceived by petition, born of legislation, and nurtured through litigation." The major intent of the law is to assure full and appropriate education for all children who are disabled between the ages of three and twenty-one.

The impact of Public Law 94-142 has been both beneficial and substantial. It has changed not only the education of children with handicaps but has had widespread influence on the entire education system. State laws and regulations have been changed, parents have become more involved in the education of their children with handicaps, advocacy groups have influenced education at the local and the state levels, and training institutions and their programs have been affected. Parents and guardians of all children who are disabled are guaranteed legal due process with regard to identification, evaluation and placement.

Public Law 94-142 has had a pervasive and profound effect on public school speech-language and hearing programs. Before the passage of the law, individual states had enacted legislation *permitting* speech and hearing services in the schools, but PL 94-142 *mandated* services for children with speech-language or hearing impairments. In addition, the law established a legal basis for services and provided financial assistance. The scope of speech-language pathology and audiology services are defined in the provisions of the law and mandate the identification and evaluation of communicatively handicapped children as well as the development of an Individualized Education Program (IEP) and its implementation. The regulations also cover the provision of appropriate administrative and supervisory activities necessary for program planning, management, and evaluation.

Legislation: PL 99-457

In 1986, President Ronald Reagan signed into law Public Law 99-457, amendments to the Education of the Handicapped Act (PL 94-142). These amendments expanded and strengthened the mandate for providing services to children with handicaps by assisting states to plan, develop, and implement statewide interagency programs for all young children with disabilities from birth through age two. The law included those infants and toddlers who are experiencing developmental delays in the areas of physical development, including vision and hearing, language and speech, psychosocial development, or self-help skills. The law also included infants and toddlers who have a diagnosed physical or mental condition that has a high probability of resulting in developmental delay, or children from birth through age two who may experience developmental delays if early intervention is not provided.

Section 619 of PL 99-457 creates enhanced incentives for states to provide a free and appropriate public education for eligible three- to five-year olds with disabilities. Parent training, family services, and variations in child programming are encouraged by law.

Legislation: PL 101-476

In 1990, Public Law 94-142 was further amended. The changed legislation is called IDEA (The Individuals with Disabilities Education Act) or Public Law 101-476. The law resulted in some major changes. Two new categories of disability (autism and traumatic brain injury) were added. In addition, "person-first" language was introduced changing all references to handicapped children to "children with disabilities." Another change mandated that schools provide transition services to support movement from school to post-school activities.

The impact of these three laws will be discussed further in Chapter Three.

Terminology: What's In a Name

The historical development of school programs in speech, language, and hearing is interestingly revealed in what titles have been used over the years. The earliest professionals called themselves "speech correctionists." Some who had previously worked in school systems in this capacity were known as "speech teachers," although they were more concerned with habilitation than with elocution. During the 1950s and the 1960s we became "speech and hearing therapists" and "speech and hearing clinicians." All these changes caused no end of trouble, especially in trying to explain ourselves to others.

During the 1970s we became known as "speech pathologists," and in 1977 The American Speech-Language-Hearing Association in a preference survey found that "speech-language pathologist" was the choice of professionals in the field.

How did we get from "speech correctionist" and "speech teacher" to "speech-language pathologist"? The answer is not simple, but perhaps a review of clinical practices may shed some light.

In the 1930s a few universities began programs to train people for clinical roles in public schools and universities. We were "speech correctionists" and "speech teachers." Stuttering problems were the major focus during the earliest days, along with articulation problems. Clinicians were aware of language systems, but problems in that area were treated as speech problems. When faced with children who did not talk, clinicians attempted to stimulate speech by targeting vocal play and babbling. Speech clinicians weren't without their Bryngelson-Glaspey Speech Improvement Cards (1941) or Schoolfield's book *Better Speech and Better Reading* (1937).

Children who did not talk or who had little speech were viewed as having "organic" problems, those related to the brain or neurologic system. Children whose problems in communication yielded to therapy were said to have had "functional" problems. Children who had even minimal vocalization, such as cerebral palsied children or hearing-impaired children, were treated as speech problems. It was at this time the titles of "speech therapist" and "speech and hearing therapist" were used.

Very young children with "delayed speech" and mentally retarded children were excluded from therapy as it was thought they had not reached the proper stage of development to benefit from treatment.

This clinical model was followed for about 30 years, until the late 1950s and early 1960s, when Noam Chomsky's "generative grammar" theories set the stage for the beginning of the profession's understanding of language and language behavior. Although Chomsky offered little help in solving clinical problems, it was at this time that B. F. Skinner's behavioral theories appeared. Speech clinicians still used the functional approach to therapy; however, they did include language-handicapped children on their caseloads for the first time.

One result of these two widely divergent schools of thought was to move the speech clinician's focus away from concentration on phonemes and articulation.

During the 1960s and the 1970s, the stimulus-response and reinforcement strategies as well as "precision therapy" methods were used to elicit language and speech. These behavior modification methods were widely accepted and speech clinicians freely dispersed rewards and "reinforcers."

Chomsky's grammar and Skinner's behaviorism systems prepared the way for the profession's move into semantics and pragmatics and the area of child language. During the 1970s the profession expanded the knowledge base and built on the foundations developed in the 1960s. This had the effect of developing new concepts about language behavior and its component parts.

During the early 1980s children previously excluded from therapy were now included. Children with articulation problems, although still a large part of the speech-language pathologist's caseload in the public schools, now included individuals with severe language deficiencies, language-learning disabilities, mental retardation, motor handicaps, and hearing handicaps. Adding impetus to this development was the passage and implementation of Public Law 94-142.

The U.S. Department of Labor (1979) uses the title "speech pathologist" as its official designation. The American Speech-Language-Hearing Association prefers "speech-language pathologist."

Although some may view the trouble with terminology as an identity crisis affecting an entire profession, it might also be construed as symptomatic of a gradual shift in focus from a preoccupation mainly with articulation problems to an interest in language-learning behavior. It also indicates a widening of the scope of services to include prevention as well as remediation, to hone and fine-tune our individual professional skills, and to see that these skills are delivered in the most efficient and effective way to the appropriate consumer.

The Emerging Role of the School SLP

Traditionally, in the United States of America, speech, language, and hearing services have been offered as a part of the school program, and the bulk of the profession has been employed in the schools. Unlike the systems in other countries where speech, language, and hearing professionals have followed the "medical model" and have provided services through health and medical facilities such as hospitals, in this country we have followed the "educational model" and provide services in the public schools. Our system is undoubtedly a reflection of our democratic philosophy of education that children have a right to education and that our function in the schools is to prevent, remove, and alleviate communication barriers that interfere with the child's ability to profit from the education offered.

Furthermore, the schools constitute an ideal setting in which to provide speech, language, and hearing services: there is an identified population who are the "consumers" of the services, there are legal mandates for implementing and carrying out the services, and there is local, state and federal financial support. Competency in oral and written communication is one of the primary objectives of the school system and today many states, with the encouragement of the federal government, have mandated assessment in these areas. Speech, language, and hearing services are the primary support systems in the achievement of these competencies. (Engnoth, 1987).

14

Chapter 1:
The Growth
and
Development
of the
Profession in
the Schools

It is probably safe to say that pathologists in the schools often have been viewed as itinerant workers dealing mainly with functional articulation problems and working with children in groups rather than individually because of high maximum caseload requirements set by state law. Unfortunately, this stereotype has persisted although the school pathologist's role is continually changing. Let us look at the roles and responsibilities of the school speech, language, and hearing specialist.

The school pathologist plans, directs, and provides diagnostic and remediation services to children and youth with communication disabilities. The pathologist works with articulation, language, voice, disfluency (stuttering), and hearing impairments, as well as speech, language, and hearing problems associated with such conditions as cleft palate, cerebral palsy, intellectual impairment, visual impairment, emotional and behavioral disturbances, autistic behavior, aphasia, and traumatic brain injury.

The speech-language pathologist in the schools serves high-risk infants and toddlers from birth to age five in school-operated child development centers, Head Start programs, special schools, centers, classrooms or home settings. Also served are children with severe disabilities in special schools, centers, classes or home settings, and students with multiple impairments, as well as elementary, middle and secondary-school pupils.

An important aspect of the school pathologist's duties is cooperation with other school and health specialists, including audiologists, nurses, social workers, physicians, dentists, special education teachers, psychologists, and guidance counselors. Cooperative planning with these individuals on a regular basis results in effective diagnostic, habilitative, and educational programs for children with communication problems.

The school pathologist works with classroom teachers and resource teachers to implement and generalize remediation procedures for the child with handicaps. Working with parents to help them alleviate and understand problems is also a part of the pathologist's function. School administrators are often the key to good educational programming for children, and the school pathologist works with both principals and superintendents toward that end.

The school pathologist may also be a community resource person, providing public information about communication problems and the availability of services for parents and families and for the personnel in both public and voluntary community agencies.

Many school pathologists are engaged in research related to program organization and management, clinical procedures, and professional responsibility. The field of language, speech, and hearing is constantly broadening, and the school pathologist must keep abreast of new information by reading professional journals and publications; attending seminars and conventions; enrolling in continuing education programs; and sharing information and ideas with colleagues through state, local, and national professional organizations.

Frequently school pathologists are asked to help university students by serving as supervisors of student teaching and by providing observational opportunities for students-in-training. The supervision of paraprofessionals and volunteers in school programs is also the responsibility of the school pathologist.

Because the school pathologist is considered an important part of the total educational program, the size, need, and structure of the local school district will have much to do with the organizational model used as well as the nature of the services provided. Many school pathologists work as itinerant persons. Some will be assigned to a single building, whereas others may work in special classes, resource rooms, or self-contained classrooms. Often the school pathologist will be either a full- or part-time member of the pupil evaluation team or a resource consultant to teachers, administrators, or other staff members. Many school pathologists are employed as supervisors or administrators of speech and language programs.

The role of the school pathologist is changing from that of an itinerant clinician who works with large numbers of children with articulatory problems to that of the specialist in communication disorders. The collaborative-consultative role is becoming more and more important, and more is required of the school pathologist in the way of diagnosis of speech, language, and hearing problems. Classroom teachers, special teachers, and personnel in other specialized fields will depend on the school pathologist to provide information on diagnoses, assessment, and treatment.

Some school SLPs may be sensitive about the term *specialist*. Freeman (1969) pointed out that the term *special* should not be equated with *superior*, as it implies no superiority over the other school personnel. The school pathologist is a professional specialist in the school, whose role is similar to that of the speech, language, and hearing specialist in the hospital or community agency.

Future Challenges

What is the future role of the speech-language pathologist (SLP) in the schools? Undoubtedly a catalyst to programs in the schools and the role of the school pathologist are the federal laws related to special education. In a study of the effectiveness of Public Law 94-142 by Hyman (August 1985), seven out of ten respondents having five or more years of experience with children in the schools agreed that the law had improved the quality of speech, language, and hearing services. Approximately 80 percent of this group believed that the law had enhanced the access to services and that it had served to augment parental involvement in the educational process.

There is reason to believe that Public Law 94-142 set the course of events toward positive goals and that there will be no turning back. There are still many problems to be solved and challenges to be met, and these need to be identified by school SLPs and the profession as a whole.

Donnelly (1984) identified several of these problems, including the following three main areas: first, the changing size and composition of the caseload and how it has led to burnout; second, the imbalance between monies generated by SLP services and those actually spent to support these programs; and third, the professionally compromising position that SLPs often find themselves in because of the school administrator who is unaware of their professional responsibilities, which often include referral to services outside the school.

Donnelly has offered some strategies for coping with these professional

16

Chapter 1:
The Growth
and
Development
of the
Profession in
the Schools

problems. In the area of burnout she has suggested that the school SLPs get out of the isolated speech therapy room and work more with pupils in their classrooms, to work more closely with classroom teachers, and to demand from school administrators smaller caseloads in order to offer to any given child the therapy required.

Regarding the amount of money generated by SLP services, Donnelly suggests that the school SLPs should keep abreast of the political information that affects their programs. Communicatively handicapped children constitute the second largest category of handicapped children, second only to learning-disabled children, and therefore generate a very substantial amount of money for school districts. These funds, however, are not always used for SLP services. Donnelly says that these facts should be brought tactfully but knowledgeably to superintendents and others who make budgetary decisions.

The third problem, that of the professionally compromising position, calls for a combination of solutions. First, the school SLP must do what is professionally appropriate and ethical. In addition, the SLP should inform the parents that if the condition in question does not interfere with educational performance, the school district is not liable for payment for treatment by an outside agency. The SLP must also assume the responsibility of educating school personnel concerning the appropriateness of the recommendation. Along this same line, the SLP needs to keep school personnel advised of the availability of services that exist outside the school.

The Future is Now

Although there are many problems to be faced by school SLPs and the profession as a whole, there are also exciting and challenging developments. It is difficult to predict how speech-language pathology will be different in the future, but we can make some educated guesses. The makeup of caseloads in the schools has already shifted from a preponderance of articulation problems to language and learning disabilities. More and more children with severe handicaps will be in regular classrooms and many of these children will have speech and/or language problems. There will be an extension of services to preschool children. It will be necessary to develop programs which meet the growing and diverse needs of our multicultural society. The role of the SLP as a collaborator and consultant will be greatly expanded, as will the role as a team member in the school in diagnosis, assessment, and placement. The school SLP will be more and more involved in overall education, in the communicative skills of reading, writing, and spelling as well as in speaking and listening. As has been true in the fields of medicine and dentistry, there will be an emergence of specialists in speech-language pathology and audiology.

Strategies for coping with these changes will have to be met by the school SLP and audiologist as well as by the profession as a whole, and certainly by the professional organization, the American Speech-Language-Hearing Association, and the state speech, language, and hearing groups.

Margaret C. Byrne-Saricks (1989) very aptly stated regarding the future of clinical services in the schools

School services require well-educated, skillful, tolerant clinicians. Whatever the nature of their roles—consulting, evaluating, or providing intervention—they must take school schedules and limited space into consideration. In addition to their expertise in communication disorders, clinicians must be knowledgeable about the social, political, and cultural backgrounds of their students. They must be skilled in using computers both for the required record keeping and for selected aspects of therapy. They need sufficient background in research to evaluate tests and intervention materials flooding the market.

Finally, clinicians must be flexible. Our responsibilities have changed since the 1950s and will continue to do so in the years ahead.

DISCUSSION QUESTIONS AND PROJECTS

1. How does an understanding of the early role of the school speech-language clinician help in understanding the current role?

2. How has the role of the clinician in the schools changed over the years? Do you think this has any relationship to the titles by which we have been and are presently called?

3. Read Swift's (1972) article. How relevant is it today?

4. Ask ten of your friends, not in the speech-language or hearing field, to comment on the titles by which we have called ourselves and what these titles convey to them. Ask the same questions of elementary education majors at your university.

5. Do you think the changes in the profession were brought about by outside pressures or by internal factors?

6. How does the role of the SLP in the schools differ from the role of the SLP in private practice? In a community clinic? In a hospital setting?

CHAPTER 2

The Professional School Speech-Language Pathologist

Introduction

The Code of Ethics of the American Speech-Language-Hearing Association has established the ground rules for the entire profession. The principles include conduct toward the client, the public, and fellow professionals. Certification is the stamp of approval issued by a responsible agency to the individual meeting specific requirements. It confers the right to practice and the right to be recognized as a professional. It also carries with it the responsibility of exemplary professional behavior.

Organizations are important links facilitating the exchange of new ideas, information, research, recent developments, materials, and professional affairs. School pathologists will need to be aware of the various organizations and their functions in order to choose the ones with which they will affiliate.

The topics of the importance of professionalism and professional behavior are discussed.

The Code of Ethics

One of the first tasks of the American Academy of Speech Correction, as the professional organization was first called, was the establishment of a Code of Ethics. Mindful of the fact that there were unscrupulous individuals who would take advantage of persons with handicapping conditions by making rash promises of cures and by charging exorbitant fees, the earliest members of the profession felt it necessary to maintain professional integrity and encourage high standards by formulating a Code of Ethics. As may be expected, it was a difficult task, and throughout the history of the organization the code has been periodically updated to meet current problems; however, it has remained substantially the same. The Code outlines the ASHA member's professional responsibilities to the patient, to co-workers, and to society. Thus, it might be said that accountability has always been one of the profession's highest priorities.

Although the Code was adopted for an association, it serves the entire profession. In the language of the code the term *individuals* refers to all members of the American Speech-Language-Hearing Association and those nonmembers who hold the Certificate of Clinical Competence.

A code of ethics defines a profession's parameters; it should also protect the rights of the consumer. The ASHA Code addresses confidentially, the use of persons in research, the supervision of paraprofessionals and of students in training, as well as other matters.

The Code has no legal basis except in states where it has been adopted as part of the licensing requirements.

The American Speech-Language-Hearing Association has established an Ethical Practice Board whose major responsibility is the enforcement of the Code of Ethics. A member of ASHA who is a holder of the Certificate of Clinical Competence and who is found guilty of noncompliance may be dropped from membership and have the Certificate revoked. A nonmember who is found guilty of noncompliance would face revocation of the Certificate. The loss of membership status and/or the revocation of the Certificate of Clinical Competence would follow procedures of due process set up by the Ethical Practice Board. There is also an appeals procedure. A copy of the Board's practices and procedures as well as the appeals procedures are printed in the Directory of the American Speech-Language-Hearing Association, 10801 Rockville Pike, Rockville, Maryland 20852. In addition, the Association's Code of Ethics is reprinted each year in the January issue of *Asha*. That issue also lists all issues in ethics statements that the Board has published to interpret sections of the Code. (At the end of this chapter is a list of problems, the solutions to which may be found in the Code of Ethics.)

Following is the revision of the ASHA Code of Ethics, January 1, 1992. Read it carefully.

Code of Ethics of the American Speech-Language-Hearing Association*

Preamble

The preservation of the highest standards of integrity and ethical principles is vital to the responsible discharge of obligations in the professions of speech-language pathology and audiology. This Code of Ethics sets forth the fundamental principles and rules considered essential to this purpose.

Every individual who is (a) a member of the American Speech-Language-Hearing Association, whether certified or not, (b) a nonmember holding the Certificate of Clinical Competence from the Association, (c) an applicant for membership or certification, or (d) a Clinical Fellow seeking to fulfill standards for certification shall abide by this Code of Ethics.

*Reprinted with the permission of the American Speech-Language-Hearing Association.

20

Chapter 2:
The
Professional
School
Speech-
Language
Pathologist

Any action that violates the spirit and purpose of this Code shall be considered unethical. Failure to specify any particular responsibility or practice in this Code of Ethics shall not be construed as denial of the existence of such responsibilities or practices.

The fundamentals of ethical conduct are described by Principles of Ethics and by Rules of Ethics as they relate to responsibility to persons served, to the public, and to the professions of speech-language pathology and audiology.

Principles of Ethics, aspirational and inspirational in nature, form the underlying moral basis for the Code of Ethics. Individuals shall observe these principles as affirmative obligations under all conditions of professional activity.

Rules of Ethics are specific statements of minimally acceptable professional conduct or of prohibitions and are applicable to all individuals.

PRINCIPLE OF ETHICS I: *Individuals shall honor their responsibility to hold paramount the welfare of persons they serve professionally.*

Rules of Ethics

A. Individuals shall provide all services competently.

B. Individuals shall use every resource, including referral when appropriate, to ensure that high-quality service is provided.

C. Individuals shall not discriminate in the delivery of professional services on the basis of race, sex, age, religion, national origin, sexual orientation, or handicapping condition.

D. Individuals shall fully inform the persons they serve of the nature and possible effects of service rendered and products dispensed.

E. Individuals shall evaluate the effectiveness of services rendered and of products dispensed and shall provide services or dispense products only when benefit can reasonably be expected.

F. Individuals shall not guarantee the results of any treatment or procedure, directly or by implication; however, they may make a reasonable statement of prognosis.

G. Individuals shall not evaluate or treat speech, language, or hearing disorders solely by correspondence.

H. Individuals shall maintain adequate records of professional services rendered and products dispensed and shall allow access to these records when appropriately authorized.

I. Individuals shall not reveal, without authorization, any professional or personal information about the person served professionally, unless required by law to do so, or unless doing so is necessary to protect the welfare of the person or of the community.

J. Individuals shall not charge for services not rendered, nor shall they misrepresent,[1] in any fashion, services rendered or products dispensed.

K. Individuals shall use persons in research or as subjects of teaching demonstrations only with their informed consent.

L. Individuals shall withdraw from professional practice when substance abuse or an emotional or mental disability may adversely affect the quality of services they render.

PRINCIPLE OF ETHICS II: *Individuals shall honor their responsibility to achieve and maintain the highest level of professional competence.*

Rules of Ethics

A. Individuals shall engage in the provision of clinical services only when they hold the appropriate Certificate of Clinical Competence or when they are in the certification process and are supervised by an individual who holds the appropriate Certificate of Clinical Competence.

B. Individuals shall engage in only those aspects of the professions that are within the scope of their competence, considering their level of education, training, and experience.

C. Individuals shall continue their professional development throughout their careers.

D. Individuals shall delegate the provision of clinical services only to persons who are certified or to persons in the education or certification process who are appropriately supervised. The provision of support services may be delegated to persons who are neither certified nor in the certification process only when a certificate holder provides appropriate supervision.

E. Individuals shall prohibit any of their professional staff from providing services that exceed the staff member's competence, considering the staff member's level of education, training, and experience.

F. Individuals shall ensure that all equipment used in the provision of services is in proper working order and is properly calibrated.

PRINCIPLE OF ETHICS III: *Individuals shall honor their responsibility to the public by promoting public understanding of the professions, by supporting the development of services designed to fulfill the unmet needs of the public, and by providing accurate information in all communications involving any aspect of the professions.*

---

[1] For purposes of this Code of Ethics, misrepresentation includes any untrue statements or statements that are likely to mislead. Misrepresentation also includes the failure to state any information that is material and that ought, in fairness, to be considered.

22   *Rules of Ethics*

Chapter 2:
The
Professional
School
Speech-
Language
Pathologist

A. Individuals shall not misrepresent their credentials, competence, education, training, or experience.

B. Individuals shall not participate in professional activities that constitute a conflict of interest.

C. Individuals shall not misrepresent diagnostic information, services rendered, or products dispensed or engage in any scheme or artifice to defraud in connection with obtaining payment or reimbursement for such services or products.

D. Individuals' statements to the public shall provide accurate information about the nature and management of communication disorders, about the professions, and about professional services.

E. Individuals' statements to the public—advertising, announcing and marketing their professional services, reporting research results, and promoting products—shall adhere to prevailing professional standards and shall not contain misrepresentations.

PRINCIPLES OF ETHICS IV: *Individuals shall honor their responsibilities to the professions and their relationships with colleagues, students and members of allied professions. Individuals shall uphold the dignity and autonomy of the professions, maintain harmonious interprofessional and intraprofessional relationships, and accept the professions' self-imposed standards.*

Rules of Ethics

A. Individuals shall prohibit anyone under their supervision from engaging in any practice that violates the Code of Ethics.

B. Individuals shall not engage in dishonesty, fraud, deceit, misrepresentation, or any form of conduct that adversely reflects on the professions or on the individual's fitness to serve persons professionally.

C. Individuals shall assign credit only to those who have contributed to a publication, presentation, or product. Credit shall be assigned in proportion to the contribution and only with the contributor's consent.

D. Individuals' statements to colleagues about professional services, research results, and products shall adhere to prevailing professional standards and shall contain no misrepresentations.

E. Individuals shall not provide professional services without exercising independent professional judgment, regardless of referral source or prescription.

F. Individuals who have reason to believe that the Code of Ethics has been violated shall inform the Ethical Practice Board.

G. Individuals shall cooperate fully with the Ethical Practice Board in its investigation and adjudication of matters related to this Code of Ethics.

It is important that you read the Code of Ethics because it is there that you will find the answers to many of the vexing problems you will encounter in your day-to-day work.

Under Principles of Ethics I is a statement that says, "Individuals shall honor their responsibility to hold paramount the welfare of persons served professionally." There is hardly a professional problem that cannot be solved by asking yourself, "What is best for the client?"—not "What is best for me?" or "What is best for the school?" Your role as a speech-language pathologist puts you in the position of a child advocate. In other words, you are on the side of the child, whose best interests are your professional responsibility and for whom you speak.

Deciding what is best means that you will have to look at the needs of the *whole* person. A communication problem cannot be separated from the rest of the individual. The educational, health, psychological, and social aspects will have to be taken into consideration. Fortunately you do not always have to make decisions by yourself because in a school system you will be working closely with the classroom teacher, psychologist, school nurse, physician, social worker, educational audiologist, and other professionals. The decision concerning what is best for the student is therefore a consensus of those in the school, who hold paramount the best interests of that individual.

Another important ethical consideration is confidentiality. You will have access to much information about the student with whom you are working and the child's family. This information is given in trust and should be regarded as confidential. The only other persons with whom you might share this information are other professionals in the school who may be working with the child. Within a school system the school policies usually state that pertinent information may be shared among interested professionals, whereas information that may be conveyed to professionals or agencies *outside* the school system must have the written consent of the parents or guardians.

"Shared information" does not mean idle gossip. A conference with a classroom teacher is not to be carried on in the hallways, over lunch in the teachers' lunchroom, or in the teachers' lounge. When I was supervising student clinicians in the schools, one of the nicest compliments from a classroom teacher about a student was the following: "We like your student teacher very much; she's friendly, professional, and gets along well with everyone, but she certainly is close-mouthed!"

Personal and Professional Qualifications

The communication disorders profession is a multifaceted one. Some members teach university courses, some supervise in clinics, some administer programs, some provide treatment, some do research, and some are diagnosticians. The SLP who chooses to work in education has the responsibility of preventing, removing, and alleviating communication barriers that may hinder a student from receiving the instruction offered in the classroom. In addition, the school

24

Chapter 2:
The
Professional
School
Speech-
Language
Pathologist

clinician is a resource person to others in the school system. Another role of the school clinician is counselor to the family of the student who has the communication disorder or to that individual.

In addition to the appropriate education and specialized knowledge and skills, what personality traits are desirable for the school SLP, who must wear so many hats? Among the most frequently mentioned are patience, understanding, honesty, adaptability, flexibility, sense of humor, warm and friendly nature, respect for others, acceptance of others, dependability, resourcefulness, and creativity.

In a career/life planning seminar, Sarnecky (1987) pointed out that speech-language pathologists and audiologists are highly trained and skilled professionals who unfortunately sometimes view themselves as having no skills beyond their current functions. Becoming aware of their skills and identifying career and life goals are important to individuals who wish to function successfully in a complicated school system.

In addition to the traditional clinical and research skills acquired through training and experience, ASHA's Committee on Career Information and Development in the early 1980s considered some skills that could be identified and developed. These skills include the following:

- *Detail/Follow Through Skills:* Speech-language pathologists and audiologists are detail-oriented, explicit in communication, and orderly in work habits. They demonstrate these skills daily through their case management and leadership.

- *Money Management Skills:* Budget planning and cost analysis is a responsibility of many speech-language pathologists and audiologists.

- *Influencing/Persuading Skills:* Speech-language pathologists and audiologists influence clients, parents, professions in related areas, physicians, state legislators, and the public about the needs of individuals with communication disorders.

- *Performance Skills:* Observation by and demonstrations to students in practicum, parents, teachers, and related professionals are an integral part of a speech-language pathologist's and audiologist's typical work day regardless of work setting.

- *Leadership:* Speech-language pathologists and audiologists demonstrate leadership skills in their place of employment, in the community, in their state association, and in their national association.

- *Communication:* The entire profession centers around communication and speech-language pathologists and audiologists are excellent communicators with clients, in the classroom, and with the public.

- *Human Relations:* Speech-language pathologists and audiologists use skills in this area not only during the times they are providing direct clinical services but also with co-workers, employees, and students they supervise in practicum or during the Clinical Fellowship Year.

- *Educational Skills:* Speech-language pathologist and audiologists teach undergraduate and graduate courses, give lectures at state association meetings and annual conventions, give presentations to parents, teachers, physicians, and other professionals, and provide other continuing education opportunities.

In addition to these skills, speech-language pathologists and audiologists frequently design, plan, market, implement, and evaluate conferences or state association meetings, publish articles in professional journals and newsletters, raise funds to purchase materials for their facility or expand their services, and work with the media to improve public understanding of the profession (Sarnecky, 1987).

Becoming A "Professional"

In a few short months, you, the student, will become a professional person with all the rights and privileges as well as all the challenges that go along with being a speech-language pathologist.

What does it mean to be "professional?" Well, for one thing, you will be earning money for doing the things you did for free as a student teacher and as a student intern in clinical practice. During that time, your hours, your therapy plans, and your therapeutic decisions were subject to possible revision by your supervisor. When you turn that corner and become a professional, *you* will be the decision maker in all these areas. Knowing who you are and what you are and where you fit in, together with your values and your attitudes, will provide the basis from which you will make decisions and plans in your professional life.

Guidelines for behavior as a professional speech-language pathologist and audiologist have been set forth in the Code of Ethics. Please note that these are only guidelines. They can only assist you in making ethical, moral, and legal decisions. There are no clear-cut answers to many of the vexing problems that arise.

There are numerous behaviors that contribute to professionalism. What sort of message do your mannerisms convey? Are they distracting, annoying, or demeaning? Do you give the appearance of aloofness? Or do you present yourself as being a competent person who shows both friendliness and helpfulness?

Your general appearance also contributes to professionalism. You may be more comfortable in what you wear when relaxing with friends, but on the job this same style of dress may convey an unintended message to parents, to co-workers, and to the individuals who are your clients. It goes without saying that cleanliness, careful grooming, and good hygiene are at the top of the list.

By dressing appropriately and conservatively you underscore respect for your client and the seriousness of your purpose. No matter what your personal preferences are, you should take into consideration the impression you are making on others. According to Moursund (1990), clothing that is comfortable, clean, and appropriate to your setting and lifestyle is another part of your therapeutic self.

Certification, Licensure, and Accreditation

Credentialing Agencies

Understanding the various forms of credentialing in speech-language pathology and audiology is part of each person's professional responsibility. To the neophyte clinician the task may seem formidable; however, some basic information may help clarify the situation.

Prerequisite to understanding is a knowledge of the types of agencies in the United States and their roles in relation to the profession of speech-language pathology and audiology.

The Voluntary Agency

Voluntary agencies have developed in countries with a democratic form of government. The voluntary agency is more clearly identified with the United States than with any other nation and has usually evolved out of an unmet need and a concern for one's fellows. The unmet need may be related to social issues, to leisure time and recreation, or to health. Voluntary health agencies may be related to specific diseases or handicapping conditions. Usually the membership of voluntary agencies is made up of both lay persons (in many cases, parents) and professionals. Examples of voluntary health agencies are the Society for Crippled Children and Adults, the United Cerebral Palsy Association, and the National Multiple Sclerosis Society.

Voluntary agencies are not certifying agencies in the usual sense of the word; however, they perform extremely vital functions for individuals with disabilities.

The Official Agency

The official agency is tax-supported and may be on the city, county, regional, state, state and federal, or federal level. Official agencies cover a myriad of categories, including health, education, welfare, vocation, recreation, and social, and they are interested in the prevention of problems, in research, and in the specific disease category. Examples of official agencies are the city or county health department and the Office of Vocational Rehabilitation. Some official agencies may be certifying bodies, such as a state department of education.

The Professional Organization

In addition to official and voluntary agencies there are also professional organizations. These, as the name implies, are made up of individuals sharing the same profession. Their goals are the establishment and maintenance of high professional standards, research, recruitment of others into the field, and the sharing of professional information. Examples are the American Speech-Language-Hearing Association, the American Medical Association, and the American Dental Association.

These various types of agencies often work together in a unique fashion, sometimes motivating each other to carry out specific tasks, often supporting each other financially and in other ways, frequently exchanging services and information and preventing duplication of services. The official agencies and the professional organizations are often accrediting and certifying bodies in addition to their other functions.

Four Types of Certification

There are four types of certification that directly affect the individual speech-language pathologist. Certification in one type does not preclude holding certification in any or all of the other three. In fact, most professionals hold more than one type.

In looking at the academic, clinical, and experience requirements of all certifying and licensing bodies, you will note that they are almost, if not completely, identical. The academic requirements follow the same pattern. Specific courses can be used to fulfill requirements of several agencies. For example, a course in articulation problems can fulfill the requirements for ASHA's Certificate of Clinical Competence, for public school certification from the state's department of education, and for a state license.

Table 2-1 may help to clarify the various forms of certification and licensing in speech-language pathology and audiology.

Certification by the American Speech-Hearing-Language Association

One type of credentialing is that issued by the American Speech-Language-Hearing Association (ASHA). Unlike licensing and state certification, it has no legal status, but nevertheless it is recognized by various states and by other professions as authenticating the holder as a qualified practitioner or supervisor. ASHA certification is known as the Certificate of Clinical Competence (CCC) and can be obtained by persons who meet specific requirements in academic preparation and supervised clinical experiences and who pass a national comprehensive examination. It may be granted in speech pathology or audiology, and some individuals hold certification in both areas. It permits the holder to provide services in the appropriate area and also to supervise the clinical practice of trainees and clinicians who do not hold certification. In 1977, it was decided that persons who were not members of the Association also could obtain the certificate by complying with the requirements.

A master's or a doctoral degree will be required for certification as a speech-language pathologist (CCC-SLP) or as an audiologist (CCC-A) by the American Speech-Language-Hearing Association by January 1, 1994. Furthermore, the graduate coursework and the graduate clinical practicum must be obtained at an institution whose program was accredited by the Council on Professional Standards of ASHA (*Asha*, 1991).

TABLE 2.1. CERTIFYING AND LICENSING AGENTS

Agency	Form	Possible Holder
American Speech-Language-Hearing Association	Certificate of Clinical Competence in Speech-Language Pathology and/or Audiology	Person who wishes to be identified by the American Speech-Language-Hearing Association as a qualified practitioner and/or supervisor in speech-language or audiology. Requires meeting ASHA standards, including a master's degree and passing an examination.
State of _____ Department of Education	Certificate to practice in the public schools of the State of _____	Person who wishes employment in the State of _____ as a speech-language pathologist and/or audiologists in an educational facility. Requires meeting state certification standards.
State of _____ Board of Speech-Language Pathology and Audiology	License to provide speech, language, and/or audiology services in the State of _____	Person wishing to practice in a voluntary or official agency (except specifically named educational facilities) or practice privately in the State of _____. Requires meeting state board standards and passing an examination.
State of _____ Board of Health or Health Occupations Council	Registration to use title of Speech-Language Pathologist and/or Audiologist	Person who wishes to use title of Speech-Language Pathologist and/or Audiologist in the State of _____. Does not bar a person from practicing but does require defined qualifications for registration.

The CCC is held by individuals who provide services in schools, universities, speech, language, and hearing centers, hospitals, clinics, private practice, and other programs throughout the United States, Canada, and many foreign countries. Information on how to apply may be obtained from the American Speech-Language-Hearing Association, 10801 Rockville Pike, Rockville, Maryland 20852.

State Certification

The speech-language pathologist who wishes to be employed in the public schools of a specific state must obtain a certificate issued by that state's department of education. The qualifying standards are set by each state and include following a prescribed course of study and fulfilling the practicum requirements. They include both clinical practice in the university clinic or one of its satellite clinics and student teaching. These experiences must be under the supervision of licensed and/or certified qualified professionals, including the clinic supervisor, the cooperating school SLP, and the university supervisor.

The passage in 1986 of Public Law 99-457, the Education of the Handicapped Act Amendments of 1986, has resulted in activities in many states to improve speech, language, and hearing services in schools by upgrading certification standards. The law, which in addition to extending services to infants and toddlers and their families and to preschoolers, also calls for personnel standards to be "based on the highest requirements in the State applicable to a specific profession or discipline."

According to Lynch (1988), states having licensure laws and the requirements of a master's degree or master's degree equivalent for private sector speech-language pathologists and audiologists, but which permit persons with a bachelor's degree to practice in schools, are the states working hardest to change state education agency certification requirements to be consistent with the academic degree requirements for licensure.

At this writing, 30 states require the master's degree or master's degree equivalent for state education agency certification. An additional eight states have adopted policies to upgrade their certification requirements by a specified future date (Lynch, 1991).*

Information on the certification requirements of each state can be obtained by writing to the office of the state's commissioner of education or its equivalent. Addresses of the various state departments of education are published periodically in *Asha*.

Licensing

A license to practice a business or profession within the geographical bounds of a specific state is issued by that state's legislature, usually through an appointed autonomous board or council. Licensing came about originally to protect the consumer from unqualified and unscrupulous persons. It is also viewed by some as a way to control growth and income of professional interest groups. Obviously, the laws to create licensure are unique to each state.

In the speech, language, and hearing profession, the licensure board may establish rules for obtaining and retaining a license, continuing one's education, and setting standards for ethical conduct; administer examinations for applicants; and enforce the license law. Usually a fee is charged for the license, which may be renewed yearly.

Another aspect of licensing is the "sunset law," which means that periodically the legislature may review the licensing agency (and other regulating agencies) and recommend whether or not it should be terminated.

Registration

An alternative to licensure is registration, a process by which an individual must meet defined qualifications in order to use a title. Nonqualified persons are not barred from practice but are prevented from presenting themselves to the public as qualified.

In some states school speech-language pathologists are not required to be licensed to practice in the public schools.

Inasmuch as laws regarding licensure change not only from state to state

*Connie Lynch, *Speech-Language Pathologist*, American Speech-Language-Hearing Association, Rockville, Maryland, (Through personal correspondence with the author).

but also from year to year, it is a good idea for the speech-language pathologist and the audiologist who plan to seek employment in a particular state to write to that state's department of education or department of health and human services to learn the current credentialing qualifications.

Accreditation of Agencies and Programs

Relevant to the administration of speech-language-hearing programs, the American Speech-Language-Hearing Association has established the Educational Standards Board (ESB), and the Professional Services Board (PSB). Accreditation by ESB assures that institutions offering educational programs in speech-language pathology and audiology at the master's level meet minimal standards. Likewise, PSB accreditation assures that minimal standards are met in school programs and clinics delivering speech, language, and hearing services to the public. Complete instructions for fulfilling ESB and PSB requirements are available from the national office of the American Speech-Language-Hearing Association.

Professional Organizations

The school SLP has a professional responsibility to keep abreast of new ideas, research, recent developments, materials, publications, and professional affairs. This is a lifelong commitment, and it is part and parcel of what being "professional" means. One way of keeping current and informed is through organizations. Organizations have meetings with speakers, publish journals and newsletters, and provide an excellent way to get to know fellow professionals. Speech-language pathologists in schools often feel isolated even though they are in daily contact with clients and school personnel. This sense of isolation comes from not having enough contact with other speech-language specialists, with whom they can share ideas, information, frustrations, and triumphs.

The oldest professional organization in the field of speech, language, and hearing is the American Speech-Language-Hearing Association, which at this writing has over 65,000 members. This organization has been one of the chief agents for growth and development in the profession.

Students are encouraged to affiliate with the National Student Speech-Language-Hearing Association (NSSLHA), which offers many opportunities not otherwise available to individuals in training. It is an affiliate of ASHA, with chapters in colleges and universities.

The Public School Caucus is an organization comprised of individuals in private and public school settings. It serves as a support group and information network that focuses on relevant school issues on the local and national levels. The group maintains a close working relationship with the American Speech-Language-Hearing Association's Ad Hoc Committee on Service Delivery in the Schools and is represented on ASHA's legislative council. PSC publishes a quarterly newsletter, holds membership meetings annually at the ASHA convention, and a PSC representative from each state is appointed to serve as an advocate for and liaison between local and national memberships. Public School Caucus members are committed to increasing the school professionals' voice in matters that concern their work and recognition of the speech-language pathologist's contribution and role. Information concerning membership may be obtained from the national office of ASHA.

Another organization with which the school speech-language pathologist may want to affiliate is the Division for Children With Communication Disorders, an associate of the Council for Exceptional Children. This organization publishes the *Journal of Childhood Communication Disorders*, holds state and national meetings, and is organized as a state group in many states. The business of DCCD is conducted by officers elected by the membership and has representation on the CEC's Board of Governors and Delegate Assembly. There are student chapters on many college campuses.

Every state has its professional organization, which holds conventions, publishes journals, sponsors continuing education programs, and offers short courses. The state organizations also publish directories of members' names and professional addresses. Listings in some professional directories authenticate the member.

In addition to the state organizations, the state may contain regional organizations. Affiliation with the regional group provides an invaluable opportunity for exchange of information and offers support to individual members. Involvement in such groups is both rewarding and enjoyable.

The national as well as state and local speech, language, and hearing professional organizations are concerned with such things as research, the study of human communication and its disorders, the investigation of intervention and diagnostic procedures, and the maintenance of high standards of performance. The professional organizations are also interested in the dissemination of information among its members and the upholding of high ethical standards to protect the consumer. There are other benefits to be derived from affiliating with a professional organization. Such a group can provide a forum for discussion of issues and can speak with a concerted voice on matters of professional interest. If the professional individual wishes to have a voice in decisions and opinions, the best way to do so is through a professional organization on the state, local, or national level.

There are a number of other professional organizations with which the school clinician may wish to become affiliated. Membership in other professional groups provides opportunities for valuable exchanges of information and enhances cooperation and understanding. Here are the names and addresses of some of the organizations you may wish to know more about:

Acoustical Society of America
335 East 45th Street
New York, NY 10010
(212)661-9404

Alexander Graham Bell Association for the Deaf, Inc.
3417 Volta Place NW
Washington, D.C. 20007
(202)337-5220

32

Chapter 2:
The
Professional
School
Speech-
Language
Pathologist

American Cleft Palate Association
Administrative Office, 331 Salk Hall
University of Pittsburgh
Pittsburgh, PA 15261
(412)481-1376

American Academy for Cerebral Palsy
1910 Byrd Ave., #118
P.O. Box 11086
Richmond, VA 23230
(804)282-0036

Association for Children with Learning Disabilities
5225 Grace Street
Pittsburgh, PA 15236
(414)341-1515

Auditory Verbal International, Inc.
505 Cattell Street
Easton, PA 18042
(215)253-6616

Autism Society of America (Nat. Soc. for Autistic Children)
1234 Massachusettes Ave., N.W.
Suite C-1017
Washington, D.C. 20005
(202)783-0125

Council for Exceptional Children
1920 Association Drive
Reston, VA 22091
(703)620-3660

Council of Supervisors of Speech Pathology and Audiology
c/o Sandra M. Uhl
Miami University
Oxford, Ohio 45056

Educational Audiology Association
Kris English, EAA Membership Chair
Dept. of Communication, C.L. 1117
University of Pittsburgh
Pittsburgh, PA 15260

International Society for Augmentative and Alternative
Communication (ISAAC)
P.O. Box 1762 Station R
Toronto, Ontario, Canada M4G 4A3

National Association for Hearing and Speech Action
814 Thayer Avenue
Silver Springs, MD 20901
(301)897-8682

National Down's Syndrome Congress
1800 Dempster Street
Park Ridge, IL 60068
(312)823-7550

National Head Injury Foundation (NHIF)
1140 Connecticut Ave, NW, Suite 810
Washington, DC 20036
(202)296-6443

National Easter Seal Society for Crippled Children and Adults
2023 West Ogden Avenue
Chicago, IL 60612
(312)726-6200

United Cerebral Palsy Association
330 East 34th Street
New York, NY 10016
(212)947-5770

DISCUSSION QUESTIONS AND PROJECTS

1. You are the school SLP. What do you do in these situations:
A parent asks you to continue therapy with a child even though the child has reached optimum improvement. The parent says that the child enjoys therapy and it would be traumatic to terminate the therapy. The parent offers to pay you for continuing to see the child.
A local hearing-aid dealer asks you to supply a list of the students in the school with hearing losses.
An elementary teacher asks if she may see the records and reports of a junior high-school student enrolled in therapy. She asks your opinion concerning whether or not the student is mentally retarded. (The child isn't.)
You are asked to do private after-school therapy with a child enrolled in a school in which you are working. The child is already receiving therapy and is on your caseload.
The parents of a student referred for medical evaluation ask you to recommend a doctor.
You are asked to do therapy in the school with a student who is currently receiving therapy at a nearby private speech, language, and hearing center. You are aware of this, but the parents did not provide you with this information.

2. Find out what your state department of education standards are in relation to what is required for certification as a speech-language pathologist in the schools.

3. Find out if your state has licensing or registration for school speech, language and hearing professionals. If so, what are the requirements?

34

**Chapter 2:
The
Professional
School
Speech-
Language
Pathologist**

4. Find out what speech, language and hearing organizations are active in your area. Check to learn how often meetings are held and what types of programs are presented. Invite an officer of a local organization to speak to your class.

5. Is there a state speech, language and hearing organization in your state? When do they hold meetings? Do they publish journals and newsletters?

6. What are the advantages in joining the National Student Speech-Language-Hearing Association?

CHAPTER 3

Foundations of the Program

Introduction

This chapter contains basic information about the factors that need to be considered in planning and organizing a school speech-language program. It should be understood that the information about the structure of the school system is general. You, as the school speech-language pathologist, should acquaint yourself with the structure of the educational system in the state in which you live and work. The same is true about the city, county, or district school system in which you are employed. In fact, if you are considering a specific site for future employment it is a good idea to learn as much as possible before you sign a contract; then continue to increase your knowledge as you go along.

Public Laws 94-142, 99-457, and 101-476 have had tremendous effects on public school special education and speech-language programming. As you read through this book you will find frequent references to these laws. Your task will be to keep abreast of the changes and requirements of federal and state laws affecting your school speech, language, and hearing program.

Public schools are supported by state and local taxes as well as federal flow-through funds. It is important to be knowledgeable about how your program is supported, how budgets are determined, and the process by which funds are allocated. In some cases the input of the SLP is required or expected and in some instances you may wish to have input. Without a knowledge of how schools and programs are financed the SLP is at a serious disadvantage.

Another factor in planning a speech, language, and hearing program is the number of students with whom you will be dealing. It would be nice if these figures were conveniently available, but unfortunately determining prevalence figures is a complex and slippery matter. The best we can do is to rely on all the current information at hand and make generalizations that apply to individual school systems. Much more attention is given to determining prevalence figures at the present time than in the past, and the developments in this area are promising.

The Organizational Structure of the School System

The Program on the State Level

Because of our democratic philosophy of education, we are committed to the idea of education for all. The major responsibility for education rests with each state rather than with the federal government. Through a state board of education, policies, regulations, rules, and guidelines are set. The laws for education in each state are enacted through the state legislatures, and money is appropriated through this body. A state superintendent of instruction is the chief education officer in each state. A state department of education is responsible for carrying out and developing policies, regulations, and standards related to schools. Figure 3-1 depicts the jurisdictional relationship between the state and the local educational agencies (Rebore, 1984).

State departments of education provide state consultants in various areas of special education. The responsibilities of the consultants in speech, language, and hearing may vary slightly from state to state, but in general the tasks are similar throughout the nation. A major task of the professional staff on the state

FIGURE 3.1. Jurisdictional Flow Chart. From Ronald W. Rebore, Sr., A HANDBOOK FOR SCHOOL BOARD MEMBERS, 1984, p. 5. Reprinted by permission of Prentice-Hall, Englewood Cliffs, New Jersey.

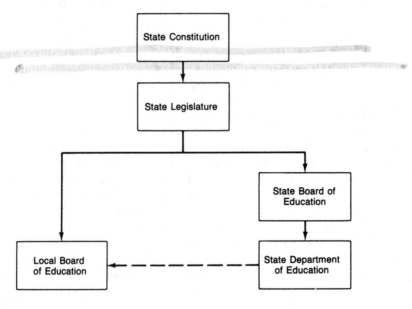

level is to monitor and enforce minimum standards of practice in local programs that are partially or fully reimbursed with state money. Along with this local programs are encouraged to approach optimal goals in serving the needs of students with disabilities. The state staff may provide leadership and assistance in identifying, developing, and maintaining optimal standards. Some examples of the ways in which professional leadership may be exerted by the state consultants in assisting local programs include the following (*Rules for the Education of Handicapped Children* 1982):

A. Professional literature and materials
   1. Establish procedures by which local materials can be exchanged.
   2. Periodically prepare a selected bibliography of significant materials.
   3. Write or prepare materials that are needed but not available.
B. Preservice education programs
   1. Identify unmet needs in university and staff program.
   2. Serve as an instructor on an emergency basis.
   3. Serve as a resource person for university students and instructors.
   4. Assist in the development of new professional curricula.
   5. Assist in the evaluation and improvement of existing professional curriculum.
C. Inservice education programs
   1. Provide professional field services.
   2. Conduct and encourage area professional meetings.
   3. Encourage and assist professional organizations.
   4. Encourage and stimulate development of appropriate non-credit workshops and courses.
D. Research studies and experimental projects
   1. Identify research needs.
   2. Initiate and conduct research studies and experimental projects.
   3. Promote and encourage research studies and experimental projects.
   4. Interpret and disseminate findings and conclusions.
E. Professional relations at the local, state, and national level
   1. Maintain membership in professional organizations.
   2. Attend meetings of professional organizations.
   3. Contribute to journals of professional organizations.
   4. Provide leadership for professional organizations.
F. Appropriate and desirable criteria for optimal special education
   1. Initiate procedures by which these criteria can be identified.
   2. Encourage schools to use the criteria in self-evaluation.
   3. Utilize criteria in professional field services.

G. Extension of present programs in special education

    1. Identify unmet needs within present standards.

    2. Assist local district in establishing new programs or expanding established programs.

H. Identification of emerging needs for new programs in special education

    1. Identify unmet needs not now provided for within existing standards.

    2. Encourage and stimulate the development of pilot studies and experimental programs.

    3. Evaluate results of studies and submit recommendations for needed modifications in existing law and standards.

Public Law 94-142 requires each state to submit an annual plan, which is to be approved by the U.S. Department of Education. Each of the components of the act is addressed in the state's plan with a description of the process by which the requirements will be met. One of the responsibilities of the state education agency is to monitor and evaluate the activities of the local education agency to assure compliance with the federal statutes.

In addition, the state education agency is responsible for the proper use of federal funds in the administration of local programming for children with disabilities. The state education agency is also responsible for the following activities in regard to PL 94-142: (1) the adoption of complaint procedures, (2) the disbursement of federal funds, (3) an annual report on the number of children served and the criteria for counting them, (4) the establishment of a state advisory committee on the education of children with disabilities, (5) a comprehensive system of personnel development, and (6) records on all the activities related to PL 94-142.

Regional Resource Centers

An important linkage between the state and the local school districts is the regional resource center. The Ohio Division of Special Education, for example, recognized that a state agency cannot relate to each individual teacher, supervisor, and school district. Under PL 94-142, Title VI-B, Amended Annual Program Plan, the Ohio Department of Education utilized the discretionary portion of Title VI-B to fund the Special Education Regional Resource Center (SERRC) system (*Operation and Management Plan for the Northwest Ohio Special Education Regional Resource Center,* 1983). The SERRCs:

Assist school systems in the initiation and expansion of programs and services for children with disabilities through joint planning and cooperation among school systems to serve an increased number of handicapped children.

Serve as the mechanism by which school systems will plan, organize and implement an effective regional identification and child find strategy to insure that all handicapped children residing in Ohio who need special education will be identified, located, and evaluated so that appropriate programs and services can be planned and provided.

Provide school systems with resources designed to improve the quality of instruction for handicapped children through a materials delivery and in-service training based on newly developed instructional materials and methodologies.

Provide school systems with technical assistance in interpreting, implementing, and complying with legislative mandates, rules and regulations.

Serve as a catalyst for product development and dissemination of information which meets the needs of special educators, parents and children.

Serve as a clearing house for information pertaining to special education.

The Program on the Local Level

On the local level, school systems are organized into school districts. In some states, these are known as intermediate units. The district, or intermediate unit, is a geographical area and may cross county lines. It is governed by a superintendent, who is the chief administrative officer, and a district board of education, which is elected by the people of the district and is responsible for developing and establishing policies.

The superintendent is the chief personnel officer for the school system in that he or she makes recommendations to the board concerning the hiring, promotion and dismissal of staff members. The superintendent is responsible for the total operation and maintenance of the school system; leadership of the professional staff; and administration of the clerical, secretarial, transportation, and custodial staffs.

The basic responsibility for each school system rests with the citizens of that community inasmuch as they elect the school board. The school board selects the superintendent, who recommends the needed staff to operate the schools.

Depending on the size of the school system, there may be assistant superintendents who have specific areas of responsibility, such as finance or buildings and grounds.

The structure of individual school systems may vary from state to state and from community to community. Usually there are directors of elementary education and of secondary education. There may be directors of pupil personnel service, instructional program services, special education services, child accounting and attendance, guidance and health services, and others.

Each principal is responsible for supervising the professional and support-services staff assigned to that building. The role and function of the elementary-school principal will differ from that of the middle- and secondary-school principal. In addition, roles and functions of principals will vary according to the unique characteristics of the community and will reflect the various cultural backgrounds of the students and their parents. The principal is responsible for managing the school's instructional program, pupil personnel services, support services, and community relations.

Figure 3-2 is a partial organizational chart of the school system on the local level.

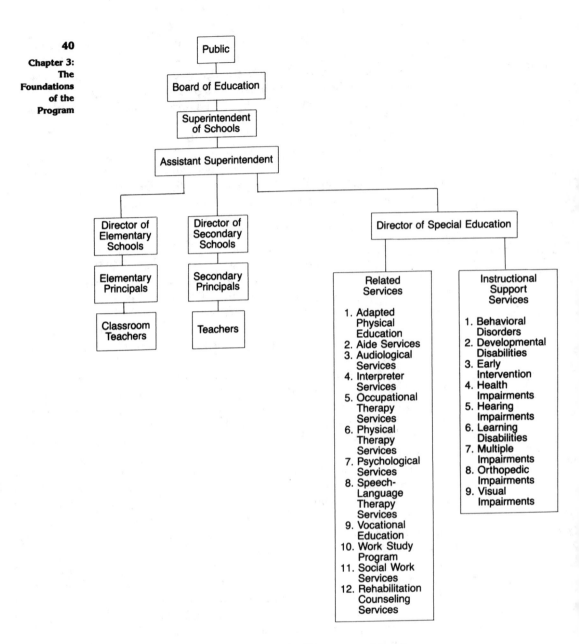

FIGURE 3.2 Partial Table of Organization on the Local Level.

An understanding of the structure of the school system is necessary for the speech, language, and hearing specialist to function effectively. Obviously there will be variations in organizational structures throughout the country; thus in addition to having a general knowledge of the school system, you, as the SLP, will need to be familiar with the educational facility in which you are employed.

The Education for all Handicapped Children Act of 1975 mandates a free, appropriate public education for all children and youth with disabilities. Special education and related services must be provided at no cost to the child or parents.

The act provides:

1. All children with disabilities and their parents are guaranteed due process with regard to identification, evaluation, and placement.

2. A written individualized education program must be developed and implemented for each child receiving special services.

3. To the greatest extent possible children with disabilities should be educated with nonhandicapped children in the least restrictive environment appropriate to the child's needs.

4. There are two priorities among children with disabilities (a) those not currently receiving any education and (b) those with the most severe handicaps within each disability who are receiving an inadequate education.

5. The federal government is committed to assuming up to 40 percent of the excess costs incurred in providing the programs for children with disabilities.

6. The local education agencies are responsible for providing the appropriate educational programs.

7. The local education agencies are responsible for periodic review and monitoring of such programs.

8. Local education agencies must file a written plan clearly stating the procedures involved in meeting the provisions of the mandatory law. These include (a) a child-find process, (b) nondiscriminatory testing and evaluation, (c) the goals and timetable of the plans, (d) guarantee of complete due process procedures, and (e) a guarantee to protect the confidentiality of data and information.

Not only are children with disabilities eligible for appropriate educational programs but they are also eligible for all extracurricular activities such as music, art, and debate. The costs of educating children are borne by the school system. When the child's school cannot provide the appropriate educational placement, the local school system must pay for transportation, tuition, and room and board if the child is enrolled in a residential or tuition-based program.

Public Law 94-142 also states that the child with disabilities has the right to a nondiscriminatory evaluation of educational needs. Tests and evaluation materials must not be culturally discriminatory and must be administered in the predominate language spoken in the home. The evaluation is administered by a team of professionals and must include the child's parents and/or guardians.

The heart of PL 94-142 is the Individualized Education Program, or as it is more familiarly known, the IEP. Essentially the law requires that an IEP be developed for *each* child with a disability and reviewed jointly by a qualified school official, the student's teacher or teachers, the parents or guardians, and when appropriate, the student. The components of the IEP are explained in Chapter Eight including a sample IEP.

Public Law 99-457

In 1986, PL 94-142 was amended to authorize early intervention programs for infants, toddlers, and preschool children who are at either biological or environmental risk for developmental delays. The amendment, known as PL 99-457, expanded the age ranges for receipt of services down to birth and increased the diversity of populations to be served by public school programs. It provided funding incentives for states to facilitate development and implementation of programs and services to children ages three to six years with handicaps. By the school year 1990–1991, states had to implement programs that ensured that the rights and protections of PL 94-142 were available to children ages three to five. State and local education agencies were to supervise the programs. To receive federal funding, school districts needed to include this population in their state education plan submitted annually.

PL 99-457 also established a discretionary program for provision of services to children birth to three years of age. States had to designate "lead agencies" to oversee the implementation of programs for infants and toddlers. In some states, schools accepted the responsibility for these programs. In other states, agencies such as the Department of Health or the Department of Maternal Care accepted the responsibility.

Because PL 99-457 is an amendment to PL 94-142, there are many similarities in the mandates of the two laws. All rights and protections of PL 94-142 are extended to infants, toddlers, preschoolers, and their families. Like PL 94-142, PL 99-457 mandated due process, services provided at no cost to families, interdisciplinary interaction and the team process, a comprehensive system of personnel development, and a comprehensive child-find and child-count system.

Just as PL 94-142 has had great impact upon the role of the SLP practicing in the schools, so will PL 99-457. Since the target populations are infants, toddlers, and young preschoolers, the focus of programming is necessarily on the family unit. This supports the understanding that family services play an important role in preschool programs and require a partnership between parents and professionals. This means that changes will be needed in service delivery models and intervention procedures employed by speech-language pathologists. They will be required to use infant and family assessment tools and interventions and to work with numerous agencies outside of the school system. In some cases, services will be provided by private practitioners, community-based program, local education agencies, or in the family's home.

As professionals increase their understanding of the needs of persons with disabilities, the federal mandates regulating the provision of education and services continue to change. In 1990, The Education of the Handicapped Act was further amended. Reflecting sensitivity to the negative effects labels often carry for individuals, the title of the law was changed to the "Individuals with Disabilities Education Act (IDEA)." It reinforces the use of "person first" language, changing all references in the law to handicapped children to "children with disabilities."

Two new categories of disability were added, "autism" and "traumatic brain injury." Another change mandated that schools provide transition services for students, promoting movement from school to post-school activities. These include post-secondary education, vocational training, integrated employment, continuing and adult education, adult services, independent living, or community participation. The law also assures that students needing assistive technology services will receive them from trained personnel. The addition of these categories and services will influence the types of students carried on public school clinicians' caseloads. The changes support developing therapy objectives and procedures which are functionally based. The law also requires the inclusion of a statement of needed transition services in the IEP for students when they reach the age of 16. Speech-language pathologists and audiologists can be expected to collaborate with other educators and agency representatives to plan transition services and recommend strategies for meeting transition objectives.

Inclusive Education

Instructing children with disabilities has always been very difficult. The practice of mainstreaming children with disabilities into regular class situations on a full-time or part-time basis was mandated in Public Law 94-142. The intent was to provide students with learning opportunities they would not have if they spent their entire day in the special class setting interacting only with other children who also have disabilities. Mainstreaming has worked well in some school systems and not so well in others. Some educators and family members did not feel that mainstreaming went far enough in meeting the full needs of children.

Recently, leaders in special education have advocated meeting the challenge to provide improved programming for children with special needs by embracing the concept of the *inclusive education*. Also referred to as *integration*, the philosophy of inclusion is founded in the belief that children shold be educated and completely involved in the activities of their neighborhood schools and within their communities regardless of the severity of their disability.

In order for inclusion to work successfully, there needs to be a great amount of support, communication, and interaction among teaching personnel. There are some who believe that the entire education system will have to be reorganized in order for inclusion to be successful. Watching educational programs spring into action and work toward the goal of implementing more effective programs for children with disabilities is very exciting. What you see are regular education and special education teachers forming partnerships and working closely together (collaborating) to plan the best teaching strategies, materials, and techniques for individual children. The objective is for educators, regardless of their discipline, to combine their knowledge and expertise to jointly develop better solutions to problems than each could have done alone. The classroom teacher maintains the primary responsibility for the student's instructional program. Specialists, including speech-language pathologists and audiologists provide support in designing and implementing special programs to meet the students' needs.

Parents as Team Members

The public laws clearly give parents a major role in making decisions regarding the education and services provided to their children.

The rights and responsibilities of the parents and school district are described under the *due process* section of the handicapped child law. Due process provides a procedure for reaching resolution when either party is in disagreement regarding the educational program for a child. Both the school district and parents have equal status at meetings. Parents have a right to question why any one procedure is necessary, why one may be selected over another, how a procedure is carried out, and whether or not there are alternative procedures. If parents disagree with the recommended procedures they have the right of review with an impartial judge. The purpose of due process is to give parents the right to have the school system explain to them and defend the recommended procedures. It does not necessarily make the parents adversaries to the system.

On the other side of the coin, the parents have the responsibility of dealing openly and honestly with the school system, accurately describing their child's behavior and reasonably and realistically requesting services (Sherr, 1977). The school district has the right to disagree with the parents.

Under due process the parents are entitled to the following procedures:

1. A written notice before any action is taken or recommended that may change the child's school program

2. A right to examine all records related to the identification, evaluation, or placement of the child

3. A chance to voice any complaints regarding any matters related to the educational services the child is receiving

4. An impartial hearing before a hearing officer or a judge in the event that the school and the parents cannot agree on the type of school program for the child

5. An adequate appeals procedure if parents are not satisfied with the due process procedure. The case may be taken to the state department of education or finally to a court of law.

Prevalence and Incidence: How Many Children Are We Talking About?

The *prevalence* figures of speech, language, and hearing problems, or the *existing* number of persons affected at a *specified* time, are difficult to obtain. *Incidence* figures, the number of *new* cases occurring during a given time period, are usually not available. When reading or interpreting reports, care should be taken not to confuse these two terms.

Why is it important for prevalence figures to be known? One of the most crucial reasons is that programs for children to 21 years of age are based on the number presently being served and those to be served in the future. Because the infusion of money into states by the federal government is based on prevalence figures, these figures should be available and as accurate as possible.

Not only is it important for planners on the state and national levels to have prevalence information, but it is important on the local level as well. The school speech-language pathologist needs to know approximately how many students in a given school population can be expected to be eligible for speech, language, and hearing services. The principal needs to know because of space requirements. The superintendent needs to know so that an adequate number of speech-language pathologists may be hired.

Unfortunately, determining the number of individuals with communication impairment is not simply a matter of taking a head count. Reports on incidence and prevalence of speech, language, and hearing problems among preschool and school age pupils have been difficult to complete for several reasons. Definitions and terminology regarding disabling conditions may vary from state to state and from person to person so that the reporting of various conditions is not consistent. There is not yet a universally accepted, comprehensive classification system for speech and language disorders. Sometimes the data reported are based on too few children, and sometimes survey results are based on reports completed by persons with little or no training in identifying speech, language, or hearing problems. Often children who are nonverbal, non-English speaking, institutionalized, school dropouts, preschool age, or in special classes are not considered in the survey collection. Many children who might have died at birth or as a result of a traumatic brain injury are today being saved through improved medical care, and this points to an increase in communication problems.

Very few prevalence and incidence studies have been completed in recent years. Therefore, a reliable data base has not yet been established. Much of the information reported in the literature is based on studies and surveys that were completed over 20 years ago. While this is not ideal, it does provide us with some insights into data available about prevalence and incidence.

A national study of communication disorders among school-age children (Hull, 1969) included 40,000 pupils and was based on a random demographic sample. It covered overall speech patterns, articulation, voice, fluency, and hearing and has provided us with important information about the communication disorders in public schools (see Table 3-1).

Phillips (1975) stated, "Based on the majority of recent studies, it is probably safe to judge that between 8 and 10 percent of the children now enrolled in school exhibit some kind of oral communications disorder." I would tend to agree with Phillips. There are even indications that the figure of 10 percent is a conservative one. There are possible reasons for this. In reporting it is often common practice to report the presence of only one handicapping condition. For example, a learning-disabled child may also have accompanying speech, language, or hearing problems, but in a survey that child is reported as being learning-disabled only.

In regard to the incidence of language problems, Jones and Healey (1973) observed, "The incidence and prevalence of language and language-learning problems are not known. Only recently has there been increased awareness of the problems many children have in using linguistic symbols in comprehension, transformation and/or expression for communication."

The issue of identifying students with language disabilities has become even more complicated as the definition of language disorders has expanded to include pragmatics, problems related to reading and written language, and nonverbal communication.

The difficulty in ascertaining the incidence of children with language delay and language deviations continues to be a problem, not only for speech, language, and hearing clinicians but also for all workers in the field of special education. As indicated earlier the number is probably larger than we suspect.

Beitchman, Nair, Clegg, and Patel (1986) conducted a study to determine the prevalence of speech and language disorders in five-year-old kindergarten children in the Ottawa-Carlton region of Canada. Their results indicated that 6.4% of the children exhibited a speech impairment without concomitant language disorder, 8.04% presented language disorders only, and 4.56% showed a

TABLE 3.1. COMMUNICATION DISORDERS IN THE PUBLIC SCHOOLS (1969)

Degree and Type of Deviation	Percent
Acceptable overall speech pattern	34.8
Mild overall speech deviation	53.1
Moderate overall speech deviation	10.6
Extreme overall speech deviation	1.5
Acceptable articulation	66.4
Moderate articulation deviation	31.6
Extreme articulation deviation	2.0
Acceptable voice	50.1
Moderate voice deviation	46.8
Extreme voice deviation	3.1
Acceptable fluency	99.2
Dysfluent	.8
Normal bilateral hearing	88.8
Reduced hearing	11.2

47

**Prevalence
and Incidence:
How Many
Children Are
We Talking
About?**

combined speech and language disorder. They identified differences between boys and girls in that age group, with prevalence being higher among the boys than girls. The authors suggested that these results be interpreted cautiously due to the many variables surrounding prevalence research. Their study also did not suggest whether the children identified would benefit from therapy. They recommended further study of these issues.

Recent research in the area of prevalence and incidence remains scant. ASHA's Research Division maintains reports on the prevalence and incidence of communication disorders. Their information is derived from a variety of sources including omnibus surveys, census statistics, the National Center for Health Statistics, and annual reports to Congress from the U.S. Department of Education Office of Special Education. Based on sources such as these, staff in the Research Division reported the following statements about the prevalence and incidence of communication disorders in children in recent years:

- More than one in 25 preschoolers suffer from some type of communication disorder.

- Sixty to 70% of the preschool children identified as having disabilities exhibit speech or language impairments.

- In 1988, over 2 million school-age children received speech-language services: over 57,000 children were classified as hard of hearing or deaf.

- Of the approximately 4.8 million children (ages 6 to 21) with disabilities served in 1987, 39.2%, or about four in 10, received services for a communication disorder.

- The number of children ages 6 to 21 with disabilities receiving services in the 1989–1990 school year declined to 23.1%. It was believed that the decline was due to several factors, including:

  1. improved and more discriminating identification procedures;

  2. provision of speech and language services outside of the special education delivery system (such as within the regular education classroom); and

  3. a current trend to identify students with language disorders as having specific learning disabilities rather than having speech and language impairments.

Number of Students Reported as Receiving SLP Services

Each year, the Office of Special Education Programs of the U.S. Office of Special Education and Rehabilitative Services in the Department of Education reports the progress being made in providing a free appropriate public education for all children with disabilities. The report includes statistical information on the number and percentage of children who received special education and related services in a given time period, the implementation of particular sections of the law, and the provision of financial assistance to state and local education agencies through formula and grant funding to support the delivery of services (U.S. Department of Education, 1991).

The system for determining the amount of funds schools receive for providing services for children with disabilities necessitates categorizing and counting children according to the disabilities they present. The data presented in the reports concerning the numbers of children served are referred to as "child count" data. States collect the information annually and these numbers are used as the basis for allocating funds to states in order to provide necessary services. Counts are nonduplicative, representing the number of children served rather than the prevalence of disability conditions.

Services provided for the primary disability are referred to as "special education" and are included in the count. Services provided for concomitant conditions are designated as "related services" and are not included in the child count. Thus, only those children whose primary handicap is speech or language can be counted as receiving speech-language services. Children with other handicaps who receive speech-language and audiology services as related services have to be counted in the category which represents their primary disability (mental retardation, specific learning disability, serious emotional disturbance, multiple disabilities, hearing impairment, and so on). Therefore, the numbers reported in the "speech-language-impairment" category are not representative of the total number of children actually served by speech-language pathologists in schools. This procedure for counting has made it difficult to determine how many children in the nation have actually been receiving speech-language services and may have resulted in underfunding for speech-language and hearing services over the past several years.

Speech-language pathologists in the schools provide services to students with a wide variety of communication impairments. Results of a 1985 ASHA Omnibus survey showed the following caseload composition in the school setting: language (52.2%), articulation (34.8%), fluency (4.1%), hearing (4.5%), voice (2.4%), and other conditions (2.0%). These findings were supported by the results of a 1988 ASHA Omnibus survey indicating that the largest portions of speech-language pathologists' caseload were language disorders (median 50.2%) and articulation disorders (median 39.7%). Informal reports by practitioners indicate that at least 45% of their school caseload was comprised of students who had primary disabilities other than speech-language and were receiving therapy as a related service.

Table 3-2 reports the number of children ages 6 to 21 served under Chapter 1 of the Elementary and Secondary Education Act, State Operated Programs (ESEA [SOP]) and Part B of IDEA (formerly EHA-B) during the 1989–1990 school year. Due to space limitations, only four of the seven disability categories of interest to speech-language pathologists and audiologists are presented. The "All Disabilities" column reports totals for all seven disability categories.

The percentage of funding generated by a particular category is derived by determining the ratio of children with a particular disability in comparison with the total number of children with disabilities. Youth with speech-language impairments (ages 6 to 21), therefore, accounted for 23% of those served in 1989–1990. Children with hearing impairments, including deafness, comprise 1.3%.

TABLE 3.2. NUMBER OF CHILDREN (AGES 6 TO 21) WITH DISABILITIES
RECEIVING SPECIAL EDUCATION SERVICES UNDER PL 94-142:
SCHOOL YEAR 1989–1990*

State	All Disabilities	Speech Language Impairment	Hearing Impairment	Specific Learning Disabilities	Mental Retardation
AL	89,916	21,528	991	32,132	26,800
AK	12,213	2,917	144	7,535	408
AZ	52,231	10,496	964	30,312	4,987
AR	42,283	6,951	527	22,653	10,657
CA	410,448	94,355	6,819	246,619	24,039
CO	50,220	81,030	774	25,029	3,041
CT	57,788	8,985	625	31,254	3,670
DE	12,208	1,769	191	6,801	1,253
D.C.	5,695	749	50	2,800	933
FL	206,124	60,858	1,371	88,909	25,627
GA	90,442	19,888	1,137	27,074	22,623
HI	11,727	2,129	243	6,679	1,153
ID	18,506	3,501	344	10,907	2,695
IL	221,505	55,1076	2,901	105,062	25,741
IN	103,219	35,491	1,159	40,060	19,573
IA	52,641	23,875	768	23,875	10,241
KS	39,628	10,531	629	16,800	5,502
KY	68,264	21,136	802	22,606	18,311
LA	63,902	17,962	1,219	26,307	10,656
ME	25,208	5,715	286	11,165	2,352
MD	80,878	22,751	1,172	41,949	5,384
MA	135,431	28,841	1,712	49,592	29,412
MI	148,332	32,743	2,388	68,630	18,698
MN	71,561	13,575	1,362	32,913	10,220
MS	54,492	17,472	486	27,057	7,905
MO	96,294	24,649	888	46,587	14,096
MT	14,507	3,680	205	8,050	1,073
NE	28,795	7,651	513	12,689	4,176
NV	15,496	3,335	145	9,226	1,112
NH	17,235	2,939	227	10,427	922
NJ	160,634	48,449	1,294	82,820	5,681
NM	31,544	9,259	473	15,180	2,024
NY	272,928	24,055	3,999	163,562	21,081
NC	109,519	23,006	1,853	49,009	21,134
ND	11,406	3,644	172	5,420	1,461
OH	189,787	49,525	2,093	74,077	42,217
OK	59,992	15,661	630	28,896	11,248
OR	51,120	12,739	1,429	26,746	4,381
PA	192,843	52,474	2,744	82,837	33,944
P.R.	33,009	1,278	1,068	10,017	16,202
RI	1,492	3,066	159	12,170	1,042
SC	69,072	17,968	961	28,280	14,408
SD	12,648	3,852	254	5,788	1,509

(*continued*)

TABLE 3.2. (Continued)

State	All Disabilities	Speech Language Impairment	Hearing Impairment	Specific Learning Disabilities	Mental Retardation
TN	93,935	22,404	1,196	49,871	12,938
TX	306,574	3,852	4,313	174,410	23,735
UT	40,585	7,253	537	18,940	3,162
VT	12,352	3,437	204	5,752	1,572
VA	97,107	22,241	1,212	50,222	12,705
WA	71,171	12,788	1,660	37,016	7,412
WV	40,089	10,035	379	18,314	8,261
WI	71,064	13,506	213	23,785	4,694
WY	9,412	2,499	138	5,175	595
U.S. TERR.	9,204	1,738	141	4,906	1,484
TOTAL	4,261,676	976,186	58,164	2,064,892	566,150

*U.S. Department of Education, (1991). "Thirteenth Annual Report to Congress on the Implementation of the Individuals with Disabilities Act." Washington, D.C.: U.S. Government Printing Office.

Other important points not shown in these tables include the following:

- Because the procedures used for identifying, classifying, and reporting students with speech-language impairments vary from state to state, the percentage of children served ranged from .9% to 4.1%.

- The educational placement (environment) for 75.9% of those students with speech and language impairments and 26.9% of those with hearing impairments was reported as being the regular class: 33.5% of the children with hearing impairments were reportedly served in a separate classroom.

- Since 1976, the number of students reported with speech or language impairments declined from 35.6% to 23.7% in 1989–1990.

- By contrast, in the 13-year time period between 1976–1989, there was an increase from 25% to 49% in the number of students classified with specific learning disabilities.

- There is a decrease in the relative proportion of children and youth identified with mental retardation. This decline has been a trend.

Funding for School Speech, Language, and Audiology

Who pays for speech, language, and audiological services in the schools? Not surprisingly the answer is that everyone who pays taxes pays for the schools and their many services. Local education agencies are supported in part from local taxes, with reimbursement from state foundation programs. In recent years the federal government through the Public Laws have reimbursed states for a portion of the expenditures for special education.

States have set minimal standards for speech education programs including speech, language, and audiology. The standards may cover such areas as person-

51

**Funding for
School
Speech,
Language,
and
Audiology**

nel qualifications, housing, facilities, equipment, materials, transportation, caseload, and case size. Failure to comply with state standards may result in the loss of foundation money to the school district.

There are three types of reimbursement to the local education agency; unit, per pupil, and special. Each state has its unique features in funding patterns, but generally they fall within these three categories.

A. Unit reimbursement
   1. Pure unit
      a. Per professional
      b. With stipulations (class size, number of regular class units)
   2. Percentage
      a. Salaries, transportation, materials, equipment, and so on.
      b. Provision for proration
   3. Straight sum
      a. Specified personnel-type allotments
      b. Provision for materials and equipment
B. Per-pupil reimbursement
   1. Straight sum
      a. Specific sum for each disability area
      b. ADA-based or ADM-based
   2. Excess cost above a base figure for each student served
   3. Weighted formula
C. Special reimbursement
   1. Instructional materials and equipment
   2. Transportation
   3. Facilities
   4. Research and experimentation
   5. Personnel training
   6. Pupil assessment
   7. Residential care
   8. Extended school year
   9. Specific personnel
      a. Administrators and supervisors
      b. Teachers and specialists
      c. Paraprofessionals
      d. Ancillary services (physicians, audiologists,* psychologists, social workers, physical therapists, occupational therapists and so on)

*In states where audiologists are not employed in the schools and services by these professionals are obtained through contractual arrangements.

"ADA-based" refers to average daily attendance, and "ADM-based" means average daily membership. The terms are identical in meaning. Because school attendance is compulsory all schools must report the attendance each day. At some point in the school year, usually in October and February, the ADA is determined.

A "unit" may be defined as a specific number of students or a special class. In Ohio, for example, (*Rules for the Education of Handicapped Children,* 1982) a unit for a speech-language pathologist may be approved on the basis of 2,000 children in "average daily membership." Therefore, a school system with a total population of 6,000 students would be eligible for three full-time SLPs. Or a school system with a population of 5,000 students would be eligible for two and one-half units, which would be two full-time and one half-time SLP.

"Per pupil reimbursement" means that the local education agency is compensated for each student receiving special education services. This could be based on ADA or ADM.

A "special reimbursement" plan usually supplements a unit or per-pupil reimbursement. For example in Ohio a special unit for speech-language pathology may be approved on the basis of 50 children with multiple impairments, hearing impairment, orthopedic and/or other health impairments in special class or learning center units. Many of these reimbursement formulae encourage high caseloads because the amount of funds generated for a local education agency increases as numbers of students served increases (Dublinske, 1988). These reimbursement procedures fail to account for the total number of students with communication disorders or the frequency and intensity of services needed.

While the intent of the laws which enable government supported education to children with disabilities is noble, the reality is that Congress has never adequately provided the needed level of funding to support services and programs. This has created financial difficulty for local school districts. Out of need, schools have had to seek alternative methods of funding programs to help defray expenses for providing education and services to students with disabilities. The regulations interpreting Public Law 94-142 indicated that states could use any sources available to pay for services included on the child's Individualized Education Program. This included state, local, federal, and private funding sources such as insurers or third party payers such as Medicaid (Kreb, 1991).

School districts had difficulty trying to collect funds from private and third party funding sources until Public Law 94-142 was amended in 1986. At that time, Public Law 99-457 required interagency cooperation and coordination of resources. It reaffirmed the obligation of third party payers to fund services delivered as part of the IEP (O'Brien, 1991).

According to Peters-Johnson (1990), school districts in some states started billing private insurance companies, health maintenance organizations (HMOs), and Medicaid for services provided. Reimbursable services included:

• audiological services;

• case management;

• mental health services;

53

**Funding for
School
Speech,
Language,
and
Audiology**

• allied diagnostic services and treatment for physical therapy;

• occupational therapy; and

• speech-language therapy.

Although billing third-party payers for services may bring economic relief to school systems, the practice is not without problems. O'Brien (1991) raised a number of questions related to third-party billing:

• Will insurance companies drop coverage of speech-language and audiology services as the number of insurance claims increase?

• Will the type of documentation required by third-party payers create hardships for speech-language pathologists and audiologists and result in reduced contact time?

• Will school systems be able to bear the expense of setting up complex billing systems?

• Will individuals currently working in the school setting have the necessary qualifications and credentials required for third-party reimbursement?

• Will unhealthy competition arise between school practitioners and private practitioners?

The answers to these questions will most likely evolve over the next several years as schools increase the frequency with which they seek third-party funding. Speech-language pathology and audiology programs will be directly effected by these funding issues since the cost of conducting these programs is high.

DISCUSSION QUESTIONS AND PROJECTS

1. Why is it necessary for the school pathologist to know the structure of the school system on the local level?

2. What questions would you ask about the structure of the school system if you were being interviewed for a position as SLP?

3. What relationship do you see between the prevalence figures for students with speech-language impairments and program planning?

4. Why are most prevalence figures for children with language disabilities difficult to obtain?

5. Public Law 94-142 states that test and evaluation materials must be non-discriminatory. Give examples of what this means.

6. Find out the minimum standards for speech-language and audiology programs in your state.

7. Find out if there is a regional resource center in your area. What services does it provide? Visit the center.

8. Interview a school SLP to find out to whom this individual is directly responsible in the school structure.

9. Invite the state department of education consultant in speech-language pathology to speak to your class. Prepare a list of questions to ask.

10. How would you explain the parent's rights and role in program planning to the parents of a child if they do not speak fluent English?

11. Why is it important to use "person first" language when referring to individuals with disabilities. Discuss some of the ramifications of referring to individuals by labels such as "mentally retarded," "learning disabled," "emotionally disturbed," "deaf," and the like.

12. What type of documentation is required in order to receive reimbursement from third-party pay sources?

CHAPTER 4

The School Speech-Language Pathologist as a Manager

Introduction

When school speech-language clinicians are asked about their programs, services, and job performances, they are quite likely to make the following responses: "We need more time to plan," "There are too many children on my case roster," "We need more staff members," "I have trouble scheduling students because of all the other school activities," "My room is too small and not well ventilated," and so on. Interestingly enough, the school clinician is generally pleased with the progress of the children in the program, and the school administration is pleased with the program. Why, then, the complaints? Very possibly the reason is that each school pathologist is constantly faced with the challenge of providing the highest caliber of services with the most efficient expenditure of time, money, and resources, including physical, technical, and human resources.

In this chapter we will examine how the school SLP, in the role of manager, may utilize time more efficiently and expand human resources more effectively to provide optimal services to students. Topics covered include planning ahead, establishing goals, managing time and paperwork, utilizing supportive personnel, and using computers to carry out administrative functions.

Management: Basic Principles

Perhaps the best place to start is to admit to ourselves that in the field of management we need to acquire new skills, new techniques, and new instruments, as well as an understanding of the principles of the management process: planning, organizing, staffing, directing, and controlling. The goal of comprehensive ser-

56

Chapter 4:
The School
Speech-
Language
Pathologist as
a Manager

vices for all children with disabilities points out the need for appropriate managerial skills at the local level as well as at the state and national levels.

Presently, there is a trend toward implementation of formal systems for program planning, development, management, and evaluation. "Total quality management" principles are gaining acceptance at national, state, and local levels. By adhering to the philosophy and processes associated with total quality management, professionals can identify their program's strengths and weaknesses and work toward better development of programmatic goals and objectives. The basic tenet of total quality management is consumer satisfaction. Speech-language pathology and audiology programs serve many consumers including students with communication impairments, teachers and other specialists, parents and family members, school administrators, and the community. Efforts to provide quality services should be supported through all aspects of the program including planning and managing time, developing program goals and objectives, scheduling, implementing assessment and treatment, reportwriting, and so on.

The need to examine closely the school programs, what they are attempting to do, how they are doing it, and how effective they are is vital. The school speech, language, and hearing clinician today and in the future will need to be acquainted with sophisticated tools and systems for evaluation and measurement of programs and personnel. A "cookbook" approach is not the answer because there is no single "recipe" for a good program.

The Management Roles of the School Speech-Language Pathologist

There was a time when most speech-language pathologists (we called them "speech therapists" then) entering the job market had to start from scratch in organizing speech, language and hearing programs in a school system. Fortunately for you, speech-language and hearing programs are already in place in most school systems thanks to federal and state legislation mandating help for children with communication impairments. And thanks, too, to far-sighted school boards and administrators who realized that children needed to communicate effectively in order to benefit from what the educational system had to offer. Last, but not least, thanks to our founding fathers (and mothers) whose foresight and concern established the professions of speech-language pathology and audiology.

Today, however, the picture is different. You, in all probability, will enter the profession in the schools in an already established program. But this condition has its own set of challenges and problems. What are some of the possible roles you may fill in a school system?

Following is a list of some of the possible roles you may fulfill when you are employed as a speech-language pathologist in a school system. This list is by no means complete and it should be pointed out that you may be fulfilling a combination of any of these roles simultaneously.

1. You may be the only SLP in a small school district and would be working in several schools using the pull-out model.

2. You may be one of a large staff of SLPs serving a large city system.

3. You may be one of many SLPs in a rural school district covering a large geographical area.

4. You may be assigned to a self-contained special classroom in one building.

5. You may be assigned as a specialist in one area of communication disorders (for example, stuttering), and providing therapy.

6. You may be a consultant in one area of specialization providing consultant services to classroom teachers and other SLPs.

7. You may be an SLP serving only special education classes.

8. You may be providing consultative services through in-class intervention in regular classrooms.

9. You may be providing consultative services through in-class intervention in self-contained classrooms. For example, a modified learning disabilities classroom.

10. You may be supervising paraprofessionals or aides.

11. You may be supervising student interns.

12. You may be the coordinator of the speech-language services in a school district, or an entire school system.

13. You may be the administrator of a department of pupil personnel services and special education.

14. You may be the administrator of speech-language services in a geographical area encompassing several school districts.

But don't be concerned that these last three will be offered to you as your first job. On the other hand, with experience and with your personal professional goals, you may sometime find yourself as an administrator. In examining all of the professional roles of a school speech-language pathologist, as we will do in this textbook, you will see that all of them require administrative and managerial skills. Your very first position out of college as an SLP will require that you have a firm grasp of the administrative hierarchy of a public school system and your place in it, as well as your managerial skills in carrying out your own program, on your own or in concert with others.

The Many Faces of Management

What is management? It has been said that management is the art of getting things done through people. It does not require doing things so much as in seeing that things get done. Even in our highly mechanized civilization, most things are done by people. The major function of management is to see that people function effectively to accomplish what needs to be done. The skills necessary to good management include the following:

• communicating effectively;
• managing time;

58

Chapter 4:
The School
Speech-
Language
Pathologist as
a Manager

- understanding the job of supervision;
- understanding leadership and developing a leadership style; and
- planning, setting goals, and measuring results.

Many colleges and universities through their continuing education programs offer courses in management and supervision. Professional organizations such as the American Speech-Language-Hearing Association offer seminars in management and supervision for credit. In addition, there are books available on the topic. Some of the publications which would be of help to speech-language pathologists and audiologists are:

- Anderson, Jean. *The Supervisory Process in Speech-Language Pathology and Audiology.* Boston: College-Hill Press, 1988.
- Coventry, W. F., and Irving Burstiner. *Management: A Basic Handbook.* Englewood Cliffs, New Jersey: Prentice-Hall, Inc., 1977.
- Flower, Richard M. *Delivery of Speech-Language Pathology and Audiology Services.* Baltimore/London: Williams and Wilkins, 1984.
- Frattali, C. M. Editor. *Quality Improvement Digest.* Rockville, MD: The American Speech-Language-Hearing Association. Published quarterly.
- Kouzes, James M. and Barry Z. Posner. *The Leadership Challenge: How To Get Extraordinary Things Done in Organizations.* San Francisco, London: Jossey-Bass Publishers, 1988.
- Oyer, Herbert J., Editor. *Administration of Programs in Speech-Language Pathology and Audiology.* Englewood Cliffs, New Jersey: Prentice-Hall, Inc., 1987.

The Management of Time

The management of time is an important factor in considering the role of the school SLP. Public Law 94-142 has been blamed for creating increased amounts of paper work in the implementation of its procedures. Although this has undoubtedly accounted for an increased expenditure of time, there are ways of managing time that can lead to increased productivity.

Let us look first at what the school clinician's job entails.

1. *Screening.* In this activity the clinician identifies children with speech, language, and hearing problems.
2. *Diagnosis and assessment.* This task includes formal and informal testing and is carried on throughout the school year.
3. *Staffing and placement.* This procedure is often carried out by a placement team and involves reviewing the data on individual students to develop individualized educational programs for each student.
4. *Intervention.* These are the actual therapy and instructional activities provided by staff members to develop, improve, or maintain communicative abilities.

5. *Record keeping.* This task includes all activities involved in maintaining information on the delivery of services to each student.
6. *Consultation and collaboration.* These activities include the exchange of information and jointly sharing responsibility with parents, teachers, psychologists, nurses, and others in regard to individual students.

Other services, not directly related to students with communication disorders, maintain, promote, and enhance the speech, language, and hearing program. These activities are of an indirect nature, but at the same time, are essential to the program. They include in-service training programs provided by the speech, language, and hearing staff, as well as in-service training received by them for the purpose of upgrading their skills. Travel to provide services is a necessary part of many school clinicians' programs, and many specialists are engaged in research related to the school programs. Time is also spent organizing, planning, implementing, analyzing, and evaluating programs. Some school specialists spend time supervising student teachers in speech pathology and audiology as well as paraprofessionals assigned to the program. Conservation and prevention programs may be carried out by the school clinicians, as well as public information activities such as talks to various groups, radio and television programs, and newspaper articles.

The roles and responsibilities of speech-language pathologists have expanded and changed in recent years. The expansion of delivery of service models to include consultation and collaboration, the increasing numbers of children served in the schools, the increasing numbers of children with handicapping conditions and severity of problems are factors which demand more time and greater expertise of the school clinicians. In addition, the SLP's role has been expanded to include the gestalt of a client's total communication system. All of this means that there must be careful planning and careful allocation of time by the speech-language pathologists in the schools.

Planning for the Year

After the school clinician has taken a good look at what the job entails, he or she determines long-range goals based on a priority list. Inexperienced clinicians in a new situation sometimes try to do everything the first year. This is not only impossible but also unwise even to attempt. The result may be spreading oneself too thin and not accomplishing anything satisfactorily. For example, the clinician may have to decide whether a teacher in-service program or a parent in-service program is more important during the first year. The clinician may then rationalize that the teachers are more readily available and need to understand the program more immediately than do the parents, so the in-service program for teachers would take precedence. During the following year, however, the clinician may decide to devote more time and energy to the parent in-service program, and that program would be given top priority.

After priorities for the year are established, the long-range program goals are written. It should be pointed out that long-range goals need to be examined periodically and modified if necessary. The goals for the year should indicate the

60

**Chapter 4:
The School
Speech-
Language
Pathologist as
a Manager**

time (or times) of the year that the goals would be implemented and accomplished as well as the amount of time involved.

Goals may be written for an entire school year, or some school clinicians may prefer to write them for a semester. A combination of the two time slots may also be utilized.

Program goals should not be confused with goals that individual clinicians establish for themselves. These clinician's goals and the program goals may not necessarily be at odds, but it should be kept in mind that although clinicians may come and go, programs, it is hoped, go on forever. Setting goals for the program, with the clinicians as the implementers, will allow smooth, continuous functioning of a program despite changes in personnel. There is probably nothing more frustrating for a school clinician who is stepping into a job than to learn that the previous clinician left no records concerning what was planned, what was accomplished, when it was accomplished, how long it took, and what has yet to be done.

In addition to establishing yearly or semester program goals based on a priority list of the tasks involved in the clinician's job, other information would have to be available, including

1. Number of speech, language, and hearing clinicians on the staff
2. Number of schools to be served
3. Amount of travel time between schools
4. Enrollment figures for each school building. This would have to be further broken down into the following figures:
   a. Enrollment by grade level
   b. Enrollment of special education classes, including hearing impaired, physically impaired, mentally retarded, emotionally disturbed, learning disabled, and trainable mentally retarded
5. Number of preschool children in the school districts based on child-find figures

The school clinician uses this information to decide on the appropriate methods of delivery-of-service and scheduling systems.

Planning for the Week

In planning for the week the key word is *flexibility*. The school clinician will have to decide how much time during the week will be spent in actual therapy and in travel if more than one school is involved during any one day. Specific blocks of time can be devoted to these activities. An activity such as screening must be carried out in a block of time, and the school clinician may want to reserve blocks of time at certain times of the year or the semester for this part of the program.

Such activities as diagnosis and assessment, staffing and placement, and consultation are necessary parts of the program, and time for these activities may be set aside in daily or weekly blocks. For example, the staffing and placement team may not meet every week, so the block of time set aside weekly could be used on alternate weeks for staffing and placement and diagnosis and consultation.

Record keeping and time spent in organizing, planning, implementing, analyzing, and evaluating the program could be scheduled at times of the day when staff members are in the school but children are not present. For example, mornings before children arrive at school and afternoons after they are dismissed could be utilized for these activities. Many school systems set aside a time usually referred to as *coordination time* for tasks of this nature.

Another important activity is that of consultant to the classroom teacher. This may be done on an informal one-to-one basis or as part of an inservice training program for teachers, school administrators, other school personnel, and parents. Because communication is the keystone of the education process and because even the most skilled classroom teacher cannot teach a child who has not developed adequate communication skills, the school speech-language pathologist has much to offer in helping to improve communication abilities. The school SLP needs to plan for time for consultation.

Providing in-class intervention in the regular education classroom may be done on a weekly basis. Be sure to check if this service delivery model is consistent with the standards of the state in which you are working.

If paraprofessionals and aides are assigned to the program, time must be planned for their in-service training programs, and time must be allowed for the supervision of such personnel.

For many of the activities mentioned, time is not planned on a regularly scheduled basis but certainly must be set aside to include these important facets of the program.

Planning for the Day

In planning time for the day the school clinician will have to know how many hours per day the children are in school. What is their arrival time and what is their dismissal time? How much time is allowed for lunch and recess?

The time that the teachers are required to be in school and the time they may leave in the afternoon is set by school policy, and school clinicians should follow the same rules that teachers are required to follow. This sometimes poses a problem for the school clinician who is scheduled in School A in the morning and School B in the afternoon, but who must return to School A for a parent conference after school is dismissed. The problem arises when the teachers in School B think the clinician is leaving school early. The problem can usually be alleviated by following the rule of always informing the principals of School A and School B of any deviation in the regular schedule.

The greatest percentage of actual therapy time will take place in the morning because the morning sessions are longer and children are available for a longer period of time. This is true in most school systems, but there will be exceptions.

The school clinician will have to decide the length of the therapy sessions. There does not have to be a uniform length, and sessions may range from 15 minutes to an hour. The length depends on a number of factors, and before

62

**Chapter 4:
The School
Speech-
Language
Pathologist as
a Manager**

determining the pattern of the sessions the clinician may want to look at the school's schedule of classes, recess, dismissal time, and so on.

Among the considerations are the number of children to be seen in total, the number in groups, and the number in individual therapy. Also, some children will be in the generalization phase of therapy and do not require as much time as children who are just beginning. It is wise to schedule the sessions a few minutes apart to allow for children to arrive on time or to allow time for the clinician to locate a child whose teacher has forgotten to send him or her to therapy. Children often assume the responsibility of remembering when to come to therapy, and for younger children who have not yet mastered the art of telling time, a clock face drawn on a sheet of paper with the hands pointing to the time of the session will allow the child to match the clock face with the clock on the wall.

In planning the daily schedule the school clinician will need to retain as much flexibility as possible. Children change and their needs change. The child who once required 30 minutes of individual therapy per day may later need only 15 minutes twice a week. Or the child who once needed individual therapy may need the experience of a group to progress. This flexibility must also be understood by the principal and the teachers, and it is the responsibility of the clinician to interpret the rationale involved in making changes in schedules.

As a result of mainstreaming and the influx of more children with serious disabilities into the public schools, the school clinician will need to allow time for working with classroom teachers of the mentally retarded, emotionally disturbed, hearing impaired, learning disabled, and multi-handicapped. In fact, any communicatively handicapped child may require direct or indirect intervention by the speech, language, and hearing pathologist in the school, and depending on the needs of the children in a specific school, the clinician will have to make allowances for the intervention in both the daily schedule and the overall scheduling of services.

Coordination Time

In most school systems, the SLP sets aside a specific time which is allotted to the numerous activities that must be carried on in addition to the time spent in therapy. This is usually referred to as "coordination time." This may be a block of time set aside during the week or it may be several periods of time during the week not scheduled for therapy. Or it may be a combination of the two.

A study was carried out involving 57 school clinicians during the 1986–1987 school year in both rural and urban areas of Erie, Huron, and Lorain counties in Ohio encompassing a total of 3,507 students with communication impairments, ages 0–22. The study kept track of the type and frequency of activities that consumed time other than direct therapy. One of the areas of concern related to whether time allocated for coordinating activities was sufficient to meet the changing demands of the speech-language pathologist's position in the public schools. (Smith, Carter, and Gilder, 1988).

Table 4-1 shows the average amount of time spent on coordination activities per speech-language unit for the 1986–1987 school year.

TABLE 4.1. AVERAGE OF TIME SPENT ON COORDINATING ACTIVITIES
PER SPEECH-LANGUAGE UNIT FOR 1986–1987 SCHOOL YEAR

Activity	Average Number	Estimated Duration (Minute)	Average Time Per Year (Hour)
Speech screenings	191	20	63
Language screenings	161	20	53
Hearing screenings	219	10	36
Speech diagnostics	46.7	20	15
Language diagnostics	45	90	67
Auditory processing diagnostics	14	60	14
Three-year re-evaluations	20	60	20
Teacher conferences	92	10	15
Administrative conferences	13	10	2
Multifactored team meetings	24	15	6
Guidance conferences	6.3	10	1
Nurse conferences	12	10	2
Parent conferences	80.9	30	40
Phone calls to parents	63.5	10	10
Phone calls to others	17.7	5	1
Annual reviews	64	10	10
Speech-language summary report	30	30	15
IEP writing	57.4	30	29
Communication status report	27	10	4
State or national conferences	0.4	—	—
Regional inservices	3.4	180	10
Local professional meetings	5	120	10
Referrals received	43.2	—	—
Classroom observations	18	30	9
Totals			432 hours

In reviewing the data collected on the division of time within a work week and considering the growing demands to expand coordinating activities while maintaining high case loads, the authors of the study recommended that the following changes be considered:

1. Time allocated for coordinating activities must be increased, particularly during that period of the day when students are in attendance. . . . One can justify easily the use of the full day permitted by state standards to conduct such responsibilities.

2. As time allocated for coordinating increases, time for direct therapy decreases. Speech-language pathologists need to re-evaluate their own caseloads, adhere to severity rating scales, and perhaps develop more strict criteria for student enrollment. Reduction of direct therapy would require the development of a variety of service delivery models. This also requires administrative support and a shift in philosophy that the entire educational team, on which the speech-language pathologist plays an important part, is responsible for communication programming.

64

Chapter 4:
The School
Speech-
Language
Pathologist as
a Manager

3. Speech-language pathologists have been strongly encouraged by their districts to maintain maximum caseloads, because caseload size directly influences the revenues coming into the districts. States may consider basing some aspect of funding procedures on types of services provided to students, in addition to caseload size.

4. Attempts should be made to increase access to support personnel. We need the services provided by secretaries, aides, and volunteers.

5. Training programs in colleges and universities need to address issues such as time management, efficient implementation of coordinating activities, interdisciplinary team strategies, and use of support personnel (Smith, Carter, and Gilder, 1988).

Personal Time Management

The school clinician must take into consideration two factors in overall time management. The first is the need to plan time on a yearly, semester, weekly, and daily basis; the second is the need for the clinician to manage his or her own time within the larger framework. In respect to both factors, planning is an essential first step. The next important step is setting priorities and sticking with them.

The school clinician who is the sole speech, language, and hearing specialist will have much greater responsibility than a person stepping into a job where there is an ongoing program with other school clinicians already involved. In the latter situation, the new clinician fits into the program that has already been set up. In the former, the clinician may be the key planner and organizer.

Time-saving techniques are not necessarily new; most people are too busy to implement them or perhaps do not know how to implement them. One technique is to make a list of things to be done *today*, then to set priorities on that list and follow them. Another piece of advice is to keep a card file containing alphabetized names and telephone numbers of persons and agencies necessary to the work. A record of incoming and outgoing telephone calls might be recorded on a sheet and later put in a loose-leaf notebook, providing a record and synopsis of the conversations. An example of this form follows:

TELEPHONE CALLS

STAFF MEMBER: (your name) _____

Date	To or from	Results
2/16/93	From Billy Jones' mother, Mrs. Henry Jones	Requested results of Billy's hearing test. Letter sent 2/16/93. See file
2/17/93	To Susan Smith, prin. Findlay Jr. High	Confirmed date to talk to teachers (March 3rd)
2/18/93	To Tommy Brown's parents, M/M Jack Brown	Requested parent conference. Agreeable. Will call me back re time

Another important factor in personal time management is not to let paper work pile up. A period of time each day or each week should be devoted entirely to this task.

It is also important to look at ways that may be wasting time, for example, attending too many meetings or allowing too many interruptions. Most school clinicians would like to add an extra hour to a day now and then or think in terms of an occasional eight-day week. Because time is scarce it must be managed with maximum effectiveness. Experts in time management tell us that selecting the best task from all the possibilities available and then doing it in the best way is more important than doing efficiently whatever job happens to be around.

No matter how one looks at it, we are dealing with that precious and fleeting commodity—time. It is scarce, inelastic, does not have a two-way stretch, cannot be stored or frozen for future use, and cannot be retrieved. It can, however, be managed with effectiveness.

Writing Program Goals and Objectives

The school SLP, although responsible to another person in the hierarchy of the administration, is responsible for the management of the school's speech, language, and hearing program. The school system may be a large urban system, a small community system, or a sprawling countywide system, and the school SLP must assess the needs in light of the local situation and plan accordingly.

If the school system employs more than one SLP, there must be coordination of their activities. If it is a large or moderately large system, one SLP may be designated as the coordinator of the program. But even the school SLP who is working alone in a small school system needs to have a plan of action.

Planning ahead is the key to a successful program. Setting goals and objectives is one of the most critical elements of the planning process. Once the goals and objectives have been determined, the next step is writing them down in such a form that they clearly communicate their intent to all the persons concerned and involved in the program.

The utilization of written goals and objectives has many potential advantages in the school speech, language, and hearing program. First, it allows for change, because through the system of periodic review, objectives will need to be revised and rewritten. Also, it creates a positive pressure to get things done. Communication among professionals will be improved. There will be more precise definitions of the roles and responsibilities of the school speech, language, and hearing clinician. A system for evaluating and assessing the overall program is inherent in the written goals and objectives. Better utilization of each staff member's time and capabilities will be encouraged. And finally, there will be a better basis for understanding the program both within the school system and in the community.

According to Coventry and Burstiner (1977), a common core of problems exists for any organization. First, there is a need to establish major objectives and major policies. What is the purpose of the organization, and how can that pur-

66

Chapter 4:
The School
Speech-
Language
Pathologist as
a Manager

pose be attained? Does everyone involved understand clearly the objectives and policies?

Second, a structure must be set up to determine the responsibilities for the various tasks that must be accomplished in order to achieve the objectives. The relationships between these jobs must be established.

Third, there must be resources such as space, equipment, furniture, staff, supporting services, and supervisors, to mention only a few.

Finally, there must be long-term and short-term programs of work that conform effectively to the objectives and policies that have been laid down.

Goals are long-term and short-term, tangible, measurable, and verifiable. They are not nebulous statements but specific statements of a desired future condition or accomplishment. Ideally, goals should be set by all person involved in the structure so there is a commitment on their part. Once the goals have been determined it is crucial to get them down in writing. The language must be clear and concise and must communicate the intent to all relevant parties.

Writing Goals for the Program

Let us look at some examples of writing goals and objectives. We will first consider writing long-range program goals, assuming that you have already evaluated the existing situation and have determined the overall needs of the program. Keep in mind that although these are long-range and broad in focus, they still need to be stated specifically and concretely.

> *Example:* One year from (date) the clinician will have developed and written a language curriculum guide for teachers of the adjusted curriculum classes in Ottawa County.
>
> *Example:* By (date) the clinician will have completed a research project related to case selection at the kindergarten level.
>
> *Example:* By (date) 90 percent of the pupils in Danbury School identified as having communication problems and needing therapeutic intervention will be receiving services.

Some goals and objectives may be narrower in focus and have a shorter time frame.

> *Example:* By (date) the clinician will have administered audiometric screenings to 95 percent of the second-grade pupils in the Port Clinton School district.
>
> *Example:* By (date) the clinician will have conducted group parent meetings for parents of all children enrolled at Lakeside School.

Some objectives are very short-term and have a very narrow focus. Sometimes they may be considered subgoals, that is, contained within a goal or objective and contributing to its attainment.

> *Example:* During the second week of school in September 19—, the

clinician will acquaint teachers at Jefferson School with referral procedures through an in-service meeting.

Example: By (date) the clinician will write an article for the local newspaper and prepare items for the local radio and television stations regarding the prekindergarten communication evaluation program to be held during the first week in May at Catawba and Danbury schools.

A *criterion,* or *standard of performance,* is the description of the results of a job well done. It should always be a number or an indication of quantity, that is, *how much* and *by when.* It should be realistic, control-oriented, and high enough so that when the task is completed it will have been of value to the program.

Example: Dismiss 30 percent of the pupils enrolled as functionally corrected and 50 percent as greatly improved by the end of the school year.

Example: By (date) the clinician will provide three demonstration language-development sessions in 50 percent of the kindergarten classrooms of Bataan School, and receive positive feedback, in written form, from 90 percent of the teachers involved.

The *evaluation* is an indication of the method to be used to determine if the goal or objective has been accomplished. An indication of the evaluation may be a report sent to the coordinator of speech-language and hearing services. Or it may be a list of post test scores, a list of referrals made, or a chart indicating that change has occurred.

Example: By (date) the clinician will have administered speech-language screening tests to 95 percent of the third-grade pupils in Marblehead School, and a report will be submitted to the school principal and the director of speech-language and hearing services.

Occasionally, objectives are difficult to measure or confirm, even though they are activities or events that when accomplished lead to the overall improvement of a situation or condition.

Example: The clinician will attempt to improve communication with the classroom teachers by
    1. Eating lunch with the teachers at least two times per week or more often if possible
    2. Inviting teachers to observe therapy sessions
    3. Attending as many school meetings and social functions as time permits.

School SLPs are familiar with the process of writing goals and objectives for the students with whom they work. Program goals are also important so that there is a clear understanding of *where* the program is going, *how* it will get there, and *how* to know when the objectives and goals are achieved. The manager of the program should be sure everyone understands the goals and, ideally, each participant should have a part in formulating them.

Quality Improvement

Another aspect of the management of school speech-language-hearing programs must be taken into consideration. This aspect is quality. The profession's commitment to quality began as early as 1959 when the American Speech-Language-Hearing Association established its accreditation program with the founding of the American Boards of Examiners in Speech Pathology and Audiology (ABESPA). Later, the name of the accrediting body was changed to the Professional Services Board (PSB). At the present time, standards and guidelines are established by ASHA for the accreditation of educational programs, certification standards for professionals, and standards for professional services. These standards and guidelines are continually reviewed and, when necessary, changed to meet current needs.

Quality Improvement of Professional Practices

The communication disorders profession is continually evolving. Our understanding of the nature and impact of disorders is improving as are our techniques and approaches to diagnosis and treatment. Consequently, it is important to monitor and review professional practices on an ongoing basis to assess the quality of service delivery and to determine adjustments needed to make improvements.

Speech-language pathologists and audiologists in various settings have begun to develop and use continuous quality improvement approaches to improve performance and service delivery in order to better meet consumer expectations and needs (Frattali, 1991). These efforts have been supported by state and local education agencies, third party payers, government regulators, and accreditation agencies.

School clinicians should establish a comprehensive quality improvement plan which is appropriate to the school setting. The plan should reflect a commitment to continual improvement. It should focus on all activities of the program. It should include a process for monitoring, assessing, and evaluating various aspects of the program's work process and service delivery such as the program *structure* (facility and staff characteristics), the *process* (methods of treatment and care), and the *outcome* (end result) (Frattali, 1990). The plan should also state the specific elements (e.g., criteria, indicators, standards, or protocols) against which aspects of quality are compared. The intent is to use performance-based and outcome-oriented measures to identify areas in service delivery in need of improvement. If deficiences are noted, then actions or steps must be taken to make improvements.

It is important that staff members work as a team in developing and implementing the quality improvement plan. This means jointly assuming responsibility for identifying problem areas and implementing change. Therefore, to be effective, the plan should incorporate procedures for peer interaction and review. It should encourage collaboration among staff and administration in a joint planning effort to improve areas where problems are noted.

The concept of continuous quality improvement crosses all health and education settings. It is a professional and ethical responsibility. Frattali (1990) recommends the following 10 steps for designing a quality assurance process:

1. Select a structure, process and/or outcome approach (e.g., *structure* (clinician qualifications, condition of test equipment, adequacy of test environment), *process* (treatment methods, selection of diagnostic measures, appropriateness of goals), *outcome* (client satisfaction, functional communication, goal attainment).

2. Define a target client population (e.g., age group, diagnosis, disorder severity).

3. Choose a method of assessment (e.g., retrospective, concurrent, prospective).

4. Select a data source (e.g., clinical records, interview, observation, questionnaire).

5. Select/develop standards against which to measure the quality of care provided.

6. Set the level of compliance.

7. Specify expectations.

8. Collect and analyze data: evaluate the quality of care.

9. Formulate corrective action if deficiencies are found.

10. Monitor care until deficiences are corrected.

Lastohkein, Moon, and Blosser (1992) developed a quality improvement plan appropriate for the school setting. As a process for review, they selected the implementation of a collaborative service delivery model within a local school district. Following is an explanation illustrating how each of the ten steps described by Frattali would be applied to evaluate and improve collaborative efforts. (See Table 4-2, Quality Improvement Plan.)

Step One (Assign Responsibility)

The first step in Frattali's model is to determine who will be responsible for monitoring the speech-language pathology program's collaborative efforts. The following individuals will most likely be involved in collaboration: the speech-language pathologist, audiologist, parents/caregivers, special education director, principle, superintendent, classroom teacher, social worker, school nurse, psychologist, and other professionals in special education.

Any of these professionals could function as the quality improvement coordinator responsible for assigning each individual with specific responsibilities and establishing a formal reporting mechanism. For the purpose of this discussion, the SLP on the team is designated as the quality improvement coordinator.

In order to determine the effectiveness of collaborative efforts and areas where improvement is needed it was necessary to narrow the focus of the quality improvement plan by delineating the scope of care in the following ways.

70

Chapter 4:
The School
Speech-
Language
Pathologist as
a Manager

Step Two (Delineate Scope of Care)

The second step, delineate scope of care, determines the who, what, where, and when of the QI process. In our school collaborative program, the following guidelines are specified:

Who: Individuals needing/requiring services in schools who may be served under a collaborative model include elementary children who are language-learning disabled with class placement in a program designated for children with learning disabilities.

What: Services provided under a collaborative model include but are not limited to the following: consulting with other professionals, inservicing the caregivers and other professionals, establishing goals and treatment plans, co-treating, maintaining and exchanging reports, teaching other individuals to implement intervention strategies, counseling caregivers/individuals regarding student's communication disorders and the impact on education.

When: Collaboration should continuously be occurring among professionals. This may take place throughout the school day, at weekly staff meetings, or at IEP meetings.

Where: Collaboration can occur in the students' learning environment, at staffing meetings, at IEP meetings, via other forms of communication exchange.

How: Collaboration can be achieved by communicating face-to-face (e.g., at staffing meetings, IEP meetings, in the classroom), via written communication (e.g., exchange written reports, memos, news letters), or via telephone.

Steps Three Through Six (Identify important aspects of care, identify quality indicators, establish thresholds for evaluation and collect and organize data, respectively)

Important aspects of care must be identified to provide a focus for the quality improvement efforts. Aspects of care required for effective collaboration include: long term planning, assigning responsibilities, improving participant's competence in specified areas, identifying case selection criteria, and addressing administrative issues such as scheduling conflicts and time constraints. For each aspect of care identified, a quality indicator, threshold evaluation, data source, collection method, and time frame are established. Table 4-2 illustrates how these steps were adapted in the quality improvement plan. To complete the process, Frattali indicates that the following four steps are necessary.

Step Seven (Evaluation of Care)

If a predetermined threshold is not met, the data should be analyzed to determine if opportunities for improvement exist.

Step Eight (Action Plan to Improve Care)

If improvements can be made, an action plan to improve care should be established. Because this step provides an opportunity to make revisions (i.e., review plan, change indicators, identify new indicators), this is a critical step in the model.

Step Nine (Assess the Actions and Document Improvement)

Procedures should be established for continuous monitoring, evaluation, and documentation of revisions specified in Step Eight.

Step Ten (Communication Findings)

Finally, a report to communicate findings is distributed to all team members involved.

TABLE 4.2. QUALITY IMPROVEMENT PLAN

Aspect of Care	Quality Indicator and Threshold Evaluation (TE)	Data Source	Collection Method	Time Frame
Administrative Issues: Time Constraints and Scheduling Conflicts	Establish regular meeting times.			
	A) Full Team TE: 90% attendance at scheduled meetings	Records of meeting dates & attendance at meetings.	100% review; Concurrent	Quarterly
	B) 2–3 Person Collaborative Partner Teams TE: 90% attendance at scheduled meetings	Records of meeting dates & attendance at meetings.	100% review; Concurrent	Monthly
Long Term Plan	All team members (as listed in Step 1) will participate in setting long term goals (e.g., goals to be met in 5 years). TE: 90% actual participation	Staff minutes and reports.	100% review; Concurrent	March 1993
	All team members will participate in setting short term goals used to achieve above long term goals. TE: 90% actual participation	Staff minutes and reports.	100% review; Concurrent	June 1993

(continued)

TABLE 4.2. *(Continued)*

Aspect of Care	Quality Indicator and Threshold Evaluation (TE)	Data Source	Collection Method	Time Frame
Participants' Responsibilities	Specific responsibilities will be assigned to each team member for completion during a specific period of time (e.g., 3 month increments over a 2 year period). TE: 85% completion of all task assigned	List of assigned tasks, activity reports, summary reports.	100% review; Concurrent	Quarterly
Team members' expertise and competence	Team members identify areas of knowledge necessary for collaborative model to be successful (e.g., knowledge of each others' disciplines, knowledge of speech and language development, impact of communication on academic success, school curriculum, process of collaborative model). TE: 85% agreement on topics selected	Topics for discussion identified by team members at staff meetings or via questionnaire.	100% review; Concurrent	Ongoing
	Team members obtain information on specified topics necessary for the collaborative model to be successful. TE: 80% participate in learning activities	Agendas and brochures from inservice programs, continued education credits, academic records, summaries of literature reviews, information received from other professionals.	Periodic review; Retrospective	Ongoing

(continued)

TABLE 4.2. (Continued)

Aspect of Care	Quality Indicator and Threshold Evaluation (TE)	Data Source	Collection Method	Time Frame
Case selection criterion	Accurate identification of language-learning disabled children to be served under the collaborative model.	Test scores of students placed in learning disability classes.	50% of caseload; Concurrent	Semi-annually
	TE: 90% agreement of team members regarding eligibility criteria and case selection			

Supportive Personnel

Ptacek (1967) suggested the use of aides to expand the services of the speech-language pathologist and audiologist in his article "Supportive Personnel as an Extension of the Professional Worker's Nervous System." The advent of PL 94-142 in 1975 presented an immediate and continuing need for increased services to children with handicaps in public schools. In 1981, the Committee on Supportive Personnel, of the American Speech-Language-Hearinge Association published "Guidelines for the Employment and Utilization of Supportive Personnel." These guidelines included the definition of supportive personnel, qualifications, training, roles, and supervision. The following issues formed the basis for the guidelines:

1. The legal, ethical, and moral responsibility to the client for all services provided cannot be delegated; that is, they remain the responsibility of the professional personnel.

2. Supportive personnel could be permitted to implement a variety of clinical tasks given that sufficient training, direction, and supervision were provided by the audiologist and/or speech-language pathologist responsible for those tasks.

3. Supportive personnel should receive training that is competency-based in character and specific to the job performance expectations held by the employer.

4. The supervising audiologist and/or speech-language pathologist should also be trained in the supervision of supportive personnel.

5. The supervision of supportive personnel must be periodic, comprehensive, and documented to ensure that the client receives the high-quality services that he or she needs.

In 1985, the National Colloquium on Underserved Populations developed a resolution recommending that the needs of the following populations be ad-

74

**Chapter 4:
The School
Speech-
Language
Pathologist as
a Manager**

dressed: American Indians, economically disadvantaged, remote/rural, linguistic minority, institutionalized, developing regions. The resolution was subsequently passed by ASHA's Executive Board. The Committee on Supportive Personnel then prepared a report which acknowledged the needs of underserved populations while stressing the importance of maintaining adequate standards of clinical service (*Asha*, 1988).

ASHA has suggested that it is necessary for supportive personnel to have a thorough knowledge and understanding of the culture and language of persons with whom they work clinically. It is also suggested that supportive personnel may be used as interpreters or translators with linguistically diverse populations if the SLP does not meet the recommended competencies to provide services to speakers who have limited English proficiency skills.

The Code of Ethics (revised January 1992) of the American Speech-Language-Hearing Association clearly deals with the issue of supportive personnel and the supervision of same in "Principle of Ethics II: Individuals shall honor their responsibility to achieve and maintain the highest level of professional competence." (Refer to the Code of Ethics printed in Chapter Two.)

In the school setting, supportive personnel have been referred to by different titles (e.g., teacher's aides, classroom aides, educational associates, and volunteer aides). Sometimes, they are paid employees or they may be volunteers. In some states, they are licensed and the background and educational levels and amount of training may vary, depending on the requirements of the school district. Supportive personnel in special education usually receive specialized training. Supportive personnel in speech-language pathology and audiology may receive training provided through formal course work, workshops, observation, supervised practicum, or any combination of these activities. Some institutions have training programs leading to state certification of paraprofessionals. Appropriate areas of training may include:

1. Normal processes in speech, language, and hearing

2. Disorders of speech, language, and hearing

3. Behavior management skills

4. Response discrimination skills including but not limited to the discrimination of correct and incorrect verbal responses along with the dimensions of speech sound production, voice parameters, fluency, syntax, and semantics

5. Program administration skills including stimulus presentation and consequation, data collection and reporting procedures, and utilization of programmed instructional materials

6. Equipment and materials used in the assessment and/or management of speech, language, and hearing disorders

7. Overview of professional ethics and their application to the assistant's activities

Some institutions have training programs leading to state certification of paraprofessionals.

As the goal of full educational opportunities for all special students is realized, the utilization of paraprofessionals by speech-language pathologists and audiologists will enable the professional to provide more services and allow more personal contact with more communicatively handicapped students.

At this point, it should be clear that while supportive personnel have been around for a number of years the professions of speech-language pathology and audiology have not addressed some of the issues. In an interview with Ann L. Carey, president of ASHA, published in *Asha* magazine in January 1992, she stated,

> We must devise new methods of service delivery. It seems inevitable that support personnel will take on greater responsibility for actual service delivery while we take on a more supervisory role. Some of the tasks we currently perform could be shared by other people. I predict that supervision of support personnel will be an integral part of our role as the collaborative model becomes the norm by the end of the 1990s. The pull-out model will be the exception, not the rule. Of course, that means that our education programs will have to change dramatically to teach our graduate students supervisory skills. ASHA's continuing education will also change to reflect this development (Asha, 1992).

Carey further pointed out that the 1992 Task Force on Support Personnel will study the present and future impact of support personnel and will be making recommendations. Undoubtedly, some of the questions regarding support personnel will be what kind of education and supervision should they receive, and how can they enhance the growth of the speech-language and audiology professions as well as the public's perception of us (Asha, 1992).

School Programs Using Supportive Personnel

A number of pilot programs utilizing communication aides have been reported in the professional speech, language, and hearing journals. One of the earliest was a pilot program undertaken by the Colorado State Department of Education. It involved ten aides working in nine school districts of metropolitan Denver for one semester. The aides observed clinicians at work for four days and worked under their assigned clinicians for two days. Instruction also covered school organization and administration; the role of the speech clinician; professional responsibilities and ethics; child growth and speech and language development; speech and hearing mechanisms; disorders of speech, language, and hearing; and identification and remediation of these disorders (Alpiner, 1970).

The majority of the aides' time was spent working with children with articulation problems; the remainder was divided between clerical duties and working with children with language disorders. The result was that these areas matched those in which the clinicians felt the aides were most helpful. In general, the communication aides were accepted by the classroom teachers, school administrators, and school nurses in the buildings in which the aides worked. Several of the clinicians had some reservations about the aides; they gave many reasons, but their major complaint was a problem in keeping the aides occupied. They also felt that the use of aides should not be mandated by the state. The majority wished to continue working with the aides but expressed a desire to interview them before employment to increase the likelihood of compatibility.

76

Chapter 4:
The School
Speech-
Language
Pathologist as
a Manager

A pilot project, reported in the Montgomery County Public Schools of Maryland (Braunstein, 1972), was designed to aid in the remediation of language problems. The aides' responsibilities were as follows:

> . . . to meet groups of children on a daily basis and conduct activities, to record daily progress, to record comments on students' behavior and responses, to tape-record weekly group sessions for evaluation, to confer with the clinician regularly, to participate in in-service activities designated by the clinician and approved by the principal, and to assist in the preparation of materials.

Each aides' caseload was made up of children with mild to moderate language problems in kindergarten through the second grade. Each aide worked with three groups of eight children for at least 25 minutes daily. The remaining time was allotted for conferences. All the materials used in therapy were part of a prepared programmed language-development series. The aides received 35 to 40 hours of training and analyzed 25 to 30 hours of audio and video tapes. At the outset of teaching the clinician and aide alternated the duties three times a week.

Another paraprofessional program involved language remediation for culturally different children in Prince Georges County, Maryland, under a program called "Operation: Moving Ahead" (Lynch, 1972). Begun in 1966, it involved children in kindergarten through the third grade. Its primary objectives included the acquisition of standard English vocabulary, increased standard English familiarity, and the use and refinement of standard English.

The aides were divided into two groups: children's aides and parent helpers. The children's aides' function was to help small groups of children by reinforcing the instruction program planned and provided by the classroom teacher. These aides were supervised by the *helping teacher,* who did the diagnoses, further planning, and evaluations. The parent helpers' functions were to help parents learn about the school program, to understand the importance of language in the child's future success in school, and to suggest ways of working with the children in the home. They primarily worked in the community by visiting homes and distributing materials. They also developed a language box for stimulating language in preschool children and a folder containing ideas for making materials and equipment from inexpensive objects found in the home.

During the 1972–73 school year, the Los Angeles Unified School District established a paraprofessional/volunteer program to supplement and expand the services of the language, speech, and hearing clinicians (Scalero & Eskenazi, 1976). These supportive personnel were intended to work with the remediation of articulation and language disorders. The aides received an intensive 70 hour preservice training course; they then worked six hours five days a week. The volunteers attended a condensed form of the training course—mainly in-group sessions which emphasized practice with the programmed materials; they then worked in two-hour blocks a minimum of two days each week.

At the outset, the speech clinicians tested all potential clients. The 15 aides and 15 volunteers then used programs designed specifically for them. They each kept a log of the pupils' performance and the particular lessons completed. The clinicians then evaluated the clients' progress and determined when they were to move to the next stage; they also supervised and rated the aides through the use of checklists and rating scales. Throughout the year the supportive personnel worked with 125 articulation cases and 136 language problems. A postinstruction evaluation of the clients revealed 90 percent of the articulation problems had 80 percent or more carry-over in 15 weeks or less of therapy. These successes were independent of the age, education, or previous training of the aides but were related to their rapport with their pupils and their ability and willingness to follow directions. The children who worked with the volunteers attained the same goals as the children who worked with the aides, but in longer periods of time.

A slight variation of the paraprofessional program was attempted in Maine to meet the requirements of PL 94-142 in the isolated rural districts without speech clinicians (Pickering & Dopheide, 1976). Instead of being trained to perform supervised therapy, these aides were to screen for communication disorders. In two separate workshops, 51 people from 20 different schools were trained; the majority of these trainees were school aides, but classroom teachers and "floating" teachers were also involved. Each workshop lasted two days and had performance-based success levels.

As a result of the screening by the paraprofessionals, 11 percent more children were identified in the first testing. Voice quality was the most difficult for the trainees to evaluate and for the instructors to define. A total of 1,700 children were screened, with the aides referring 35 percent of the children tested and the teachers referring 28 percent; of these referrals one-third needed remediation. The program significantly reduced the amount of time the language, speech, and hearing clinicians had to spend in screening children.

Some school speech, language, and hearing programs utilize the services of volunteers or unpaid aides. These individuals have been used in assisting with hearing screening programs. The school clinician must train the volunteers in the specific tasks they are to perform. Often mothers of schoolchildren will serve as the volunteer aides in the screening programs.

Strong (1972) reported on a program in northern Minnesota designed to utilize supportive personnel in screening school populations for speech problems and managing direct therapy with children over eight years of age who exhibited frontal or lateral distortions of sibilant phonemes or distortion of the phoneme /r/. The program was carried on in a rural area, and the results indicated that the use of supportive personnel allowed the school clinician to devote more time to the more severe cases.

Galloway and Blue (1975) described a program in Georgia which was carried out over a period of three years. The paraprofessionals were trained to administer programmed materials to first- through fifth-grade students who had articulatory errors. The errors exhibited were in the mild to moderate range of functional articulation problems. The findings suggested that paraprofessionals using a preplanned program and materials can enhance the program carried out by the school pathologist by allowing more time for problems that require greater expertise.

A model for training and using communication assistants was developed by Jimenez and Iseyama (1987) and used to train aides in Migrant Head Start centers. After all students were screened and assessed by the SLP and necessary referrals were made to other professionals, a therapy program was designed for

78

**Chapter 4:
The School
Speech-
Language
Pathologist as
a Manager**

each child. Prior to implementing the program, the selected communication assistants participated in pre-service training sessions which included four steps:

1. orientation;

2. demonstration;

3. participation; and

4. implementation.

Orientation included providing the assistant with information pertaining to behavior modification, techniques for charting responses, guidelines for following lesson plans, and maintaining daily records. The SLP described the nature and causes of the identified disorder, the therapy program designed for each child, and the rationale.

In the second step, demonstration, the SLP conducted therapy while the assistant observed. Throughout the session the SLP described and demonstrated the therapy techniques and identified correct and incorrect target responses. The assistant was able to ask questions and receive information during the discussion that followed each session. The demonstration sessions were concluded when both the SLP and the assistant agreed that the assistant had an adequate understanding of the procedures.

During the participation sessions both the SLP and the assistant were actively involved and the child's responses were charted by both, independently. Additional discussion followed each session and a point-by-point comparison was made of the charted responses until agreement was reached on 85% of the responses and the student met minimal performance levels.

Implementation was the final step in the model. The assistant actively conducted the therapy sessions and the SLP acted in a supervisory capacity. In addition to the therapy, the assistant charted target behaviors and maintained daily logs. Follow-up procedures, consultation, report writing, conferences, referrals, and the determination for student dismissal were the responsibility of the SLP (Jimenez and Iseyama, 1987).

A pilot program for training and utilizing communication aides in Head Start programs in Wyoming was reported by Jelinek (1976). According to Jelinek benefits other than the statistical inferences were realized from the program. The aides became skilled in the delivery of language programs and more knowledgeable in child development and behavior management. "Project staff were able to develop a liaison with Head Start staffs, parents, and other professionals in the community which might not have been possible without the development of the pilot program. Because of the success of the pilot communication aide program, this model has been expanded to include all Head Start centers in Wyoming."

Costello and Schoen (1978) studied the effectiveness of paraprofessionals in an articulation intervention program in California using programmed instruction. The results indicated that paraprofessionals using a clearly written, previously tested programmed instruction format compared favorably with the results obtained by a fully qualified speech clinician. The use of audio- and video-tape aids ensured a standard quality program and reduced the responsibilities of the paraprofessionals. Costello and Schoen suggested that a possible future role of the speech clinician would be that of a program writer, program researcher, trainer, and supervisor of a paraprofessional staff. This would leave more time for clients with special and more complex needs, and would also enable the program to serve larger populations more effectively.

Future Use of Support Personnel

Paraprofessionals have been used effectively in the health, education, and human service fields for many years. In our profession, school SLPs have used aides in hearing screening and conservation programs and in speech and language programs as described in this chapter. The Code of Ethics of the American Speech-Language-Hearing Association has provided guidelines for the preparation and supervision of paraprofessionals. In some states, registration and licensing is required. The need for supportive personnel in our fields undoubtedly will increase in the coming years. As a profession it is incumbent upon us to determine the competencies, preparation, and use of paraprofessionals in order to more effectively and efficiently deliver our services.

Computers

The growing use of the computer in education, business, and everyday life has become a reality on the American scene. The practitioners in speech-language pathology and audiology in the public schools have been slower to use the computer than their colleagues in other settings. However, many of those who have been dragged kicking and screaming into the computer age have, like new converts to a religion, become its most vocal advocates. School SLPs who use computers have discovered that they are able to save time, conserve energy, increase benefits to clients, and cut down on that greatest of all time-thieves, paperwork.

The potential applications of computers to enhance therapy is beginning to be addressed in the curricula of university programs in communication disorders. A study at Portland State University (Paul, 1990) suggested that limited hands-on instruction in the context of already required coursework may serve to make students more amenable to employing computers in a variety of settings.

In order to assist speech-language pathologists and audiologists in learning about computers for clinical, educational, and administrative purposes, ASHA has developed instructional software packages known as "Project IMPACT." The project was developed by ASHA with grant support from the U.S. Department of Education. It focuses on six subjects: overview of microcomputer applications, administration, assessment, intervention, audiology, and software evaluation. Further information may be obtained from ASHA Publication Sales, 10801 Rockville Pike, Rockville, MD, 20852.

Using the Computer to Develop and Maintain Reports

School clinicians are finding that computers can be invaluable tools for managing program information and as an adjunct to intervention. Much of the SLP's

80

**Chapter 4:
The School
Speech-
Language
Pathologist as
a Manager**

workload involves paperwork and reporting tasks. Clinicians are finding that computers can provide a number of advantages: saving time, conserving energy, and increasing benefits to clients. Software programs which permit word processing, data management, and spreadsheet functions enable SLPs to communicate with other professionals, store and manage important information, and prepare reports with efficiency. Computers can help clinicians accomplish tasks such as storing data about students, maintaining records, preparing reports, developing IEPs, and storing data for administrative and research purposes (Dustrude, 1990 and Seaton, 1991).

Krueger (1985) describes numerous ways a computer can be used for program management. An analysis of computer data can help identify trends such as increases in the caseload size, disorder type, or a population shift within the school district. Accurate caseload figures, demographic figures, and disorder and severity data can promote more efficient use of school personnel and program development. Required reports can be compiled more quickly, efficiently, and accurately. According to Krueger, in the past therapy sessions had to be cancelled for one or two weeks to allow time for clinicians to complete yearly progress reports. Computerization now permits clinicians to prepare reports which are comprehensive, easier to read, and more professional in appearance. In addition, the time saved can be used for an extension of direct therapy time.

A centralized computer system can store a large number of data. Test results, pertinent medical information, referral sources, and follow-up information unique to each student can be added at any time. Retrieval of results is usually facilitated by typing a student number at a computer terminal rather than searching through files for a result. Information is accessible to personnel at remote terminals throughout the district.

Sorting options for producing printed reports are numerous. For example, a report can be printed for the school nurse, alphabetically listing students' hearing screening results by grade and room number for a given school. Results may also be sorted according to those students enrolled in a special education program, or as a compilation of students with a particular type of disorder.

This type of program eliminates time-consuming, cross-checking tasks and provides accurate records for studying screening, testing, and therapy data. Comprehensive programs such as these also provide tallies on a continual basis, allowing time to correct errors before year-end statistical compilation.

Software programs have been developed that can save clinicians considerable time and effort in dealing with the deluge of paperwork involved in developing Individualized Education Programs. Computers can be used in the generation of IEPs and for documenting completion of steps necessary for compliance with due process. According to Krueger (1985), the memory capacity of the computer allows storage of a virtually unlimited number of items in the goal and objective bank. In addition, items may be added to the bank for students who are not adequately described by existing statements or whose team members request additional objectives. Examples of a computerized data bank of IEP intervention objectives are provided in Appendix B.

The stumbling blocks to computer usage in the schools include lack of familiarity with computers, financial restraints, fear of learning how to use a computer system, and a dearth of speech-language professionals who understand its potential applications. In a survey to determine computer usage by speech-language pathologists in public schools, Houle (1988) found that frequent users had several factors in common. They had access to funds for purchasing hardware and software, their schools sponsored inservice training in computer use, computer hardware, and software were dedicated for use in the speech-language pathology program, and there were secure facilities for storage of equipment. Many of these impediments are being overcome through continuing education programs, seminars, workshops, and short courses on computers. There are excellent books on the market that provide good basic and advanced information on computer usage.

Computers may be purchased by a school system for use by the speech, language, and hearing staff. Before purchasing a computer system and software programs, identify your needs and the applications you plan to use. Take into account the type of service delivery model employed: itinerant, consultative, resource room, or self-contained program.

Krueger (1985) outlined six major steps followed by the Great River Area Education Agency 16 to make a decision regarding the purchase of a computer system:

1. *Targeting the needs.* The decision was made to focus on administrative tasks rather than remediation. At this point a decision should be made regarding who will do the actual work on the computer, as it requires computer skills and a commitment of personnel time.

2. *Gaining access to equipment.* Three choices usually exist: leasing equipment from a computer vendor; using a computer service, which does all the work at set rates; or purchasing equipment.

3. *Obtaining equipment.* Before making the financial investment it is wise to visit a program with an operational system. The next steps included choosing the data format, setting up the format, programming, and preparing an item bank.

4. After the system is prepared *each step is thoroughly tested* to reveal possible shortcomings in the system.

5. When thorough testing indicates that the system will function as planned, *implementation* may begin. During the implementation period, staff training must be thorough. After the system has been tested and implemented, the system should be used "as is" through one entire cycle. If changes have to be made it is more efficient to make them simultaneously rather than one at a time.

6. The final step is a *systematic evaluation.* It was suggested that the system should be evaluated after six months, one year, two years, and five years of operation.

The school SLP contemplating the purchase of computer software (a list of instructions to tell the computer how to perform a specific task) is faced with a bewildering array of information and material. Beginning in the March 1985 issue of *Asha,* the Materials Section began publishing a review of currently available computer software. The Educational Technology Committee of ASHA

82

Chapter 4:
The School
Speech-
Language
Pathologist as
a Manager

(1985) developed the review checksheet in Table 4-3 to assist in the evaluation of computer software.

The use of the computer as a management tool in the school setting has already been demonstrated by many school-based SLPs in:

- screening data;
- case management information;
- therapy materials;
- therapy logs;
- statistical data for accountability to school administrators, boards of education and state departments of education; and
- the storage and quick retrieval of records and reports.

Throughout this book we will examine the ways that you, a future school speech-language pathologist, can use the computer.

TABLE 4.3. SOFTWARE REVIEW CHECKSHEET

1. Poor	2. Fair	3. Good	4. Excellent	5. Not Applicable

1. Program Description
   a. Is the purpose of the program clearly defined? _____
   b. Is the manner in which the program works clearly described? _____
   c. Are the instructions for getting started with the program clearly described? _____
   d. Are the instructions for storing and retrieving data clearly described? _____
   e. Are hardware requirements clearly stated? _____
2. Program effectiveness
   a. Is the software program logical and reasonable? _____
   b. Will the program produce consistent results in various settings under various conditions? _____
   c. Is there a reprint of an article, a technical report or other information describing the results of a study(ies) of effectiveness? _____
3. User Friendliness
   a. Is the program easy to enter, e.g., a turnkey system? _____
   b. Is the program easy to exit? _____
   c. Are the instructions displayed on the screen easy to understand and complete? _____
   d. Are the input responses to the machine familiar (such as "Y" for "yes" and "N" for "no")? _____
   e. Are program options displayed as "menus"? _____
   f. What does the program do if the user strikes a wrong key (does it give a prompt reminding him of the correct options and disregard the error)? _____
   g. Can input errors be easily corrected? _____
   h. Are data outputs easily retrieved? _____
   i. Are data outputs complete and attractively formatted? _____
4. Support/Documentation
   a. Is the documentation complete (does it tell you everything you need to know)? _____

(*continued*)

TABLE 4.3. (*Continued*)

b. Is the documentation concise (does it tell you more than you want to know)? _____

c. Is the documentation written in terms you can understand? _____

d. Is the documentation well organized (can you find answers to specific problems by referring to an index or table of contents)? _____

e. Does it adequately describe the hardware needed and any special instructions for its use? _____

f. Are hardware and software options clearly explained? _____

g. Is there a source for help (someone to call or write if you have a question)? _____

h. Are back-up copies provided (if not, are instructions for making back-up copies included)? _____

i. Can the program be returned if the user decides that it is not appropriate for his setting? _____

j. Can replacement copies be obtained at a reduced rate if the originals become damaged?

k. Can updated program revisions be obtained at a reduced rate? _____

SUMMARY OF RATINGS

1. Program Description* _____
2. Program Effectiveness* _____
3. User Friendliness* _____
4. Support/Documentation* _____
5. Overall Rating** _____

*Summaries of ratings are the averages of items in each category.
**The overall rating may be different from the average of the summary ratings.

DISCUSSION QUESTIONS AND PROJECTS

1. What are some yearly program goals you, as the SLP, might develop?

2. What are the advantages of written program plans and goals?

3. Is there state licensure in your state for paraprofessionals? If so, are there requirements for training, education, and supervision?

4. How could paraprofessionals be utilized in an audiometric screening program?

5. Are there training programs for paraprofessionals in your state? Where are they?

6. Check with the school SLPs and audiologists in your area to find out whether or not computers are available to them in their school systems. If yes, inquire about how they are used.

7. Find one computer program that is applicable to each of the following areas: management, intervention, and assessment.

8. Read the articles on quality assurance in the January, 1990 issue of *Asha* magazine. Following Frattalli's 10 step protocol for developing a quality assurance plan, develop a plan for a school program.

Tools of the Trade: Space, Facilities, Equipment, Materials, and Records

Introduction

It is important that adequate facilities and equipment are available to school speech-language pathologists so that students are appropriately served. Additionally, comprehensive accountability procedures and efficient recordkeeping practices can assist the clinician in documenting responsible service delivery. Space, facilities, equipment, materials and reports may be considered the tools of the trade. Just as a carpenter needs good tools, so does the SLP. In this chapter, we will consider the basic needs and how they can be met.

Physical Facilities

There is at the present time a wide variation in the quality of work space available to school SLPs. The reasons for this are not always clear. Some schools are overcrowded, and the school clinician is in competition with other school personnel for the available space. Many school districts are financially strapped and can't provide the space. School buildings, new as well as old, have not been planned with the speech, language, and hearing services taken into account. In some cases the school administration is either unaware or apathetic about the issue of adequate working space. On the other hand, increasing numbers of school systems provide excellent facilities.

Minimal Standards for Facilities and Space

Appropriate facilities are necessary to provide an adequate atmosphere for performing responsibilities and implementing program goals. There are state and federal guidelines which stipulate that the workspace for the delivery of speech-language-hearing services be suitable and appropriate. The Professional Services Board (PSB) of ASHA has recommended minimal standards of operation for programs offering speech-language and hearing services. As a general guideline, the standards suggest that the physical facility should be barrier-free, in compliance with all applicable safety and health codes, and suitable for the conduct of those activities required to meet the objectives of the program (Asha, 1984).

In many states, minimal standards for facilities are established by the state board of education. These do not necessarily describe superior facilities, but they do provide a standard below which schools may not go. There is sometimes confusion about this issue, and the school clinician needs to be aware of exactly how the standards are worded. Some local school districts and professional organizations (such as the Pennsylvania and Virginia Speech and Hearing Associations) have also developed recommendations for physical facilities and equipment necessary for operating programs effectively.

The beginning school clinician needs some sort of "yardstick" by which to evaluate and define adequate facilities. The checklist presented in Table 5-1 can be used as a reference when observing a school speech-language-hearing program, selecting a site for your student teaching experience, or interviewing for a job. If several elements are inadequate, don't be afraid to discuss them with program administrators. While it is not wise to be confrontatious, questioning an administrator based on sound information and a desire to provide the best services possible can result in improved understanding of the speech-language hearing program and an improved environment for service delivery.

TABLE 5.1. PROGRAM ENVIRONMENT OBSERVATION CHECKLIST

ROOM
  Location
  _____   Quiet, private enough to permit confidentiality; free from distractions
  _____   Easy to locate; accessible for individuals who are nonambulatory or exhibit severe learning disabilities
  _____   Near students' classroom and restrooms
  _____   Designated for exclusive use by the SLP program during all times when the speech-language pathologist is on site
  _____   Easy access to emergency exits
  _____   Secured for storage of equipment and materials
  Lighting
  _____   Suitable for reading and manipulating pictures and objects

  Power
  _____   Adequate number of electrical outlets for operating program equipment (e.g., tape recorders, computers, amplification systems, augmentative devices, typewriters, and the like)

(continued)

86

Chapter 5:
Tools of the
Trade: Space,
Facilities,
Equipment,
Materials, and
Records

TABLE 5.1. (Continued)

Size

_____   Adequate to meet safety standards for the maximum number of persons who will be in the room at a given time

Temperature

_____   Adequate ventilation, heating, and cooling; thermostatic control available

Safety Devices

_____   Audible as well as visual safety devices (fire and smoke alarms)

FURNITURE
Chairs

_____   Appropriate size and number to accommodate clinician, students, and observers; matched to the table size and space

Desk

_____   Office style with lockable drawers

File Cabinet

_____   Lockable

_____   Appropriate size for number and type of files used for the program

Tables

_____   Appropriate height and number to accommodate a broad range of students' sizes and ages

_____   Adequate support for equipment (typewriters, computers, and the like)

Shelves

_____   Adequate number and structure for storage of books and therapy materials

EQUIPMENT AND MATERIALS
Audiometers

_____   Appropriate for testing pure-tones and immittance

_____   Properly calibrated

Amplification
Devices

_____   Appropriate to meet individual and group needs

Augmentative Communication Systems

_____   Appropriate for various age and functional communication levels

Computers

_____   Available according to need

_____   Suitable for word processing, and data storage

_____   Appropriate software for program management and intervention

_____   Accessories necessary to operate uniquely designed programs

Expendable materials

_____   Conveniently located

_____   Easily accessed

(continued)

TABLE 5.1. (Continued)

Physical Facilities		
Mirror		
_____	Appropriate size for viewing faces and bodies	
_____	Constructed of safety glass	
Tape Recorder		
_____	Designated for exclusive use by the speech-language program	
_____	Ample supply of tapes	
Telecommunication display device		
_____	Available if needed to meet the needs of students who are hearing impaired	
Telephone		
_____	Available when needed; located in a private area where confidentiality can be maintained	
Typewriter		
_____	Available and easily accessed	
Video recording and viewing equipment		
_____	Available and easily accessed	

Pleasant, Comfortable, and Functional Space

In establishing criteria for evaluating physical facilities, the factors of "realism" and "idealism" must be taken into account. Although it might be ideal for the speech-language clinician to have a room used exclusively for the speech, language, and hearing program, it may not be realistic; the speech pathologist may be on an itinerant schedule, and the space could be utilized by the reading teacher, for example, on the alternate days.

Another factor to consider is the existing facilities (things as they are today) and the potential facilities (things as they might be with some modifications), particularly in setting up a new program. It is important that there is a set of criteria which indicate that although the existing facilities may not be satisfactory, they could and should be modified in the future. In assessing this aspect of the program the policies of the school must be known. For example, is the supervisor of the speech, language, and hearing program involved in the planning of new facilities or the modification of existing ones? Are staff members included in the planning? Are alternative plans considered, such as the use of mobile units, remodeling of areas of buildings, or rental of additional space? What are the budgetary allowances and constraints?

According to Scarvel (1977), the following questions should be asked:

1. Are the facilities of adequate size or space to permit total program flexibility? (The Key Term is Total Program Flexibility.) Can this be used by both Speech and Language Clinicians and Itinerant Hearing Clinicians?

2. Is the facility relatively free from extraneous noise? The Key Word is Relatively in being realistic in terms of the existing physical plant. For example,

88

Chapter 5:
Tools of the
Trade: Space,
Facilities,
Equipment,
Materials, and
Records

one set of criteria required acoustically treated walls and acoustic tile on ceilings. This is fine; however, we may find ourselves in a room not having this, but still free from extraneous noise because of its location.

3. Are there adequate furnishings for the type of services offered? (The Key Word is Adequate.) Ideally, maybe there should be more than those appearing on this list; but we're looking for *adequate* furnishings.

4. Are sufficient electrical outlets provided? (Key Word-Sufficient) This depends upon the type(s) of services to be delivered and/or equipment utilization necessary (rather than specifying an exact number).

5. Is the lighting adequate and the facility properly heated or cooled? (The Key Word is again Adequate.) For example, one source mentions the use of artificial light in addition to natural light; specifically, at least one window is needed.

6. Are facilities accessible to physically handicapped students? This criterion would apply only in those instances where students who are disabled need to be serviced in a particular facility. As with the other criteria, those criteria not applicable to a program, or to the specific services provided, would not be used.

In addition to evaluating the room itself, there are other considerations. First, the room must be accessible to pupils who are disabled and located in an area of the building convenient to all who use it. It should not be too far from the kindergarten and first-grade classrooms because these children sometimes have difficulty finding their way to and from the room.

Space is often at a premium in school buildings, and many buildings are old and not well planned for present-day needs. With a little imagination and resourcefulness, however, some simple remodeling and rejuvenation can transform unused space into completely adequate facilities for the school pathologist. For example, a portion of a large entry foyer may be partitioned and utilized for the speech-language and hearing program.

If a new building a being contemplated, the speech-language clinician will need to be in on the planning stages to insure adequate space allotment. School architects are not always well informed about the space and facility needs of the program, and the school pathologist can be of invaluable assistance in providing needed information.

The policies of the school in regard to space must also be known when planning physical facilities. For example, the school pathologist should know how space is assigned in a building and whether or not staff members are consulted when the assignments are made. The school pathologist should also know whether or not there are provisions for modifying the room. If space is to be shared, staff members should know the procedures for obtaining input from all the persons sharing the room.

Most people feel better and do better in surroundings that are attractive, comfortable, and pleasant. Children are no exception. Color, adequate lighting, and comfortable furniture are conducive to good results in therapy. A child who is seated on a chair that is too big for him or her is going to be very uncomfortable. In a short time the child will begin to squirm and wriggle and will be unable to focus on whatever the clinician is presenting. The child may seem like a discipline problem to the unseeing clinician, but in reality the little boy or girl may simply be attempting to find a comfortable position.

One of the most attractive therapy rooms I have seen was in an old school building in a rural area. The whole building sparkled with cleanliness—wooden floors were polished, walls were painted in soft colors, and furniture was in good repair and arranged harmoniously. The therapy room was pleasant, with a carpeted floor and colorful draperies. A bulletin board served both a useful and decorative purpose. The obvious pride in the surroundings was reflected by the way the children treated the therapy room and its furnishings. The clinician reported that everyone in the school, including the custodian, the principal, the teachers, and the children were proud of their attractive building and worked to keep it that way.

Space Allocations

The space allocations in schools have been improving in recent years, perhaps because SLPs now spend more time in each school and more schools have full-time or nearly full-time therapy programs. Also, school administrators are becoming more aware of the importance of speech, language, and hearing programs, and the needs of the programs are receiving more attention. Nonetheless, it is of vital importance that the school SLP assumes the responsibility of making the needs of the program known to the principal, director of special services, and superintendent. The school pathologist must be assertive and forthright in this endeavor. The student with a hearing loss, language-learning disability, fluency problem, voice disorder, or articulatory problem cannot benefit from therapy in the nurse's station, where there are constant interruptions and exposure to illnesses; in a room next door to where the band practices; or in a storage room that is inadequately lighted, ventilated, and heated or cooled.

Overcrowded schools and substandard space within school buildings have prompted some pathologists to look elsewhere for the solution to the problem. Mobile units and stationary trailers located on the school grounds have provided solutions for many clinicians. Howerton (1973) cited a number of advantages in using mobile units: They contain everything necessary for the program, thus eliminating gathering up and storing items every day; equipment is better cared for when it remains stationary and doesn't have to be transported in the trunk of a car; they provide quiet facilities for hearing, testing, and screening; and they represent a saving in tax dollars in comparison to the cost of building permanent facilities.

Special Considerations for Special Populations

Careful thought and planning should go into designing, organizing and decorating your therapy room. Keep your students' special needs, ages, learning capabilities, and interest levels in mind. Decor should be attractive and motivating. Care should be taken to avoid arranging the room in a way that is distracting or condescending to students' ages or intelligence. Certain groups require special considerations.

90   Infants, Toddlers, and Preschoolers

Chapter 5:
Tools of the
Trade: Space,
Facilities,
Equipment,
Materials, and
Records

As a result of Public Law 99-457, school districts are now responsible for providing services to a younger group of children than they have accommodated previously. Many school buildings are not designed for such a young group. Room location, furniture size, and equipment selection is of utmost importance. The environment must be bright and stimulating. Children in this age group do not learn by sitting quietly at a table and taking turns talking. Learning quite often takes place on the floor or while the child is in motion during play. Therefore, the atmosphere and materials should invite manipulation, creativity, movement, and interaction. Toys are appropriate, especially if they can be used to encourage investigation, experimentation, imitation, and questioning. Because of the way in which children play with toys, they will need to be cleansed frequently and maintained in proper working order.

Adolescents

Obviously, facilities for intermediate and high-school students will be different than those for elementary and preschool students. The size and type of furniture as well as the arrangement of the classroom should facilitate group discussions and lessons. The typical classroom or rows of desks is not conducive to the type of learning that takes place in a typical situation. The use of carrels and learning centers provides the opportunity for independent work. Activity centers related to specific learning skills could incorporate vocabulary cards, work sheets, and learning games. Learning centers might include tape recorders, manipulable objects, and microcomputers. A library center might have reading materials, books used for book reports, story wheels, and writing materials. A career education center might contain materials related to various occupations, job application requirements, and forms.

Children with Severe and Multiple Impairments

There is likely to be wide variation in skill levels, capabilities, mobility, sizes, and intervention needs for children with severe and multiple impairments. Consequently, facilities for this group of children need to be designed so that easy adaptation is permitted throughout the day. Furniture should be of sturdy construction, adjustable, and easily moved to meet positioning requirements. Treatment materials should be selected to permit teaching important concepts and skills while still being motivating. Augmentative and alternative communication systems are valuable assets to children whose communication skills are severely restricted.

Some children with severe and multiple impairments become easily distracted auditorally and visually. Children with sensory problems, problems related to brain dysfunction, or developmental delay may have difficulty functioning in a room that is too stimulating or distracting because of garish colors or busy patterns. To accommodate these childrens' needs while still providing a bright, stimulating environment for other children on the caseload, the clinician may wish to arrange one section of the therapy room in such a way that all potentially distracting materials are out of the child's range of vision.

Facilities for Observation

The school clinician may want to invite parents, educators, and school administrators in to observe diagnostic and intervention services. This would provide opportunities for involving valuable members of the child's world in the therapy program, teaching others about the profession, and promoting collaboration.

One way to facilitate observation is to invite persons to join you during the session. If the presence of others would distract the students, one-way mirrors and intercom systems are methods which enable observation without interruption. Through observational experiences such as these, parents and teachers can learn important speech/language stimulation and correction techniques. Team members such as school psychologists can observe the child's communication skills under optimum conditions to obtain valuable diagnostic information. Administrators can learn about the scope and services of the speech-language program.

Often school clinicians hear the comment from others, "But what do you actually do in a therapy session?" Having people observe would take some of the mystery out of therapy and would make vividly clear the role they can play in the therapy process in the home or classroom. This would ultimately help the child generalize what he or she has learned.

Equipment and Materials

In addition to the therapy room and its furnishings, several types of equipment, materials, and supplies are needed for a successful program. Equipment and materials should be appropriately selected to meet the needs of the students and types of disorders being served. Appropriate schedules of maintenance and calibration should be followed to ensure that equipment remains in proper working order.

Equipment is an item that is nonexpendable; retains its original shape, appearance, and use; usually costs a substantial amount of money; and is more feasible to repair than to replace when damaged or worn out. Materials and supplies, on the other hand, are expendable, used up, usually inexpensive, and are more feasible to replace than to repair when damaged or worn out.

Using Technology

In the past, speech-language pathologists' equipment use was limited to audiometers, acoustic immittance instruments, tape recorders, and simple amplification devices. Many clinicians are now integrating technology into their programs. It is not unusual to see students with communication disorders wearing assistive listening devices, practicing language exercises at a computer or using a voice synthesizer to express their needs. Today's clinicians are using technology to manage program information and develop their students' communication skills.

Computers

In addition to the management applications discussed in Chapter Four, computers are valuable for assessment and direct intervention. Results of speech, lan-

92

Chapter 5:
Tools of the
Trade: Space,
Facilities,
Equipment,
Materials, and
Records

guage, and audiological screening programs can be maintained with computers, as can the analysis of diagnostic data. Available treatment programs are usually based on computer-assisted management (CAM), computer-managed instruction (CMI), or computer-assisted instruction (CAI) applications (Schetz, 1990).

If software is selected properly, it can be used to facilitate drill practice, encourage transfer and generalization of learned skills, and permit individualized practice and self-correction. For example, treatment for students who are hearing impaired can be enhanced through computer programs that use interactive learning and synthesized speech. The computer is also valuable to students as a means of access to information and visually oriented training and instruction.

Henoch, Scott, and Balentine (1986) caution that computer-assisted instruction may be limited for use in communicative disorders because of "the inability to use voice input effectively; the poor quality of synthesized speech to provide speech modeling; and the inability to edit software to individualize lessons." They suggest that speech recognition technology will offer solutions to these problems in the future.

Computers won't replace competent clinicians but the use of computers by SLPs and audiologists in the schools can make a positive difference in the delivery of services to students with communication impairments.

Assistive Listening Devices

Students' success in the classroom and in therapy is often limited by their inability to monitor their own speech or hear, attend to, and discriminate others' speech during conversations and classroom discussions (Flexer, 1992). Audiologists and speech-language pathologists are finding assistive listening devices (ALDs) to be very useful tools for working with students who have hearing impairments as well as students with other types of communication and learning impairments (Flexer, 1989). Assistive listening devices include various products which provide solutions to problems created by noise, distance from the speaker, or room reverberation or echo. These problems cannot be solved with hearing aids alone (Berg, 1987 and Leavitt, 1987). ALDs offer effective means for sound amplification by improving the intelligibility of the speech signal by enhancing the signal-to-noise ratio (Flexer, 1992, 1991).

Two types of devices, personal FM units and hardwire ALDs, can benefit individual children in the therapy situation or groups of children in the classroom setting (Flexer, 1989). To use these units, the teacher/clinician wears a microphone transmitter and the student wears a receiver unit equipped with insert earphones.

The cost and design of this equipment varies, but inexpensive portable devices can be assembled without much difficulty (Sudler and Flexer, 1986). The amount of amplification needed is dependent on a number of factors and individual needs for amplification vary greatly. There is some risk of damaging a child's auditory system if an inappropriate sound level is used. Therefore, the advice of an educational audiologist familiar with the performance potential and benefits of various types of assistive listening devices should be sought when recommending units for particular children or classroom situations.

Perhaps the most exciting result of advanced technology is the increased opportunity for persons with severe impairments to communicate with others in their world. Speech-language pathologists are teaching persons with disorders such as dysarthria, verbal apraxia, aphasia, glossectomy, dysphonia, mental retardation, autism, traumatic brain injury, tracheostomy, and deafness to interact with their families, peers, and teachers via augmented and assisted-communication systems (Silverman, 1989). Augumentative communication refers to communication systems that supplement speech. This can be accomplished through common techniques such as writing, gestures, and pictures or via more specialized techniques including electronic aids (Vanderheiden and Yoder, 1986).

Today's clinician needs to know how to work with students' families and professionals representing a broad range of educational, medical, and technological disciplines to help select augmentative and alternative communication systems which will be optimally suited to the student's needs (Silverman, 1989; Yorkston & Karlan, 1986). Vanderheiden and Lloyd (1986) describe several dimensions professionals can use to determine the usefulness or advantages of particular augmentative communication system components for meeting functional communication requirements. They group these dimensions into three broad categories:

1. functionality/ability to meet needs;

2. availability/useability; and

3. acceptability/compatibility with the environment.

After selecting the device, the clinician is then involved in instructing the student and incorporating the communication system into classroom and social communication activities.

The school clinician interested in incorporating augmentative and alternative systems into the speech-language program is faced with an important decision-making task. There is great variability in capability and complexity in the devices available on the market. Cost can be high. Sometimes, it is necessary to help the student's family seek financial assistance. The Prentke Romich Company (a company which develops, manufactures, and distributes augmentative communication systems) suggests that there are numerous sources which can be sought for funding the purchase of devices including:

• insurance companies and Medicaid programs;

• vocational rehabilitation programs;

• school system equipment funds;

• private corporations;

• trust funds;

• service clubs;

• fundraising agencies; and

• organizations which grant wishes to people with specific needs (Prentke Romich Company, 1989).

**Chapter 5:
Tools of the
Trade: Space,
Facilities,
Equipment,
Materials, and
Records**

During recent years, there has been an increase in commercial materials. Some of them are excellent and some of them are not useful for the purposes they claim to accomplish. On the other hand, there are many excellent homemade materials. These have the advantage of being inexpensive, and because many of them are designed for a specific purpose, they are useful.

Without decrying the use of materials, homemade or commercial, the clinician would do well to evaluate them from another point of view. Do they accomplish a goal in therapy for the child, or do they serve as a prop or a "security blanket" for the clinician? This letter from a staff member at Shady Trails, a camp for speech, language, and hearing handicapped children, illustrates the point:

> Before I went to Shady Trails Speech Improvement Camp in Michigan they sent me a list of things to bring along. I didn't notice any mention of therapy materials. Should I take some along? I had been working as a school clinician and had therapy materials of my own. What should I do? Well, if they didn't tell me to bring any, perhaps they furnished staff members with them after you got there. When I got to camp no materials in sight! What was I expected to do for therapy! I panicked.
>
> Within a very short time we were plunged into the camp program and things moved along at a fast clip. Suddenly, in the middle of the summer, I realized I had been doing therapy for several weeks and hadn't even missed any therapy materials. How could this be! In analyzing the situation I realized we had been using the life experience situations at camp, the activities, the surroundings, the educational programs and the other people in the camp as our "materials." The therapy grew naturally out of the environment.

Perhaps we often overlook the most obvious source of materials—the school itself. If therapy in the schools is to be meaningful to the child it must be a part of the school program. The school clinician needs to know what is going on at various grade levels in the way of instruction and should then tie the therapy to the classroom activities. Looking at the books children read, talking with the teacher about the instructional program, becoming familiar with the school curriculum, and looking about the classroom itself will help the school clinician become more familiar with classroom instruction and will suggest ideas for therapy techniques and motivational devices.

In most states there are regional resource centers, which provide local school districts with resources designed to improve the quality of instruction for handicapped children. Instructional and diagnostic materials are available on a loan basis to school clinicians. The instructional resource centers provide other services with which the school clinician will want to become familiar. Visiting the resource center gives the clinician an opportunity to examine a large number of tests, materials, and books before making a decision on which ones to purchase for the school. Personnel at the resource centers are also helpful in discussing the use of various items of material and equipment.

Regional, state, and national meetings of speech, language, and hearing pathologists usually include displays by commercial companies of equipment, materials, and books. Demonstrations of equipment are carried on by company representatives. This is also a good opportunity to get on the mailing lists of commercial companies. The school clinician may want to maintain a file of company brochures and current prices.

Evaluation of Materials

At the present time there are numerous speech and language development and remediation programs on the market. Unfortunately many of them have not been field tested on a variety of populations. The clinician who purchases them may have no information concerning their effectiveness, validity, or reliability. Connell et al. (1977) have suggested that clinicians should not obtain language programs unless the information necessary to evaluate their usefulness is available from the company publishing them. They recommend that the information should minimally include:

1. experimental analysis of mean or median trials to criterion and variance for each program step;
2. percentage of clients who completed each program step;
3. precise description of all the clients who were used in obtaining data; and
4. experimental analysis of the generalization of trained language behaviors.

The same cautions should be applied to the anticipated purchase of testing materials. New tests in particular should be evaluated carefully before they are purchased. Advertising brochures should not be the only criterion for selection, and the clinician should seek the pertinent information by querying the publishing company directly.

Prior to purchasing programs, tests, or equipment, clinicians should request to use the materials on a trial basis. This will provide opportunity for clearly determining the applicability to specific populations, the capability for meeting your program objectives, and to predict the durability, frequency of use, and maintenance requirements.

Shared Purchasing of Equipment. Another way to become familiar with materials and equipment is to discuss them with other clinicians in the area or with university staff members, if there is a university training program nearby. School clinicians in a geographical area may want to consider joint purchase of expensive pieces of equipment that could be shared. Or one school district may purchase one item which could be loaned to a neighboring district, while that district may purchase another item with the idea of setting up a reciprocal loan system. Time-sharing policies and insurance considerations would have to be worked out in advance.

Portability. The portability of materials should also be taken into consideration. The clinician on an itinerant schedule should keep in mind the bulk and the weight of the materials. Lugging materials and equipment in and out of build-

96

Chapter 5:
Tools of the
Trade: Space,
Facilities,
Equipment,
Materials, and
Records

ings, not to mention up and down long flights of stairs, several times a day requires the stamina of a pack horse and has caused more than one school clinician to trim down the amount of materials used.

Activity File

Usually students enrolled in clinical practica classes start to collect their own materials and ideas. Many students have found it useful to start a file box of various intervention and motivational ideas. If the file is well organized it can be expanded and ideas can be added during student teaching and beyond.

The file should be organized in such a way that material can be easily retrieved and replaced. It is suggested that information be consistently put on a uniform size card or file.

Some students have found it convenient to color code the file, whereas others have preferred to alphabetize the information under headings such as *consonants, vowels, expressive language, receptive language, stuttering, voice, hearing,* and others.

Here are some suggestions for the ingredients of a file for treatment materials and motivational ideas:

1. Various ways to teach a child to produce a consonant or a vowel
2. Lists of words containing sounds in initial, medial, and final positions (Take from the student's spelling, reading, mathematics and science books.)
3. Sentences loaded with specific sounds
4. Ideas for auditory discrimination
5. Ideas for tactile and kinesthetic production of sounds
6. Poems, riddles, and finger plays
7. Flannel board ideas
8. Worksheets for home practice
9. Exercises for tongue and lip mobility
10. Ideas for teaching-unit topics (for example, astronauts, early American Indians, baseball, good nutrition)
11. Role-playing ideas
12. Relaxation techniques
13. Ideas for language and speech stimulation techniques that could be done at home by parents
14. Progress sheets or charting methods
15. Bulletin board ideas (These could be related to seasons or holidays or be of general interest.)
16. Word lists and pictures related to holidays
17. Puppets for use in therapy and diagnostics
18. Laminated picture cards illustrating nouns or verbs
19. Lists of records and books for children

20. Lists of suggestions for parents and teachers
21. Ideas of movement activities that could be tied to therapy
22. Ideas for speech development and speech-improvement lessons in the classroom

The card file can serve a number of useful purposes. It can be an inventory of available materials and publications; it can aid in lesson planning; and the cards can be easily removed from the file and used during the sessions. In addition, it can serve as an aid when consulting with classroom teachers in speech and language development and improvement and serve as a source of ideas when working with parents. Plus, it is concise, easy to construct, convenient to use, and inexpensive.

Expendable Materials

Supplies, such as paper, crayons, chalk, and some materials that can be used only one time, are usually supplied by the school; however, it does not necessarily follow that the school clinician has access to an unlimited supply. These items may be rationed or budgeted to the clinician on a yearly or semester basis. The clinician should be aware of the school's policy in regard to supplies. It should also be pointed out that because clinicians may function in several different schools within the same system, each school may have its own policy in regard to the availability of supplies.

Sometimes budget allowances are made on the basis of pupil enrollment. Both money and supplies may be determined in accordance with the total number of children enrolled or the number enrolled at any given time. Because budgets must be made out in advance, the figures may be dependent on last year's enrollment or on the estimated enrollment for the next year.

Budgeting for Materials, Equipment, and Supplies

Materials, supplies, and equipment are purchased by the schools. In some schools the clinician is given a fixed sum of money each year to spend for these items. In considering the purchase of equipment, it should be kept in mind that although the initial expenditure may be great, it may not have to be replaced for many years. There is, however, the matter of repair, maintenance, and general upkeep to be considered. For example, an audiometer needs yearly calibration. This should be taken into account before the purchase of the audiometer and discussed with the company representative.

Commercial therapy materials are subject to wear and tear if they are used frequently and may have to be budgeted for periodically. Considerations in the purchase of therapy materials might be whether or not they can be adapted for a variety of uses and occasions and whether or not they serve the purpose for which they are being purchased. They must be appropriate to the age, maturity, and interest of children.

Another matter to be considered is insurance on audiometers, computers, language masters, and other items of electronic equipment—a figure that

98

**Chapter 5:
Tools of the
Trade: Space,
Facilities,
Equipment,
Materials, and
Records**

should be in the budget. Also, if equipment is to be rented, the rental costs will have to be included in the budget.

When budgeting for a program, don't forget to account for ongoing material needs such as office supplies (disks, paper, pens, paper clips, and the like).

Budgeting for Professional Materials and Activities. Professional books may also be considered part of the school clinician's equipment and therefore would be justifiable budget items. The clinician may want to add to his or her own library of professional books, and these, of course, would not be a part of the school budget. The same is true for dues for professional organizations.

Budgeting for Travel. Some school systems allow travel money and expenses for personnel who attend professional meetings. It is wise for the new clinician to check the policy in regard to this matter.

If a clinician must travel between schools as part of the job, a travel allowance is available. Some school clinicians are paid a flat amount for a specified period of time, whereas others are paid by the mile. Some school systems make up for this difference by paying the clinician a higher salary that the person whose job does not entail travel between schools during the working day, for example, the classroom teacher.

Inventory Records

It is a good idea to maintain a systematic record or inventory of materials and equipment purchased for the program. This will facilitate sharing materials between several clinicians, locating articles when needed, and replacing articles should they become misplaced or damaged. The inventory record should include the name of the article, the manufacturer's name, address and phone number, the date purchased, the cost, serial numbers if applicable, the intended use, the storage location, and dates equipment was repaired or calibrated. Computerized data management systems often include programs which can be used for developing inventory records and reports.

The storage of equipment during the months when school is not in session, or equipment is not in use, is a matter to be determined by the SLP and the administration.

Records and Recordkeeping

There are good reasons for maintaining a comprehensive record and report system on the language, speech, and hearing program. Although it has always been done by clinicians, the reasons today are somewhat more compelling and the goals more inclusive.

Federal mandates such as Public Laws 94-142 and 99-457 place tremendous emphasis on accountability in the school system. Accountability has made it urgent that special services in the schools develop a method of reliably and accurately reporting data on children with handicaps.

Historically, the school clinician maintained written records to inform, to keep track of the services provided, to provide continuity both to the program and to the child's progress in therapy, to serve as a basis for research, to coordinate the child's therapy with the child's school program, and to serve as a basis for program needs and development. These reasons remain valid; however, there are additional reasons why an accounting system is needed today.

There are ethical, legal, and fiscal reasons. Parents occasionally question the nature and quality of the educational program their child is receiving. Their concerns may include special service programs such as speech and language intervention. As a result, they may request detailed information about the goals of therapy and techniques used. On rare occasions, they may disagree enough with placement decisions and the education professional's practices to pursue legal recourse in order to implement changes.

Several court decisions in the past few decades have ruled in favor of the parents' concerns about the school's failure to provide appropriate education or services. In these cases, the school districts have incurred large financial obligations. This can be financially detrimental to a school district and professionally damaging to the professional. The clinician who keeps detailed records of diagnostic findings, treatment procedures, and outcome of therapy will be in a better position to explain and defend the clinical decisions she has made.

Another legal issue relates to professional qualifications. Many states have licensing for speech-language pathologists and audiologists. This implies a legal responsibility for service delivery and the need for accountability becomes greater (Caccamo, 1973).

In recent years, laws have been passed which enable school districts to seek reimbursement for services from third party payers such as Medicaid (Peters-Johnson, 1990). In order to obtain funds, documentation of services must be provided including the diagnosis, rationale for therapy, treatment procedures, short- and long-term goals, and duration and frequency of treatment.

There is increasing competition for tax dollars. As a result, government agencies are requiring statements of accountability prior to awarding funds to programs. Local, federal, and state agencies want to know what results are being obtained for the tax money spent.

Schools must demonstrate compliance with federal and state department of education rules and regulations. Appropriate records and documentation can provide the proof needed during the program review process.

O'Toole (1971, pp. 24–25) posed some questions for school speech-language pathologists in regard to accountability:

How appropriate is speech therapy for each student in your program? Does each one belong in therapy? Have you established goals which, if accomplished, will make a difference? Is therapy time so well used as to justify taking students away from their academic subjects? Do you know how much progress each of your cases is making? Is that recorded? Are you aware of the rate of change? If progress is very slow or nonexistent, are you seeking additional help? How many cases have you followed through either to complete remediation or to the greatest degree of compensation that can be expected? If not very many, why not? Are you using therapy time as efficiently as possible? Is your coordination time justifiable because it is

100

Chapter 5:
Tools of the
Trade: Space,
Facilities,
Equipment,
Materials, and
Records

being used for the ultimate benefit of your student? Are you making use of all the knowledge and resources available? Are you moving children along as fast as they can go, or only as fast as is comfortable for you? Are you adapting to student needs, or are they suiting yours? Does your immediate supervisor understand what you do and the type of students you can and should see in therapy? Does he understand that if results are expected, the quality as well as the quantity of therapy is important?

In addition to the impetus added by federal mandates for record and report keeping, it makes good sense for the clinician to keep an account of a child's progress in therapy simply because the clinician is dealing with a large number of children and it would be impossible to remember all the facts and details pertinent to each of them.

Case Management Records

In order to be useful, record and report systems should permit quick retrieval of information regarding the status, disposition, and intervention of individual students as well as the collective data that must be recorded to report program statistics. Wing (1975) developed a concise form to help itinerant school clinicians who are responsible for managing caseloads of between 75 and 150 children throughout a school year. Wing reports that although the caseloads, exclusive of mass screenings, have been reduced, there is increasing demand for accurate record keeping, case management reporting, and statistical data for accountability to school administrators, boards of education, and state departments of education. Figure 5-1 shows the data-recording form used in the Great Falls, Montana, speech, language, and hearing program.

A school clinician going into a program that has been established will probably find a record and report system already set up and in operation, whereas a clinician who starts a program will have to develop his or her own. In both instances it will be necessary to evaluate and monitor the system continuously and make the necessary changes in the forms. The confidentiality of information makes it imperative that the storage of records and reports be a major consideration. The policies regarding security measures should be established and in writing. The same is true of the availability of such records and reports to other school personnel, administrators, referral sources other clinicians on the staff, and parents. Policies and procedures for sharing information should be in writing and should be adhered to once agreed upon. For example, parents should be asked to give written permission for you to release or obtain information about their child.

The abundance of records and reports essential to a program should be taken into account on the clinician's weekly schedule. One of the most time-consuming tasks is filling out reports, keeping up to date on information recorded, and filing and retrieving material. The task is a daily one for much of the information, and when weekly, monthly, or yearly reports are involved, a large chunk of time is needed. Some of the work can be assigned to an aide and some of it might be given to the school secretary; however, there are usually

School year 19__

School __Edison__

Clinician __Mrs. Johnson__

Student's Name	Grade	Referral Date and Source	Evaluation Dates	Outside Referral	Classification	Etiology	Severity	Therapy Dates	Prescriptive Program Dates	Resource Room	Ongoing Assessment Dates	No Program	Waiting List	Parent Conferences	Teacher Conferences	Recommendation
		Cases						Disposition								Recommendation
Ondick, Johnny	3	9/14 T, 9/15 9/25		1	F	II	✗ 3/18, 7/18 5/25				10/1 12/1	I	III			Reevaluate in Sept.
Smith, Billy	1	9/16 T, 9/18		1	I	I	12/3 2/16 4/7						III			
Doornink, Edna	3	9/20 T, 9/20 10/6, 10/8 ENT	2	A	II	10/26 1/15						IIII	III			Reevaluate in March
Monroe, Brian	K	9/20 Cl, 9/22 9/24 10/5, Phys 10/7	1 2	B	III	10/15 5/25						IIII II	IIII			Continue next year

Referral source: T (teachers), Cl (clinician). *Outside referral:* ENT (ear, nose, and throat specialist), phys. (physician), sch. psyl. (school psychologist), and so on. *Classification:* 1, articulation; 2, phonation; 3, rhythm; 4, language; 5, no problem (any appropriate classifications may be used, listed in order of significance). *Etiology:* A, organic pathology; B, cleft palate; C, cerebral palsy; D, mental retardation; E, hearing loss; F, dental anomalies; G, emotional factors; H, environmental factors; I, developmental factors; J, undetermined (any appropriate classifications may be used, listed in order of significance). *Severity:* I, mild, II, moderate; III, severe. *Note:* slash marks are used to indicate change of status in any category. This form can be stenciled on standard 8½×11″ paper with spaces to accommodate seven to nine student names.

FIGURE 5.1. Data recording form for speech and hearing services

many demands on their time as well. A large program may need some secretarial help, either on a part-time or full-time basis, depending on the size and scope of the program. Most of it, however, will be up to the school clinician, and if this is the case, scheduled time should be allotted for it.

Most school systems provide a central office for the school clinicians and in this way a uniform filing, retrieval, recording, and security system can be utilized. A central office system has another advantage in that secretarial or aide assistance can be pooled.

School clinicians will have to abide by the policies of the school system in regard to how long records and reports on individual children should be retained, which records should be retained, and how records are transferred from school to school as well as from school system to school system. Statistical information in relation to program management and incidence figures can be very useful to clinicians in planning future programs and serving as a basis for research. The retaining of this type of information might be decided by the school clinical staff. Provisions for the storage of such information would have to be made.

In an effort to improve information systems for the school speech, language, and hearing programs, a Task Force on Data Collection and Information

102

Chapter 5:
Tools of the
Trade: Space,
Facilities,
Equipment,
Materials, and
Records

Systems (Healey, 1973) was appointed to study the issue. Among recommendations made to school systems, the following steps were considered essential:

1. Formulate a school-wide policy.
2. Develop a general framework for planning.
3. Determine a policy relating to information gathering and distribution.
4. Provide a clearinghouse and a meaningful circulation system.
5. Assure checks for control of information.
6. Protect individual privacy and insure confidentiality.
7. Develop uniform nomenclature.
8. Select computer language if necessary.
9. Determine what output is desired.
10. Insure accuracy and quality of the data input.
11. Determine the categories of information needed for measurement.
12. Ascertain the action that will be taken once the data have been collected.

Table 5.2, on pages 103 and 104, is an outline suggesting the type of information that should be included in documentation of program and case management records. The school speech-language clinician and educational audiologist might consider this outline as a framework for developing the record and report forms necessary to the program. Such an outline also could be used as a framework for evaluating clinician behaviors in the clinical process as well as analyzing program data to effect changes in program design and practices.

Risk Management Plan

Because speech-language pathologists and audiologists in educational settings work closely with children, they are at risk for contracting chronic, contagious diseases such as Acquired Immune Deficiency Syndrome (AIDS), Hepatitis B virus (HBV), herpes simplex, and cytomegalovirus (CMV). It is wise to take precautionary measures to manage these risks and prevent transmission of disease. School clinicians should have a risk management plan outlining infection control procedures.

The ASHA Committee on Quality Assurance (Kulpa et al., 1991) recommended several administrative considerations for clinicians interested in developing a risk management plan for their school. They also suggested supplies necessary for implementing a risk management plan and infection control procedures for decreasing the possibility of transmitting disease through treatment materials, skin contact, and contact with materials and body fluids. Tables 5-3, 5-4, and 5-5 provide an outline of a risk management plan, supplies needed, and procedures to be followed. These procedures are adapted from the Universal Precautions developed by the Center for Disease Control and are applicable to the educational setting.

The intent of using such procedures is to prevent transmission of diseases; protect the health of students and professionals; and ensure individuals' rights to privacy.

TABLE 5.2. RECOMMENDED OUTLINE FOR DOCUMENTING PROGRAM AND CASE MANAGEMENT RECORDS

I. SPEECH-LANGUAGE OR AUDIOLOGY PROGRAM INFORMATION
   A. Schools served
      1. Names
      2. Locations
      3. Demographic information
         a. Composition of student body
         b. Number of students
         c. Economic/cultural status
      4. Travel time between buildings
      5. Schedule for servicing each building
      6. Student-clinician ratio
      7. Facilities
      8. Projected need for services
   B. Caseload size and composition
      1. Types of disabilities served
      2. Ages
      3. Severity levels
      4. Numbers of students served
      5. Number of continuing cases; number of new cases

II. SPEECH-LANGUAGE PATHOLOGIST OR EDUCATIONAL AUDIOLOGIST INFORMATION
   A. Names of individuals providing speech-language or audiological services to students
   B. Licenses and/or certification held and numbers of each
   C. School designated as home-base or office location
   D. Schools assigned to serve
   E. Areas of specialization and/or interest

III. SERVICES PROVIDED
   A. Screening
   B. Assessment
   C. Treatment/Intervention Service Delivery Models
   D. Consultation
   E. Collaboration
   F. Inservice programming

IV. CRITERIA OF CASE SELECTION
   A. Eligibility criteria
   B. Severity rating criteria
   C. Prioritization criteria

V. COMPONENTS FOR STUDENT RECORDS
   A. Identifying information
      1. Student's name and address, phone number, chronological age, social security number
      2. Caregiver's name and address
      3. School district; building; grade or placement; homeroom
      4. Identification number (if applicable)
      5. Referral source, date or referral

(continued)

**Chapter 5:
Tools of the
Trade: Space,
Facilities,
Equipment,
Materials, and
Records**

B. Student History
   1. Medical history and/or diagnosis
   2. Educational history
   3. Communication disorder diagnosis (behaviors observed)
   4. Prior functional communication status
   5. Prior treatment for speech, language, hearing problems and outcomes of that treatment
   6. Frequency, length, duration of treatment in prior settings
C. Description of current status (communicative and educational)
   1. Date or multi-factored evaluation
   2. Current functional status
      a. Baseline testing (standardized, nonstandardized procedures); observations
      b. Interpretation of test scores and results
      c. Other relevant clinical and educational findings (contributed by other specialists)
      d. Statement of potential for rehabilitation; estimate of student's abilities based on findings
D. Treatment Plan
   1. Date treatment plan is established
   2. Long- and short-term functional communication goals
   3. Treatment objectives
   4. Recommended service delivery model, frequency, and duration or treatment
E. Documentation of Treatment
   1. Date treatment is initiated
   2. Number of times treatment was provided to date
   3. Objective measures of communicative performance (use functional terminology; compare performance against original measures)
   4. Significant developments that might influence rehabilitation potential
   5. Changes in treatment plan
   6. Recommendations for follow-up treatment or continued service
   7. Record of consultation and/or collaboration with other individuals and outcomes
F. Documentation of clinician and qualifications
   1. Signatures (including titles on all reports and records)

TABLE 5.3. RISK MANAGEMENT ADMINISTRATIVE CONSIDERATIONS:
A CHECKLIST

_____ School policy in place for risk management.
_____ Person designated responsible for implementation of policy.
_____ Committee established at the building level for identifying risk management policy and procedures, as follows:
    _____ Identifying risk management needs
    _____ Developing risk management procedures for implementing precautions
    _____ Implementing precautions
    _____ Assessing effectivness of precautions
    _____ Modifying precaution policy, as indicated
_____ Mechanism established for purchase of required materials to implement infection control procedures.

TABLE 5.4. INFECTION CONTROL SUPPLY CHECKLISTS

A. The following materials are needed to implement proper infection control procedures.

_____ Latex gloves
_____ Alcohol/antiseptic wipes
_____ Soap
_____ Access to sink/running water
_____ Paper towels
_____ Disinfection solution (1 part household bleach to 10 parts water)
_____ Spray bottle (to mix water and disinfectant solution)
_____ Tissue
_____ Plastic bags that seal (e.g., Ziploc)
_____ Trash bags
_____ Household bleach
_____ Hand lotion
_____ Absorbent powder for bodily secretions

B. In addition, these infection control materials should be used when implementing procedures that could expose the professional to blood, semen, or other bodily secretions that _contain visible blood_ (e.g., oral peripheral examinations, procedures involving tracheostomy tubes, etc.)

_____ Mask
_____ Goggles
_____ Gowns
_____ Red trash bags (for disposal of materials that _could be harmful_ if handled casually)

TABLE 5.5. INFECTION CONTROL PROCEDURES

Decreasing the possibility of transmitting disease through treatment materials.

What to Disinfect	When to Disinfect	How to Disinfect
• Evaluation and treatment materials (e.g., toys*, games, storage boxes, therapy materials).	• Clean tabletop and materials after each use.	• Use soap and water or a 1 to 10 solution of household bleach to water, spray, and wipe thoroughly.
• Work surfaces.	• If materials, work surfaces, electronic equipment or seating surfaces contain visible blood, use Universal Precautions.	• Use disposable materials (e.g., latex gloves, etc.) when possible.
• Electronic equipment and accessories.		
• Seating surfaces.		
• Materials, supplies and instruments to examine oral mechanism.		

*Note: Toys made of fabric and fur should be avoided due to the tendency to harbor microorganisms.

Decreasing the possibility of transmitting disease by disposing of materials and body fluids appropriately.

Decreasing the possibility of transmitting disease via skin contact.

What to Do	When to Do It	How to Do It
• Wash hands (effective if skin is intact).	• Before and after seeing each client.	• Use vigorous mechanical action whether or not a skin cleanser is used.
	• After removing gloves.	• Use antiseptic or ordinary soap under running water.
	• Immediately if in contact with potentially contaminating blood or body fluids.	• Wash for 30 seconds or longer if grossly contaminated.
		• Dry hands thoroughly with a paper or disposable towel to help eliminate germs.
		• Put on hand lotion so hands do not become chapped.
• Use gloves (to give protective barrier) if your skin or client's	• Before touching blood or other body fluids, mucous mem-	• Put gloves on.

The skin is broken.

- branes, or non-intact skin of *all* clients.
- When performing an examination of the oral speech mechanism using laryngeal mirrors, middle ear testing, handling or fabricating earmolds and other prostheses.
- When you have a cut or abrasion.
- When client has a cut or abrasion.

- If a glove is torn or other injury occurs, remove gloves, wash hands thoroughly and use new gloves.
- After removing gloves, wash hands immediately. See instructions above.
- Discard gloves.
- Change gloves after each client.

What to Dispose of	*When to Dispose of It*	*How to Dispose of It*
• Dressing and tissues.	• Immediately.	• Place used dressing and tissues (e.g., diapers, gauze, towelettes, alcohol wipes, gloves) in plastic bag and tie securely. • Discard bags carefully.
• Urine, feces, sperm, vaginal secretions, menses.	• Immediately.	• Wear gloves. • Flush urine and feces down the toilet. • If it is necessary to use a portable urinal, potty chair, etc., empty it into the toilet and thoroughly clean and sanitize before replacing it or returning it to storage.

DISCUSSION QUESTIONS AND PROJECTS

1. Visit several school speech-language programs and rate their facilities using the Program Environment Observation Checklist in Table 5-1.

2. Are mobile units used in your state? What are their advantages and disadvantages? Under what conditions would you use one?

3. You are the school clinician. The principal has assigned you to a small former storage room with no windows but a convenient location. You are not satisfied with the room. Would you try to have another room assigned or would you modify the assigned room? Outline the steps you would follow, using either alternative.

4. Collect five advertisements from publishing companies of speech, language, and hearing materials and equipment. They can be brochures or advertisements in professional journals. Analyze the advertisements by using the Connell et al. (1977) evaluation system.

5. Start an activity file. Justify the method you have chosen to organize it.

6. Interview a SLP to find out how he or she budgets for equipment and materials and how the materials are procured through the school system. How are maintenance and insurance handled?

7. Draw a plan for your ideal therapy room (1) for an elementary school and (2) for a high school.

8. Why are school programs in speech, language, and hearing accountable? To whom are programs accountable?

9. Start a collection of record and report forms used in the schools. How would you organize report forms for a school system?

10. Discuss procedures you should take if you learn that a child has a communicable disease. Who should you contact? What precautions should you take? Should services for the child be discontinued?

11. Technological assistance is needed to select appropriate ALDs and augmentative communication devices for intervention. Make a list of 10 questions you might ask of persons who have technological expertise with these devices.

CHAPTER 6

Case Finding, Case Selection, and Caseload

Introduction

One of the most challenging areas for the school speech-language pathologist is decision making in caseload, case-finding, and case-selection procedures. The ultimate task of the SLP is to identify and treat the student whose communication problem interferes with his or her educational achievement. The SLP makes decisions about how students are to be identified, how they are to be assessed, and which children should receive treatment. These processes are the cornerstone of accountability.

School SLPs are expected to comply with federal and state standards in screening, diagnosis, case selection, caseload, and delivery of service. At the same time they are accountable to the local education agency requirements as well as the professional code of ethics. In districts where funding is contributed by a number of pay sources, the clinician is also responsible for meeting the requirements established by the payers. Sometimes these requirements are in conflict. The information in this chapter is presented to help the school SLP formulate the many decisions that must be made in these areas.

Defining the Process

Case finding (or case identification) refers to locating the preschool and school age students who demonstrate communication impairments or who are at risk for educational or social failure due to inadequate communication skills. Where it is not in conflict with state law and practices and court order, case finding would also include those aged 18 to 21. Case finding in schools is accomplished by referrals and screening programs.

110

Chapter 6:
Case Finding,
Case Selec-
tion, and
Caseload

Case selection refers to the process of determining which students are eligible for speech, language, or hearing services. Not all students referred nor all students who fail screening criteria may necessarily be candidates. Those who exhibit communication problems are determined through the following steps:

1. *Obtaining appropriate background information,* that is, a case history, including onset, past development, present status and other relevant information from parents and teachers
2. *Appraising* the problem by observing, interviewing, describing, and testing when appropriate
3. *Diagnosing,* which includes making a tentative identification of the problem and determining probable causes

It should be pointed out that the SLP must use judgment in determining how rigorously these steps are followed.

For example, the third-grader who exhibits what appears to be a serious voice problem may be suffering from a cold and sore throat. That information would preclude interviewing parents or obtaining a case history.

Caseload and composition refer to the size of the caseload, or the number of students comprising it, and the range of communication problems represented in it. Caseload sizes are often mandated by state and local education agencies to serve inordinately high numbers of students. In addition, there is little or no agreement at this writing among state and local education agencies concerning what is an appropriate caseload size.

Let us now look at each of these issues in greater detail and in the chronological order in which these procedures would be carried out by the school SLP.

Case Finding

Case finding is usually accomplished by utilizing two procedures, either singly or in combination—*referral* and *screening*. The purpose of both referral and screening is the identification of the student with the communication problem. In many school systems referral is becoming widely used because of its perceived efficiency and effectiveness. In some situations, however, it may be more efficient to utilize screening, for example, on the kindergarten or first-grade level.

Referral

Let us look first at the process of referral. The school clinician needs to be aware that a particular child might have a communication problem. The clinician, in the final analysis, is the one who is responsible for determining if such a problem exists; however, referrals can be made by anyone who has the child's welfare in mind and suspects a problem. This would include the child's parents, teachers, family doctor, school nurse, school counselor, principal, or the child. Outside the school, the social service agencies within the community, physicians, health care specialists, and voluntary agencies such as United Cerebral Palsy, Easter Seal Society, the National Head Injury Foundation, and others may all be considered valuable referral agencies. The school clinician will need to know and comply with the school system's policy regarding referrals. The process for referring students for speech, language, and audiology services should be clearly defined and consistent throughout the school district. Referral forms should be made available to school staff and other individuals.

Referrals should not be discouraged even though the clinician may sometimes feel that the classroom teachers overrefer or refer children who have problems other than those in speech, language, and hearing. The door should always be kept open for referrals. Educators should be encouraged to refer any child they feel might have a problem. Because of staff turnover and changes in service delivery requirements and eligibility criteria, the procedures and opportunities for referral should be presented to the teachers periodically. The school clinician will soon learn which teachers in a school are able to identify the child with a communication impairment with a high degree of accuracy.

Following the initial referral, and depending on the information about the child gathered from the referring agent, the speech-language clinician will have to make a decision about whether the student is to receive a battery of screening tests or a more complete assessment. In addition, parental/guardian permission must be obtained before testing is undertaken.

Helping Educators Make Referrals. Educators and communication disorders professionals can work together to identify children who exhibit inadequate communication skills. If others are to function effectively as referral sources, they will need to gain an awareness and understanding of how speech and language skills develop and of communication impairments. They should know the behaviors and characteristics associated with language, articulation, stuttering, voice, and hearing problems. They need to learn the definitions and terminology used by professionals to discuss these disorders. It is extremely important for educators to understand that communication is the basis for learning and the negative impact speech, language, and hearing impairments can have on classroom performance.

The quality of referrals will be improved if teachers become skilled at observing students and relating their communication problems to learning difficulties they may be experiencing (Lass et al., 1985; Blosser and Tomi, 1985). Miller (1989) reported that speech-language pathologists in the Fayette County School District in Lexington, Kentucky conducted inservice training sessions prior to initiating the referral program. Teachers were informed about communication disorders by viewing a videotape designed especially for classroom teachers. Following the tape presentation, staff speech-language pathologists answered teachers' questions. The quality and accuracy of referrals made by teachers improved substantially in comparison with results from previous mass screening efforts.

Some colleges and universities offer courses in speech, language, and hearing problems to students majoring in education. Others integrate information about communication development and disabilities into other coursework on topics such as human development and learning or characteristics of children with special education needs. It would be helpful to the school clinician if all teachers were to learn about communication impairments during their preprofessional training, but this is not always the case. The school clinician may

112

**Chapter 6:
Case Finding,
Case Selec-
tion, and
Caseload**

want to consider offering an inservice course to teachers. This would give the clinician the opportunity to define and describe the various types of communication problems as well as discuss their impact on learning and referral procedures. Following is an outline of topics which might be discussed during an inservice presentation to teachers and other referral sources.

1. Normal speech-language-hearing development.
2. Nature and causes of speech-language-hearing impairments.
3. Terminology used by speech-language pathologists and audiologists to describe and discuss children with communication impairments.
4. Impact of communication disorders on academic and social performance.
5. Factors communication disorders professionals consider when evaluating students' communicative performance.
6. Referral procedures to be followed.
7. Collaborating with speech-language pathologists and audiologists.

Such a presentation would be enhanced by demonstrating the disorders. As a prospective clinician, are you able to imitate or simulate various kinds of problems? A library of tapes of various types of problems would be helpful for demonstration. Regional resource centers and universities may have audio or videotapes available for loan to school clinicians for teacher inservice programs.

Referrals can be initiated in person, by telephone, or in writing. The teacher is able to observe children in a variety of communication-based learning activities. Consequently, the information she has to offer regarding performance is valuable. It is helpful to provide a simple questionnaire or checklist to assist teachers and others in describing the communication behaviors they observe, their concerns, and their reasons for referring. Figure 6-1 is an example of the type of checklist teachers might find helpful when observing a child's communication skills. The initial referral form should be brief so it can be quickly completed by busy teachers. More extensive information can be obtained through guided teacher observation as part of the evaluation process once the child has been identified as having a communication impairment.

Referrals on the Secondary-School Level. Case finding on the middle and high-school level is carried out more often by teacher referral than by screening (Neal, 1976). School clinicians, while recognizing the need of improved case-finding procedures at this level, point out the difficulties of a screening program because of the inflexibility of high-school class schedules and the greater mobility of high-school students, who are changing classes.

Another factor that would hinder both a screening program and a teacher referral program on the secondary level was pointed out by Phillips (1976). The study indicated that the higher the grade taught, the less aware the teachers were of speech disorders. She suggested that this might be a result of the fact that an increasing number of universities are requiring coursework in disabilities of elementary-education majors but not of secondary-education majors. It may also be related to the demand and structure of the secondary curriculum. Secondary teachers often do not see students for as great amount of time as elementary teachers see their students. In addition, in many classes, communicative interaction is limited because teachers use a lecture style for teaching.

FIGURE 6.1. TEACHER'S REFERRAL FORM

Teacher's Name: _____

Grade: _____

Read the following statements and (√) if the child's speech, language or hearing behavior is described	CHILD'S Name & Age				
1. Voice quality is noticeably different from other children (hoarse, breathy, nasal)					
2. Speech is nonfluent (hesitant, jerky, repetitive, prolonged)					
3. Child is noticeably frustrated if unable to get message across					
4. Articulation is difficult to understand					
5. Child is unable to ask and/or answer simple questions					
6. Child cannot carry on a conversation (relay events, give explanation)					
7. Child cannot formulate 5 and 7 word sentences; grammar and vocabulary are not age appropriate.					
8. Generally nonverbal					
9. Has frequent colds or runny nose					
10. Attends to speakers face more than other children do					
11. Frequently responds to statements or questions with "what?" or "huh?"					
12. Does not follow simple directions					

English and language arts teachers are good referral sources because they are sensitive to communication and they have greater opportunity to hear students communicate during classroom activities. Guidance counselors, coaches, and teachers who sponsor extra-curricular activities also converse with students in informal situations with great frequency.

On the high-school level, self-referrals or parental referrals are often good sources of identifying individuals with communication problems. High-school students who have a speech, language, or hearing problem will have to know about the services offered if they are to refer themselves. This means that the clinician will have to find ways of letting students know the services are available, as well as make it easy for them to refer themselves.

Students can be informed of the times and days the speech-language clinician is in the school building through announcements over the public address system, through the school newspaper, or through signs posted on bulletin boards throughout the building. The message should inform students about the

114

**Chapter 6:
Case Finding,
Case Selec-
tion, and
Caseload**

services offered by the speech-language pathologist and/or educational audiologist. It should provide brief explanations of speech, language, and hearing behaviors which may cause them concern and which they might want to "check out." It should also describe how to schedule an appointment. In some districts, students may have to inform the guidance counselor of their interest and obtain a hallpass. Middle school and high school students are sensitive about other people knowing they experience difficulties. Therefore, discretion is advised about the testing appointment, location, results, and recommendations. One way to encourage participation is to stress the "self-improvement" aspect of the speech-language program.

Paul-Brown (1991) provides a compilation of various methods which can be used to identify communication problems in adolescents. She includes assessment tools, classroom observation procedures, and methods for obtaining teacher referrals. By providing instructions and guidelines for making referrals during an inservice program, you can develop a systematic referral program with a core group of teachers who see every student in the building. Reed and Miles (1989) have developed a video inservice program for secondary level educators, providing guidelines for referring adolescent students. They provide teachers with instructions for considering the students' skills in the following areas:

Thinking (organizing and categorizing information; identifying and solving problems; finding, selecting, and using information; and thinking about ideas and events)

Listening (understanding complex sentences and words; understanding main ideas and events; following complex directions; and listening effectively)

Speaking (planning what to say; organizing information in a logical sequence; using grammatically correct sentence structures; using language to give directions, make reports, tell stories; providing relevant and complete answers)

Survival language (demonstrating language skills necessary to cope with daily living situations)

It is suggested that you work with the principal and guidance counselors to determine the best method for finding secondary students with communication problems in your school district.

Screening

The clinician must decide when and where the screening will take place and which children will be screened. There are some general factors to be considered before making these decisions.

Answering the following questions can help determine how to implement the screening program so the screening time can be used in the best way possible:

• What are the goals of the speech-language-hearing program?
• Will there be new service delivery models or populations served in the coming school year?
• Is the speech clinician new to the building, district, or community?

- Will the screening program be conducted by SLPs independently or will there be a team approach involving aides or clinicians from other school buildings?
- Are there unique aspects related to the student population (socio-economic status, mobility, cultural diversity, special education needs)?
- Have there been significant changes in school personnel or resources?

When the answers to these questions have been obtained, the goals of the screening program can be established. It is important that these goals are not only established, but also in writing and made available to the school administration. When the goals are established, the procedures for carrying out the screening program can be made. The procedures should also be in writing and should be available to the superintendent, the director of special education, the elementary and secondary supervisors, the principals of each school, and the teachers in each of the schools to be screened.

It is inefficient and it creates ill will to collect data through screenings in schools and classrooms where the SLP does not expect to conduct therapy. Screening on the kindergarten and first-grade levels of schools to be serviced, however, may be the best way to identify children in need of further evaluation. This method is almost always combined with teacher referrals on these levels as well as parental input.

The purpose of screening is to determine (1) if a problem exists, (2) if further evaluation is needed, and (3) if referral to other professionals is needed.

The first step in a screening process serves to identify children with communication impairment. A second screening would be made of those children identified by the first screening or by referral as having possible communication problems. The second screening would be somewhat more extensive and would help the clinician pick out those children who are candidates for therapy. The third step would be complete diagnostic evaluation for children who need therapeutic intervention and/or referral to other professionals.

A procedure used successfully by many clinicians is to take three children at a time. While one is being tested the other two can observe and will know what to do when their turn comes without the clinician having to explain. As each child is finished he or she goes back to the room and gets the next child in the row. There is no interruption of the teacher's schedule, and the classroom activities go on as usual. A class of 25 children can be screened in approximately 30 to 40 minutes.

The same general screening procedures may be applied to small groups of children. The clinician takes a group of six to eight children to the therapy room where the screening is carried out, returns the group, and gets the next group. If aides are available, they may take the children to and from the classroom.

In many school systems a team approach is used in the preschool screening program. The team members often include the school nurse, psychologist, speech pathologist, audiologist, and other specialists who test vision, hearing, speech and language, motor coordination, dentition, general health, and physical well-being. Paraprofessionals or volunteer aides also assist in this type of screening program. If using assistants in this way, they should be trained and supervised by certified, qualified professionals.

116

Chapter 6:
Case Finding,
Case Selec-
tion, and
Caseload

General Considerations. Because the purpose of the rapid screening is detection, not diagnosis, the clinician will have to resist the temptation to spend more time that is needed with a child who obviously has a problem. Also, the clinician will have to tactfully discourage a talkative child from telling a lengthy, complicated story.

The results of the screening task should be recorded immediately after each individual is seen. All absentees should be noted, and arrangements should be made to screen them later.

Screening Procedures. Let us look at the rapid or first screening procedure. Several models can be utilized and some general principles can be applied for the rapid screening for speech, language, and hearing problems. The major purpose is to determine whether or not a problem exists. Ideally, all children enrolled in the school are screened. The screening must be done quickly and accurately; that is, it must be done with a maximum degree of professional expertise and with a minimum expenditure of time, money, and professional energy. Planning is absolutely essential. In addition to a general plan, there must also be a plan to encompass all the details of the screening.

Much of the screening is carried on during the first few weeks of school, but it may be done at any time of the year. Many clinicians prefer to screen the upper elementary classes early in the school year and the kindergarten and primary grades later. This allows the classroom teachers to become better acquainted with the children, and the very young child to become more accustomed to school. In some schools preacademic children are screened during a preschool roundup in May or August, just before enrolling in school.

Federal regulations do not require written permission of the parents prior to a group screening program; however, some states and some school districts do require that parents be notified. This can be done by letter sent home with the children or by announcements in the school newsletter or local newspaper.

Screening programs can be carried out by one clinician, by a team of clinicians, or by a team composed of clinicians and trained aides. If the school system is small and employs few clinicians on its staff, those individuals may want to team up with clinicians in adjacent towns or counties to accomplish the screening in both school districts more quickly. If more than one person is involved in a screening program, the procedures should be clearly understood by all to insure uniform administration and greater reliability.

Class Survey Method of Screening for Speech and Language. The class survey method of screening can be used with any grade level and can be carried out by one clinician or by a team of clinicians. It is done within the classroom or just outside, preferably as close as possible to the classroom. The clinician makes arrangements through the principal and arranges a time schedule so that teachers know when to expect the screening to take place. The clinician explains the procedure to the teacher and also prepares the children by giving them an explanation at their level of understanding. Young children are sometimes fearful and may not be as cooperative as the clinician would hope unless they are prepared.

The class survey can be carried out so there is little interruption of the classroom routine. The teacher supplies the clinicians with a roster of the children and indicates which ones are absent that day so the clinician can screen them later. If the roster is in the form of a seating chart, the clinician can take the children in order of their seating. In this way the clinician will not take up too much time trying to figure out the identity of very small children who have difficulty saying (or remembering!) their last names.

Keeping Teachers Informed. Teachers should be informed in advance of the screening program procedures and schedule. This will help them prepare their students and plan for the interruption in their teaching schedule. Below is an example of the type of memo you can send teachers to announce the screening program.

MARK YOUR CALENDARS TODAY!
SPEECH-LANGUAGE SCREENINGS
WEEK OF SEPTEMBER 7, 1993

Children in your building will be screened for speech and language impairments during the week of September 7.

Prior to that time, please observe the children in your class closely. Refer all children whose communication skills (speaking, listening, writing) concern you. Return the teacher referral form to my mailbox by September 3.

Children referred by their teachers plus all children in Grade 1 and the Special Education classes will be screened individually.

I will confirm the testing schedule with you after reviewing the referral forms.

If you have questions about behaviors which are significant or about the screening program, please let me know.

I'm looking forward to working with you this year.

Cordially,

Emily Butler
Speech-Language Pathologist

Screening Tests. Clinicians use a variety of methods for screening children ranging from observing informal conversations to using formal, standardized screening tests. There are advantages and disadvantages to each. For example, through observation during informal conversation, one can observe the child's overall intelligibility and the impact of the child's communication skills on communicative interactions. However, this method reduces the quantifiable information which can be obtained, reduces accountability, and may miss children who are reluctant participants or shy (Westman & Broen, 1989). Formalized methods have the advantage of enabling the clinician to compare the child's performance to others of the same age, implementing the testing consistently across children, and facilitating documentation and accountability.

Instruments for assessing communicative abilities during a screening program differ according to the ages of the children. The instruments should be easily administered and should identify quickly those children needing further testing. In a school screening, whether one clinician or several are involved, the

118

Chapter 6:
Case Finding,
Case Selec-
tion, and
Caseload

screening devices should be the same, and the standard for judging the results should be consistent from one tester to another. The screening procedures should also take into account differences in ethnic and socioeconomic backgrounds of the children being tested. The examiners need to keep in mind that they are attempting to detect differences in speech, language, voice quality, fluency, or any other problems in communication that might be potentially handicapping to the child's ability to learn in school or function as a useful member of society.

It will be necessary for the school SLP to (1) become familiar with the various speech and language tests; (2) find out what the test *purports* to measure and what it *actually* measures; (3) utilize the most appropriate test or tests for the particular situation and the students tested; (4) check the reliability, norms, and standardization of the test; (5) know the difference between "norm-referenced" tests and "criterion-referenced" tests; and (6) utilize clinical judgment and expertise in synthesizing the information from the tests.

A comprehensive screening battery carried out by the speech-language specialist or as a part of a comprehensive screening program could include the following:

1. Audiological evaluation
2. Articulation/phonological process appraisal
3. Intelligibility appraisal
4. Voice appraisal
5. Fluency appraisal
6. Language appraisal (receptive and expressive) on the
   a. Semantic level
   b. Syntactic level
   c. Phonological level
   d. Morphological level
   e. Pragmatic level

Screening procedures on any age or grade level are subject to some degree of error. Some children will slip by undetected, and others may not be identified correctly. School clinicians and classroom teachers must work together to recognize any of these children.

Teacher Interview Screening. A method that combines screening and teacher referral was developed by Finn and Gardner (1984) at Heartland Area Education Agency 11, Ankeny, Iowa. Known as the Teacher Interview Screening, it is comprised of two processes: mandatory teacher in-service programs and the teacher interview. It was developed to utilize the teachers' expertise in observing communicative behavior. (Refer to the flow chart, Figure 6-2). According to Finn and Gardner,

the speech and language clinicians were required to inservice, as a minimum, all second grade teachers, but preferably all of the teachers in their assigned schools in order to improve the quality of all referrals. Second grade was targeted to screen as it was felt that this would eliminate most developmental articulation errors. To facilitate the inservice, a Communication Competency Screening Scale (Figure 6-3) which describes communication skills was developed and lighthearted overheads made available.

The teacher inservice was held in the fall so that the teachers had a semester to observe their students' speech and language skills prior to the teacher interview in January or February. During the teacher interview, each second grade teacher was asked the following questions for each member of the class. "Considering the skills outlined on the communication competency scale, do you feel this child's communication skills are adequate when compared to his/her classmates?" The teacher and clinician then had three options available to them.

They could pass the child who had adequate skills, fail the child

FIGURE 6.2. Teacher Interview Screening Method

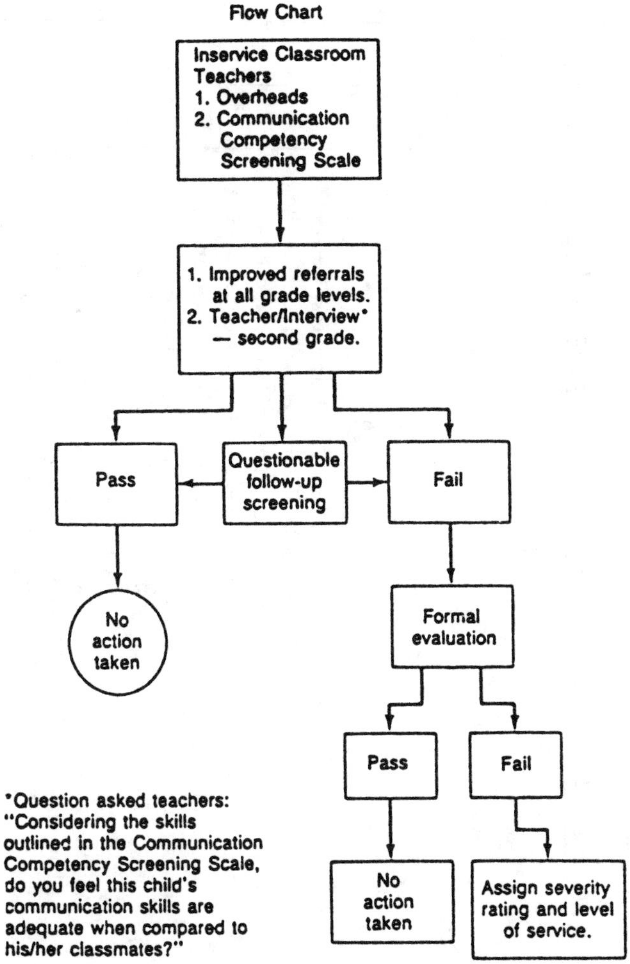

Flow Chart

*Question asked teachers:
"Considering the skills outlined in the Communication Competency Screening Scale, do you feel this child's communication skills are adequate when compared to his/her classmates?"

FIGURE 6.3. COMMUNICATION COMPETENCY SCREENING

	POOR	POOR	ADEQUATE	SUPERIOR	SUPERIOR
Skill in communication	limited awareness of listeners; speaks with little effort to evoke understanding from others; pace of words and inflection of voice not adjusted to listeners				adjusts pace and inflection to listener; is aware of need to make self understood and can adjust content to listener's needs and responses
Organization, purpose and control	rambles; limited sense of order or of getting to the point; rattles on without purpose; cannot tell a story in proper sequence				plans what is said; gets to the point; controls language, can tell a story in proper sequence; speaks fluently
Wealth of ideas/amount of language	seldom expresses an idea; appears dull and unimaginative; doesn't originate suggestions or plans during play periods; seldom talks; rarely initiates; needs to be prompted to talk				expresses ideas on different topics; makes suggestions on what to do and how to carry out class plans; shows imagination and creativity in play; talks freely, frequently and easily

Vocabulary	uses a meager vocabulary, far below that of most children this age; uses ambiguous words		uses a rich variety of words, has an exceptionally large and growing vocabulary
Quality of listening	demonstrates poor comprehension of spoken language; inattentive; easily distracted		superior understanding of spoken language; attentive
Quality of sentence structure	omissions of structural elements, including word endings; uses only simple active, declarative sentences; word order difficulties in question formations		includes all structural elements; mature sentence patterns; maintains constant tense reference within a paragraph or story; mature use of phrases and clauses and conjunctions
Articulation	child is difficult to understand due to speech sound errors; speech draws attention to itself		all speech sounds are produced appropriately
Voice	distracts listener from meaning of the message; denasal or nasal quality; frequent loss of voice; recurrent hoarseness		voice is pleasing to the listener; does not draw attention to itself
Fluency	frequently repeats parts of words and whole words; demonstrates long periods of silence while attempting speech; demonstrates struggle behavior		speaks smoothly

Adapted by: Heartland Education Agency from LOBAN'S ORAL LANGUAGE SCALE

122

**Chapter 6:
Case Finding,
Case Selec-
tion, and
Caseload**

who obviously had inadequate skills or for those children whose skills were questionable, the clinician conducted a followup screening. The followup screening consisted of a classroom observation or a more traditional one-on-one screening depending upon the areas of concern (Figure 6-4).

In order to evaluate the effectiveness of the teacher interview, results were compared to the traditional method in terms of cost, reliability and compatibility with current philosophies.

In terms of the cost comparison, a two year study was conducted. During 1980–81, data was gathered on the cost of using the traditional screening method with 4645 first graders. The following year data was gathered on 7292 students using the teacher interview method of screening. The results indicate the total time spent by the staff doing the new screening method was 100 hours and 42 minutes or approximately 13 working days. The traditional screening method took 897 hours or approximately 120 working days. At a perdiem salary of $90.00, this amounts to a significant savings. Reliability was examined by selecting one second grade classroom from one-half of the Area Education Agency's clinical speech services staff. Each clinician was trained in the use of a traditional screening tool. This was specifically designed to delineate the same skills as the Communication Competency Screening scale used by the teachers. Each child who failed either the traditional screening or Teacher Interview Screening was evaluated and the results were compared.

Interpretation of the data shows 84% agreement between the teacher interview and traditional methods of screening. There was 63% rate of false failures using the teacher interview method of screening compared to a 72% rate of false failures using the traditional method.

Even though both groups had a high rate of false failures the teacher interview method did a better job than the traditional method. It should be noted that there were no disordered students, those having a severity of 4, that were missed by either group. Also in the group missed by the teacher interview method, there were no students with a severity of 3, while there were 2 in the group missed by the traditional method.

Finally, compatibility with current pragmatic philosophies, which demand that communication be observed in a meaningful environment, has been met.

With the completion of this project it was felt that there is a better way to screen students for speech and language impairments. Using a well developed teacher interview procedures screening can:

a. be efficient,

b. sample a student's communication skills in his natural environment, and

c. utilize the skill teachers have or can develop to identify students in need of our services.

COMMUNICATION COMPETENCY SCREENING

School: _____ Grade: _____

Teacher: _____ Inservice Dates: _____

Clinician: _____ Screening Dates: _____

Student	Pass	Fail	Conversational Skills	Sentence Structure	Articulation	Voice	Fluency	Comments

CC: White — Teacher
Pink — Clinician
Yellow — Office

FIGURE 6.4. Communication Competency Screening

The Communication Competency Screening scale reported in this study did not include a clear category for reporting students who present hearing or listening difficulties. It is suggested that such a component be added either by adapting an instrument such as this, devising unique statements, or using a

124

**Chapter 6:
Case Finding,
Case Selec-
tion, and
Caseload**

commercially available screening questionnaire. During the in-service meeting, teachers should also be informed of those behaviors which could indicate problems with hearing, listening, or auditory processing.

Screening for Phonological Disorders in Primary Grades. According to studies, children in kindergarten, first grade, and second grade exhibit many phonological errors. Some of these children will overcome their errors through the process of getting a little older and being exposed to the school environment; however, there are children in this group who will not improve without intervention. Differentiating between these two groups creates a dilemma for the school clinician. Obviously, because of the large numbers, all these children cannot be included in the direct service program. Through prognostic and predictive testing school clinicians will be able to sort these children into two general groups: those who need therapeutic intervention and those who would benefit from a general speech-language improvement program.

Numerous prognostic factors related to phonological errors have been explored including rate of change toward correction, number, type, and/or consistency of errors observed, and specific sounds or phonological processes exhibited.

Van Riper and Erikson (1973) developed the Predictive Screening Test of Articulation (PSTA) to identify among primary-school children who have functional misarticulations at the first-grade level, those who will and those who will not have acquired normal mature articulation by the time they reach the third-grade level. The PSTA has of 47 items, requires no special testing equipment, and is available from the Continuing Education Office, Western Michigan University, Kalamazoo, Michigan, 49001. The PSTA assesses the child's degree of stimulability—the ability to repeat sounds, nonsense syllables, words, and a sentence; the ability to move the tongue independently of the lower jaw; the ability to detect errors in the examiner's speech; and the ability to follow the examiner in a handclapping rhythm. In a study by Barrett and Welsh (1975), the PSTA was found to be a valuable speech-adequacy screening device for a first-grade population. The test was able objectively to substantiate, with approximately 90 percent accuracy, the opinion of the speech clinician that a child's speech is normal. Steer and Drexler (1960) reported that the most effective and reliable predictive variables appear to be the total number of errors in all positions within words, errors in the final position, errors of omission in the final position, and errors on the /f/ and /l/ consonant groups.

Westman and Broen (1989) disagree with the use of number of errors as a predictor. They describe a procedure for scoring childrens' errors. They conducted a study to identify children who might require intervention and to predict eventual enrollment in a therapy program. Westman and Broen and Peterson and Marquardt (1990) state that the persistence of specific types of error patterns are more important as predictors than the number of errors. There are several error patterns which are characteristic of children who are unintelligible or phonologically delayed (Westman and Broen,1989; Hodson and Paden, 1981; Weiner and Wacker, 1982). These include errors involving deletion of phonemes or syllables, change in the manner of phoneme production; substitution of more anterior sounds for more posterior sounds, and change in the phonotactic structure of the word.

Another factor related to the predictability of the correction of functional phonological problems is the inconsistency of errors. It has been generally accepted that the more inconsistent the child's phonological errors, the more possibility there is that he or she will outgrow them. The rationale is that the child may be able to produce the sound correctly sometimes but has not learned the appropriate times to produce it. Children exhibiting inconsistent error patterns or phonological processes inappropriate for their age should be further tested with instruments that provide more comprehensive and systematic testing on the way sounds are produced in all possible phonologic contexts. Instruments which would yield helpful information are tests such as the McDonald Deep Test (1964), The Assessment of Phonological Processes by Hodson (1986), and the Khan-Lewis Phonological Analysis (Khan & Lewis, 1986).

Issues related to predictability are important because frequently children are enrolled in a therapy program unnecessarily. If given time to mature, they would not have been considered to have a problem. It requires a good deal of clinical competency, knowledge of normative development, and accurate test measures to determine which children may still present significant phonological patterns by the time they enter the third grade.

A number of picture articulation tests can be used for screening. For example, the Templin-Darley Screening Test (Templin and Darley, 1969) contains 50 of the most common consonants and blends in the English language. The Photo Articulation Test (Pendergast et al., 1966) can be used as a developmental articulation test. The Picture Articulation and Language Screening Test (PALST) (Rodgers, 1976) is designed to be used in the classroom. It is easy to administer and score, and the clinician may also make note of any anomalies such as dental deviations, tongue thrust, or characteristics of hearing. The Goldman-Fristoe Test of Articulation (1969) tests phonemic proficiency in words and sentences.

Hodson (1986) includes an instrument for screening for phonological processes in her Assessment of Phonological Processes Test. The Bankson Quick Screen of Phonology (1990) provides estimates of the number of correct productions expected for children at various age levels from age three to eight. Spontaneous speech samples will yield information on the overall intelligibility of the child, but to be used effectively, the tester must have an understanding of expectations at each age.

To make informed clinical decisions, SLPs must be familiar with normative development. Lawrence, Katz, and Linville (1991) surveyed the literature on suppression of phonological processes. A chart summarizing their findings is presented in Table 6-1.

Screening for Phonological Disorders in Older Elementary Children. In older elementary children, speech and language screening can be accomplished by having them give their name, address, and telephone number, by counting to 25, by naming the days of the week or months of the year, or by responding to pictures of objects designed to test sounds. The best screening test is spontaneous speech because it is most likely to yield a sample of the child's habitual speech and language. If the child is asked to read words, sentences, or paragraphs, the clinician must be sure that the material is within his or her reading ability.

TABLE 6.1. AGES OF SUPPRESSSION OF PHONOLOGICAL PROCESSES (Lawrence, Katz, Linville, 1991)

Phonological Processes	Grunwell	Lowe	Haelsig & Madison	Ingram	Kahn-Lewis
Deletion final consonants	3:2		4:6	3:0	Suppressed first
Deletion initial consonants					Non-developmental*
Consonant deletion (includes initial, final)		4:0–4:5			
Syllable reduction	4:2	5:0–5:5	Beyond 5	4 and after	Suppressed first
Cluster reduction	3:9	6:0–6:5	4:6		Suppressed last
Cluster substitution		6:0–6:11			
Reduplication	2:5			1st 50 words	
Consonant harmony (assimilation)	2:10			3:0–4:6	Intermediate suppress
Initial voicing				4 and after	Suppressed first
Final devoicing			4:0		Suppressed last
Context-sensitive voicing	3:0	3:0			
Fronting		5:6–5:11	3:0		
Velar Fronting	3:3			Early	Intermediate suppress
Palatal fronting				Early	Suppressed first

Phonological Process		3:0–3:5	4:0	
Backing to velars				Non-developmental*
Stopping of fricatives, affricates		6:0–6:5	4:0	Suppressed last**
/f/	2:8			
/v/	3:6			
/θ/	2:8			
/s/	3:0			
/z/	3:7			
/ʃ/	2:9			
/tʃ,dʒ/	3:1			
Affrication		3:0–3:5	3:0	
Deaffrication		4:6–4:11		Suppressed first
Labialization		8:0–8:5		
Alveolarization		6:0–6:5		Suppressed last
Liquid simplification (includes gliding, vocalization)				
Gliding of Liquids	Beyond 5	6:6–6:11	5:0	
Vocalization of Liquids		6:6–6:11	4:6	
Glottal replacement			4:0	Non-developmental

*Non-developmental: not usually frequent in normally developing phonological systems

**Age of suppression inflated by late use of b/v and d/ð in normal phonological development

128

**Chapter 6:
Case Finding,
Case Selec-
tion, and
Caseload**

Screening for Language Disorders. The identification of language disorders in the preschool and school-age child is a complicated, difficult, and often frustrating task. A thorough knowledge of speech and language development is required of the examiner as well as an appreciation of the fact that both the identification and the assessment of language disorders is a continuous process shared by the persons who are best able to observe the child in many situations. These persons are the parents and the teachers as well as the speech-language pathologist.

The amount of information on language is overwhelming, while at the same time, much of it is inconclusive. Professional speech, language, and audiology journals contain many reports of studies comparing language tests and measurements, which simply means that more is being added to the body of knowledge.

In the schools many behaviors are dependent on language abilities: reading, spelling, speech, writing, mathematics, problem solving, creative thinking, comprehension, and others. An intact language system is important in the learning process. The SLP plays a necessary role in the identification, assessment, and treatment of the student with a language disorder.

Keeping in mind that screening is an identification process, we therefore need to *identify* the student with the language disorder. The facets of language are reception (decoding) and expression (encoding). The components of language are phonology, morphology, syntax, semantics, and pragmatics. A complete language evaluation should include all of these aspects. On the screening level it is important to ascertain whether or not the language behavior is adequate and commensurate with the age of the student. The in-depth diagnosis would follow after the individual has been identified.

Language screening may include the following tests but need not be limited to them:

1. Zimmerman, Steiner, Evatt, *Preschool Language Scale.* Assesses skills in auditory comprehension, verbal ability, and articulation. (45 min.)

2. Stephens, *Oral Language Screening Test.* Identifies children in need of more detailed evaluation. (10 min.)

3. Carrow, *Screening Test for Auditory Comprehension of Language* (STACL). Identifies children in need of more detailed evaluation. (10 min.)

4. Rodgers, *Picture Articulation and Language Screening Test* (PALST). Designed to be used in the classroom. (5 min.)

5. *Bankson Language Screening Test.* Based on expressive modality but can be used to test receptive verification. (40 min.)

6. Mecham et al., *Utah Test of Language Development.* User may find it necessary to develop regional norms. Screening items include nursery rhymes, colors, sentences, forms, and pictures. ($2^{1}/_{2}$ min.)

7. Fluharty, *Preschool Language Screening Test.* Ages 2–6. Standardized from four racial or ethnic groups, three socioeconomic classes, and varied geographical areas. Assesses vocabulary, articulation, and receptive and expressive language. (6 min.)

One of the most important steps in the identification process is to obtain information from the teacher about how the language impairment may be impacting upon academic performance. Valuable information can be gained by asking teachers to observe their students and respond to a few key questions relating language skills to classroom performance. Figure 6-5 illustrates a simple observation checklist designed to guide teacher's observations and descriptions.

Screening Secondary School Students. Sommers (1969) along with O'Connor and Eldredge (1981) suggested that screening English classes is one way to observe a

---

STUDENT _____   DATE _____

TEACHER _____   GRADE _____

TO THE TEACHER: Read each of the following statements. Indicate those statements which are representative of the student's behavior. Refer children who cause you to be concerned to the speech-language pathologist for further testing.

1. _____   In your opinion, the student demonstrates a noticeable communication problem which may be affecting educational performance.

2. _____   The communication problem is most noticeable during:

    _____   Comprehension tasks (Written ___ Verbal ___)

    _____   Classroom discussion

    _____   Social communication

    _____   Mathematics

    _____   Language arts

    _____   Spelling

    _____   Oral reading

    _____   Other

3. _____   The student has difficulty understanding subject-related vocabulary.

4. _____   The student has difficulty understanding subject-related concepts.

5. _____   The student has difficulty following written or spoken directions.

6. _____   The student does not understand figurative language.

7. _____   The student has poor reasoning and problem solving ability, showing difficulty with cause/effect relationships.

8. _____   The student's response to questions is inappropriate.

9. _____   The student has difficulty participating in class discussions.

10. _____   The student has difficulty expressing ideas or relating stories and experiences.

11. _____   The student's sentence structure, word choice, or sentence organization interferes with his ability to clearly express the message.

12. _____   The student's speech production (articulation, voice, fluency) makes the conversation difficult to understand.

13. _____   Other students in the class seem to have difficulty understanding the student.

FIGURE 6.5. Observation to Determine Language Functioning in the Classroom

130

Chapter 6:
Case Finding,
Case Selec-
tion, and
Caseload

large number of students in a brief amount of time. The English classes are ideal because in most school systems, all students must take this subject. The screening procedure should be planned cooperatively with the English staff. Arrangements can be made in advance for each student to read or recite a specific passage which would enable the clinician to obtain a quick impression of the student's communication performance. If a sufficient number of clinicians were available, the task of screening the English classes on the junior-high and high-school levels could be accomplished in a short period of time. Another alternative for reaching students is to screen with the school nurse during the hearing and vision screening program because there will usually be a small private room available.

Screening devices for adolescents often include reading short passages, answering questions posed by the examiner, and recounting events. Voice quality can be noted at the same time. Spontaneous speech can be elicited by asking questions, which will give the examiner some information about expressive language.

The examiner needs to be aware of the possibility of fluency disorders during the screening. Verification would have to be made by consultation with the teachers who would be most likely to have heard the student in an informal speaking situation. These teachers might include the physical education teacher, the English teacher, the guidance counselor, and other people active in extracurricular activities.

Few screening tests for adolescents have been developed at this writing. One is the Screening Test of Adolescent Language (STAL) by Prather et al. (1981). The STAL is a screening instrument designed to measure receptive and expressive language skills through vocabulary comprehension and use, auditory memory span, language processing, and, explanation of proverbs. The test is appropriate for junior and senior high-school students, and the administration time is six to eight minutes. Another instrument available is the Test of Adolescent Language (TOAL) by Hammill et al., 1987.

Comparing Screening and Referral Methods

Unfortunately, the efficacy research comparing screening versus referral methods for case finding is limited. Finn and Gardner (1984) recommend using teacher interviews in combination with screening procedures. Miller's (1989) data supports teacher referral over mass screening programs for the elementary level. No longer under state regulation to conduct mass screenings, clinicians in Fayette County, Kentucky decided to initiate a teacher referral-based model of case finding. The quality of referrals was good and showed improvement as teachers practiced the method over a two-year time period. Miller states that the "secret ingredient" to the success of their program was giving information to teachers about communication disorders in a simple and understandable way through beginning of the year in-service meetings.

A study described by Matthews et al. (1984) contradicts these findings for the high school level. The study was started in 1974 and compared screening to teacher referral methods on the ninth grade level. During the five years of district-wide screening, between 5,000 and 6,000 freshmen were screened each year. Of those screened, approximately 5 percent were found each year to have speech-language defects. During the two years of the teacher-referral procedure only .7 percent of the freshmen in the district were referred each year for testing.

According to Matthews et al., a comparison of the results of the screening versus the referral process revealed

1. There was a significant decrease in the number of students identified with speech-language problems since the teacher-referral process was initiated.
2. Fewer students with voice or fluency disorders were identified because they were not being referred.
3. There was a decrease in the number of mainstreamed students identified with speech-language problems. Referrals were primarily special education students.
4. The referrals received from teachers were not always appropriate.

The results also revealed that the teachers on the high-school level preferred the screening process and did not feel qualified or comfortable in identifying speech-language problems.

In a telephone conversation with Matthews on January 10, 1985, she indicated that although screening on the high-school level did not save time it did yield better information about the students and seemed to be a more accurate method of identification. Referrals from teachers are always encouraged, but high-school teachers may be less likely to refer than elementary teachers. The speech-language pathologists in the Phoenix system felt that under the referral system students with voice, fluency, and language problems were often missed.

The difference in findings between the Miller and Matthews et al. studies may be related to the adequacy of teacher preparation for the referral process.

Case Finding: Children with Hearing Impairments

Approximately 1.4% of the school-age population (or 14/1000 children) demonstrate a significant hearing impairment relative to verbal communication, social and emotional growth, and academic achievement (Matkin, 1991). These figures can be further interpreted as follows: 1/1000 children have severe or profound bilateral sensori-neural hearing impairment, 7/1000 children have mild or moderate bilateral sensori-neural hearing impairment, 2/1000 school age children have permanent unilateral hearing impairment, and 4/1000 school-age children have significant speech-language delays associated with a history of recurrent otitis media and conductive hearing impairment (Matkin, 1991). These figures may actually underestimate the magnitude of the problem. Flexer (in press) believes that there may be as many as two-thirds of the children in kindergarten and first grade classes who have persistent conductive hearing losses.

The early identification of children with hearing impairments, whether the hearing loss is mild, moderate, or profound, is of concern to the educational

132

**Chapter 6:
Case Finding,
Case Selec-
tion, and
Caseload**

community. Flexer (1992) uses a computer analogy to describe the potentially negative effects of any type and degree of hearing loss on academic performance. She states, "data input precedes data processing." In other words, in order to learn, children need to have information or data. In the classroom, the primary way information is entered into the brain is via hearing (Berg, 1987). If data are entered inaccurately the child will have incomplete or incorrect information to process and their performance will be affected.

Downs (1991) defines a hearing loss in children as "any degree of hearing that reduces the intelligibility of a speech message to a degree inadequate for accurate interpretation or learning." The term "hearing impaired" implies a hearing loss of at least 15 dB HL. A person with a loss of 70 dB or more is considered to be deaf. Two to three million school aged children may demonstrate some form and degree of hearing impairment (Berg and Fletcher, 1970; Ross & Giolas, 1978).

There are numerous causes of hearing loss in children including middle ear infections, genetic causes, bacterial infections and viruses, prenatal causes, and noise exposure (Flexer, Baumgarner, Wilcox, 1990). The Joint Committee on Infant Hearing Screening (Downs et al., 1982) identified the following factors as placing infants at risk for hearing loss:

- family history of childhood hearing impairment;
- congenital perinatal infection;
- anatomic malformations involving the face, head, or neck;
- low birthweight (less than 1500 grams);
- hyperbilirubinemia (jaundice) at levels exceeding indications for an exchange transfusion;
- bacterial meningitis; and
- severe asphyxia.

Educationally, children with even mild and intermittent losses due to middle ear infection can have difficulties in the classroom. A position statement of the ASHA Ad Hoc Committee on Extension of Audiologic Services in the Schools (1983) discussed three ways in which school children are affected by hearing loss:

1. Delay in development of communication skills.
2. Poor academic achievement.
3. Social isolation and poor self-concept due to reduced ability to understand and interact with others.

Skinner (1978) suggests that there are a number of problems a child may encounter in language learning if a mild hearing loss exists:

- Difficulty abstracting the meanings of words due to inconsistent categorization of speech sounds.
- Confusion with segmentation and prosody affecting ability to detect plurals, intonation and stress patterns.

- Difficulty hearing in environments where there is ambient noise.
- Difficulty discriminating speech sounds.
- Difficulty perceiving meanings resulting in confusion in word naming, developing classes of objects, and understanding multiple meanings.
- Problems abstracting grammatical rules, identifying relationships between words and understanding word order.
- Problems detecting the emotional content of speech including the rhythm and intonation patterns.

Referrals for Hearing Problems

Teachers and parents are excellent referral sources for hearing problems. As with identifying speech and language disabilities, the quality of the referral will be increased if groundwork is layed in advance. They must have an understanding of the importance of hearing for learning, those behaviors which might be representative of hearing problems, referral procedures, and follow-up recommendations. If a hearing loss is detected, the parent should be notified immediately of the results and recommendations. If warranted, the parent will be responsible for seeking medical assistance and informing school personnel of the results of any evaluations.

Information about signs and symptoms individuals should consider of significance needs to be disseminated through inservice meetings or written materials. Educators and parents can be encouraged to refer children who display the following behaviors (The Ohio Department of Health, 1990):

A. Appearance—mouth breathing, discharge from the ear canal, malformation of the ear, ear wax impaction, damaged or poorly maintained hearing equipment.
B. Behaviors—constant tilting the head toward the sound source, inability to follow verbal directions, inattention, pulling or rubbing the ears frequently, asking for repetition of words or phrases, misunderstanding conversation of others.
C. Symptoms—poor language development, buzzing or ringing in the ears, soreness or pain in or about the ears.

Screening for Hearing Problems

Because of the importance of hearing to learning, school communication disorders professionals need to establish an ongoing identification program which will enable them to screen all children periodically during their school years. ASHA's Ad Hoc Committee on Extension of Audiologic Services in the Schools (1983) and the ASHA Guidelines for Screening for Hearing Impairment and Middle-Ear Disorders (1990) recommend that the identification program include pure-tone and acoustic-immittance screening protocols and procedures for follow-up testing, making referrals, and monitoring children found to ex-

134

Chapter 6:
Case Finding,
Case Selec-
tion, and
Caseload

hibit problems. The committees further suggested that appropriate assessment of the school age population include, but not be limited to:

- Compiling and interpreting audiometric information.
- Determining the need for further pre-assessment information, including otologic consultation.
- Administering, scoring, and interpreting a complete audiologic assessment.
- Selecting, administering, scoring, and interpreting tests determining the benefits of amplification.
- Determining the influence of the hearing loss communication and learning.
- Identifying co-existing factors that may require further evaluation.
- Referring for assessment and/or treatment using both the school and community resources (including assessments related to cognitive, academic, visual, and motor skills, emotional status, the need for financial assistance in the purchase of a hearing aid, and vocational interest and aptitude).

Hearing Screening Protocol

Screening programs need to include procedures for detecting impairments of auditory sensitivity as well as peripheral auditory disorders. The goal is to identify individuals with hearing impairments that will potentially interfere with communication and/or individuals with potentially significant ear disorders that have been undetected or untreated. Children who fail the screening should have a complete audiological evaluation and medical examination.

The recommended guidelines for a hearing screening protocol include four components:

1. case history;
2. visual inspection;
3. pure tone audiometry; and
4. acoustic immittance measurements (static admittance equivalent ear-canal volume, and tympanometric width).

The screening protocol requires an otoscope, a pure-tone audiometer, and an acoustic immittance instrument. All equipment should be appropriately calibrated.

The history can be obtained by requesting information from parents in the letter sent to inform them of the screening program and schedule. Typically, the pure tone audiometric test is given in which the frequencies 1,000, 2,000, and 4,000 Hz have been presented at 20 dB HL to each ear of the child being tested. Failure to respond to any frequency constitutes failure of the audiometric screen. The volume must not be raised to accommodate room noises. If testing conditions are unreliable or questionable, a quiet environment should be found. Refer to the methods described in the ASHA Guidelines for Screening for Hearing Impairment and Middle-Ear Disorders (ASHA, 1990).

Immittance testing is very important for identifying middle ear pathologies. The following criteria can help you decide when to refer the child for a medical evaluation (ASHA, 1990):

Referral Criteria

I. History
  - A. Otalgia
  - B. Otorrhea

II. Visual Inspection of the Ear
  - A. Structural defect of the ear, head, or neck
  - B. Ear canal abnormalities
    1. Blood or effusion
    2. Occlusion
    3. Inflammation
    4. Excessive cerumen, tumor, foreign material
  - C. Eardrum abnormalities
    1. Abnormal color
    2. Bulging eardrum
    3. Fluid line or bubbles
    4. Perforation
    5. Retraction

III. Identification Audiometry—Fail air conduction screening at 20 dB HL at 1, 2, or 4 kHz in either ear (ASHA, 1985; these criteria may require alteration for various clinical settings and populations).

IV. Tympanometry
  - A. Flat tympanogram and equivalent ear canal volume (Vec) outside normal range
  - B. Low static admittance (Peak Y) on two successive occurrences in a 4–6-week interval
  - C. Abnormally wide tympanometric width (TW) on two successive occurrences in a 4–6- week interval

As with the speech-language screening program, mandates requiring that specific age or grade levels be tested vary from state to state. It is a generally accepted practice to screen preschoolers prior to school entrance, children in kindergarten, first, third, fifth, and ninth grades, all new students, transfer students, teacher and parent referrals, and students at risk for hearing loss due to noise exposure or other conditions. Given the importance of hearing for learning, the clinician could consider testing additional students if time and resources permit.

Figures 6-6 and 6-7 show examples of forms testers can use to report results of screening tests and track follow-up information. These formats help the professional who is responsible for screening many children monitor find-

FIGURE 6.6.

HEARING SCREENING TEST BLANK

School __Lake Elementary__   City __Uniontown__   County __Stark__

Grade __1__   Teacher __De Pompei__   Room __101__   Tester __Shackelford__

The names of the pupils may be filled in prior to the day of testing.

The tester screening the children and using the ANSI standards will screen the frequencies 1000, 2000 and 4000 Hz at 20 dB and 500 Hz at 25 dB. The volume must not be raised to accommodate room noise. Testing under these conditions is unreliable and a quieter environment must be found.

If the child responds to all frequencies at the specified loudness levels, the technician should write (P) for pass under R and L (right and left ears). If the child fails to respond to any frequency at the specified loudness levels, an (F) for fail should be placed under either or both R and L, whichever applies.

Those children failing the test on the first screening should be given a second screening in about four to six weeks. A failing score on the second screening must be followed immediately by the administration of a threshold test and completion of an audiogram.

1	2	3	4		5	6		7	8
NO.	NAME OF STUDENT (List alphabetically)	ABSENT	FIRST SCREENING		DATE	SECOND SCREENING		DATE	REFERRED FOR THRESHOLD TEST*
			R	L		R	L		
1.	Blosser, Renick		P	P					

2.	Blosser, Trevor		P	P									
3.	Butler, Paul		P	P									
4.	Conner, Colleen		P	F									
5.	Gibbons, Jeff		P	P									
6.	Gibbs, Brandon		P	P									
7.	Hill, Jenny		F	P									
8.	Pelland, Cheryl		F	F									
9.	Prinzo, Mary		P	P									
10.	Romsey, David		P	F									
11.	Siladie, John		P	P									
12.	Vargas, Denise		F	F									
13.	Zimmerman, Barbie	✓											
14.													

Developed by The Ohio Department of Health Hearing Advisory Committee (1990). Reprinted with permission.

FIGURE 6.7.

HEARING FOLLOW-UP RECORD FORM

HEALTH or SCHOOL DISTRICT __Lake Elementary__   DATE __10-30-92__

The names of children failing the hearing test should be listed. A check mark should be placed in Column 3 or 4, status of case; 5 and or 6, type of referral; and in the appropriate columns under follow-up results. (*This form is designed to help local health departments and schools in evaluating their hearing conservation program.*)

1.	2.	STATUS OF CASE		TYPE OF REFERRAL		FOLLOW-UP RESULTS					
		3.	4.	5.	6.	7.	8.	9.	10.	11.	12.
NO.	NAME	NEW CASE	PREVIOUSLY KNOWN CASE	MED.	ED.	NO MEDICAL FIND.	TREATMENT OBTAINED	EDUC. OR REHAB. SERV. OBTAINED	NO INFORMATION	FURTHER ACTION	CASE CLOSED
1	Gibbs, Heather	✓		✓			✓				
2	Hill, Kirk		✓		✓	✓					✓
3	Richards, Wayne	✓		✓		✓	✓	✓			
4	Burditt, Sue	✓		✓		✓	✓				✓
5	Belcastro, Bonnie		✓	✓			✓	✓			

Developed by The Ohio Department of Health Hearing Advisory Committee (1990). Reprinted with permission.

ings and recommendations over the course of the school year (Ohio Department of Health Hearing Advisory Committee, 1990).

Hearing Testing Procedures for Preschoolers and Students with Severe and Profound Developmental Disabilities. According to Bergman (1964), with some individual exceptions, children from ages three to five years are ready for the application of monaural low-intensity screening tests.

A recent unpublished study of over 3,800 preschool children in New York City Day Care Centers demonstrated that the simple handraising responses to the test tones, as employed with older children, is a quick, efficient method for large-scale testing of children from three to five years. A key aspect of such screen testing of three-year-olds is the instruction and preparation of the children in groups. Ideally this is accomplished by the regular nursery teacher, who has been instructed by the test supervisor. In this way the test becomes a familiar game for all the children. The preparation involves group handraising responses to soft chirp sounds produced by the teacher, followed by individual children (first the more confident ones, then the more timid), each demonstrating to the rest of the children how well and how quickly he can raise his hand in response to the sound. On the day the tester arrives one, two, or three screening audiometers and testers are installed in one room of the nursery. The children come to the audiometers in groups of three for each instrument, are briefly reinstructed and two sit quietly by as one is rapidly screened. Each child, therefore, has had the benefit of previous instruction, reinstruction and observation while two of his peers performed the test task. With such preparation, from 85 to 95 percent of three-year-olds can be successfully tested on each ear with the simple pure tone screening audiometer. Approximately 96 percent of four-year-olds and 99 percent of five-year-olds can be thus screened in a nursery or similar group situation even with less preparation.

Infants, toddlers, young preschool children, and students with multiple, severe, and/or profound developmental disabilities are unable to respond to traditional audiometric testing procedures. Testing of these groups should be conducted by an educational audiologist familiar with methodologies for assessing children who are difficult to test. In addition to information supplied by family and teacher observers, the testing is accomplished through multiple behavioral and objective testing procedures. (Flexer, Baumgarner, and Wilcox, 1990; Jerger 1984; Northern and Downs, 1984).

Examples of tests which might be used are Conditioned Play Audiometry, Auditory Brainstem Response (ABR), Immittance Audiometry, Behavioral Observation Audiometry, Visual Reinforcement Audiometry, and Conditioned Orientation Reflex Audiometry.

Responsibility for the Hearing Screening and Testing Program

Who carries out the program of identifying children with hearing deficits in the schools? In a survey by Wall et al. (1985) of audiometric practices and

140

Chapter 6:
Case Finding,
Case Selec-
tion, and
Caseload

procedures, it was found that the threshold testing part of the program was done by technicians (12.89 percent), nurses (46.47 percent), speech-language pathologists (25.89 percent), or audiologists (19.78 percent).

Public Laws 94-142 and 99-457 require the completion of an Individualized Education Plan or Individualized Family Service Plan for all children with special needs. This, of course, includes children with hearing impairments. The Wall et al. survey (1985), "The American Speech-Language-Hearing Association Guidelines for Screening for Hearing Impairment and Middle-Ear Disorders" (1990), The ASHA Guidelines for Identification Audiometry" (1985), "The ASHA Guidelines for the Audiologic Assessment of Neonates, Infants, Toddlers, and Young Children" (1990) and "The ASHA Audiological Services in the Schools Position Paper" (1983), strongly recommend that identification and management programs for children with hearing impairments be carried out by an educational audiologist. However, in many school systems educational audiologists are not available, nor do the school systems have access to audiological services in the community. In some states school and public health nurses are licensed to conduct screenings in the schools. In many school systems the screenings are carried out by SLPs, nurses, or the cooperative efforts of both, often augmented by volunteers and aides. The personnel who administer the screening program should be adequately trained in the screening and referral procedures to ensure that the results they obtain are accurate and reliable. Ideally, the screening program should be at least supervised by an educational audiologist.

Regardless of who implements the actual testing (educational audiologists, speech-language pathologists, or volunteers and aides), it must be implemented according to accepted standards of practice for identification audiometry. This means that appropriate equipment which is calibrated to American National Standards (ANSI) specifications is used; the ambient noise level does not exceed acceptable levels; the testing is conducted by a person with appropriate training in audiological screening procedures; the screening procedures are administered uniformly by all examiners with specified test frequencies, screening levels, and criteria for failure; rescreening is conducted within a reasonable period of time (four to six weeks); immediate comprehensive assessment is conducted for all students failing the rescreening; and appropriate medical and educational referrals are made for children who fail.

The role of the SLP, in regard to children with hearing impairments, is to promote an understanding of hearing and the impact of hearing loss, aid in screening programs, provide remediation, monitor the functioning of hearing aids and assistive listening devices, and help teachers employ educational management strategies which improve classroom performance. Where there are no audiological services available, the SLP often assumes the responsibility of the hearing-conservation program, including the screening program. Other options include contracting for educational audiology services or sharing service providers with nearby school districts.

Hearing Testing Facilities

School clinicians encounter a number of problems in screening programs. One major problem is the lack of a room sufficiently quiet to produce reliable test results. It would be extremely unusual to find a space with an ambient noise level below 51 dB, as recommended by the Model Regulations (Jones & Healey, 1973). Testing in unsuitable rooms results in a large number of rescreenings, and eventually, in overreferrals. This can be translated into time wasted by the clinician and both time and money wasted by parents.

In order to overcome noisy testing conditions, some testers try to compensate by raising the dB HL level above 20 or 25. As shown by Melnick et al. (1964), this may result in serious limitations in identifying children with slight conductive hearing losses. Middle-ear problems are often associated with slight conductive losses, so it is a possibility that many children with middle-ear pathologies will not be detected if there is not strict compliance with recommended screening procedures.

The school clinician should insist on good testing facilities in the school. Sometimes this means demonstrating to the principal and administration what is meant by a quiet room by actually measuring the ambient noise and comparing it to the recommended standards for testing.

Mobile Testing Units. When good testing facilities are not available within the school buildings, some schools and communities have attempted to solve the dilemma by taking the service to the client. Mobile testing units have been used with success in many parts of the United States and Canada. These vehicles are often custom designed. They are self-contained units with their own water supply systems, heating and cooling systems, electrical power generators, and other necessities needed in such laboratories. The vehicles are fitted with soundproof rooms; noise-reduction barriers in the walls; clinic areas with desks, tables, and chairs; storage space for records; testing equipment; electronic calibrating equipment; and space for therapy equipment supplies and other materials needed.

Mobile hearing and speech units are often joint cost-sharing projects of local school systems, local health departments, voluntary civic organizations, and universities. Many areas are served by these units, which test preschool children and are also used in the testing of adults and in industrial hearing conservation programs.

Further Readings. You, as a potential school SLP, need to become familiar with several articles published in *Asha*, which provide detailed information on audiological practices in educational settings.

Further references on this topic are

Berg, F. S. (1976). *Educational Audiology: Hearing and Speech Management.* New York: Grune & Stratton, Inc.

Clark, J. G. (1980). *Audiology for the School Speech-Language Clinician.* Springfield, Ill.: Charles C Thomas, Publisher

Jerger, J. (Ed.). (1984). *Pediatric Audiology.* San Diego: College-Hill Press.

Northern, J. L. & Downs, M. P. (1984). *Hearing in Children (3rd ed.).* Baltimore: Williams & Wilkins Company.

Ross, M., Brackett, D., Maxon, A. (1982). *Hard of Hearing Children in Regular Schools.* Englewood Cliffs, N.J.: Prentice-Hall, Inc.

Case Finding: Special Populations

Many classrooms in schools throughout the United States are comprised of students representing varying levels of learning capability and diverse cultures. Children who present developmental, physical, or mental disabilities such as learning disabilities, mental retardation, cerebral palsy, and emotional disturbances may go undetected because the other handicapping conditions are more obvious. In some instances, children may have been misdiagnosed as having a particular type of learning disability when in reality their primary problem is a hearing or speech-language impairment. Communication problems in children who do not speak English may be particularly difficult to identify if the clinician is unable to speak the child's language or an interpreter is not available.

It is important for the school clinician to be aware of these children and apply the appropriate screening and diagnostic evaluations. The school SLP needs to be sensitive to differences in children when selecting screening or evaluation instruments. Children's performance may be affected by the selection of test items and materials, performance requirements (e.g., cognitive, motor, and communicative), the verbal style used by the tester, or the testing situation itself (Adler, 1973; Peterson and Marquardt, 1990).

Children receiving special education services or being considered for placement in special education classes should receive a speech-language and hearing test as part of the multi-factored assessment process. When facilities for further evaluation of these children are not available in the school, they should be referred for services to a university clinic, community hearing and speech center, or hospital clinic.

Many city and county school districts and regional resource centers have centralized diagnostic facilities. These programs accept referrals from education and health professionals within the district as well as from parents. The benefits of such a centralized service are that the time which is needed to conduct a comprehensive evaluation can be taken and recommendations for treatment can be derived from input from professionals representing a variety of disciplines.

Appraisal and Diagnosis

According to Public Law 94-142, all children with disabilities must be assessed before placement in a special education program or before receiving related services. This assessment cannot be discriminatory based on race, cultural diversity, or disability. In 1991, ASHA's Task Force on Clinical Standards established a draft of "preferred practice patterns" for the professions of speech-language pathology and audiology (Task Force on Clinical Standards, 1991). The document specifies the "professionals qualified to perform the procedure, the expected outcome(s), clinical indications for performing the procedure, clinical processes, environmental and equipment specifications, safety and health precautions, and documentation aspects" (p. ii). Several recommendations for practice (regardless of setting) are addressed.

Assessment procedures must assess the communication behavior and delineate strengths, deficits, contributing factors, and functional implications. As an outcome of the assessment, the clinician should develop a statement of the diagnosis and clinical description of the disorder, make recommendations for intervention, and make appropriate referrals. Safety and health precautions such as infection control procedures should be followed. Documentation of procedures, findings, recommendations, and prognosis should be prepared. If treatment is indicated, recommendations of the frequency, estimated duration, and type of service required should be included.

Assessments must be administered in the child's preferred communication or linguistic system and consider the child's age, medical status, and sensory status. If these steps are not taken, the student may not be accurately assessed and the results will not honestly reflect the child's true achievement and aptitude level. Valid testing methods, standardized and non-standardized, should be used. The materials, equipment, and environment selected for testing should be appropriate to the student's chronological and developmental age, physical and sensory abilities, education, and cultural/ethnic and linguistic background. For example, testing for a child who does not speak English should be conducted in the child's native language. Public Law 94-142 defines *native language* as the language used by the child, not necessarily by the parents. A child who uses English at school but Spanish at home could be evaluated in English. However, if it is obvious that the child is more competent in Spanish, the testing must be done in Spanish.

Multifactored Assessment

Public Law 94-142 indicates that each handicapped child should be assessed in more than the suspected area of deficit. According to Dublinske and Healey (1978),

> The communicative status of all school children should be assessed. However, some state and local school agencies do not require the participation of speech-language pathologists or audiologists on child assessment teams. As a consequence, the ASHA School Services Program recommends that all pupils suspected of being handicapped be screened by a speech-language pathologist and audiologist to determine the presence or absence of communicative disorders. If the screening results suggest disorder, appropriate assessment should be completed and presented *at the child staffing by qualified personnel.*

Diagnostic-educational teams provide a comprehensive *multifactored assessment* for children with potentially significant problems, including children with communication problems. Clinicians work in collaboration with other professionals. The composition of the team may vary from district to district. The following personnel may be represented on teams: adapted physical education teachers, audiologists, guidance counselors, occupational therapists, physical education teachers, physical therapists, physicians, principals, reading specialists, regular classroom teachers, regular education supervisors, school nurses, school psychologists, social workers, special education supervisors, special education teachers, speech-language pathologists, and vision specialists. Parents, of course,

144

Chapter 6:
Case Finding,
Case Selec-
tion, and
Caseload

contribute much to the evaluation process because they possess knowledge about their child's educational, social, and medical history.

Not all children with speech, language, or hearing impairments necessarily require a comprehensive evaluation, but such an evaluation of children with concomitant psychosocial or learning problems can be important in determining their placement and intervention follow-up. Many types of assessment procedures should be used to gather data during the multifactored evaluation process including:

—Administration of norm-referenced measures, criterion-referenced measures, standardized tests, and developmentally based tasks;

—Observation of performance in different situations;

—Completion of interviews with significant persons;

—Analysis of classwork samples; and

—Review of family, school, and medical history

The data gathered is used to determine eligibility for special education or related services. Several steps must be followed during the multifactored assessment process including:

1. Appointing a multidisciplinary team to conduct the assessment.
2. Developing of an assessment plan that addresses obtaining a comprehensive description of the problems the student is demonstrating; specifying the information needed; and selecting appropriate evaluation instruments.
3. Conducting the multifactored assessment.
4. Analyzing the results.
5. Preparing a report of findings and reviewing the findings with other team members and the child's parents.
6. Determining recommendations for placement and intervention.
7. Developing a plan for an individualized education program.

After all team members have completed their evaluation procedures and analyzed their findings, the information gathered by each member should be integrated and synthesized into one report. A comprehensive multifactored evaluation report (see Figure 6-8) illustrating the extensive amount of information that was gathered and analyzed in order to plan an individualized education program for a student is provided for your review (Ohio Statewide Task Force on Language, 1991).

Speech, Language, and Hearing Clinicians' Responsibility in Diagnoses. The speech, language, and hearing specialist in the school system has the responsibility of providing diagnostic services for children referred by the multifactored assessment team (of which the specialist may be a member), as well as all the children picked up by the speech, language, and hearing screening program and referred by teachers, nurses, parents, and others.

A minimal diagnostic appraisal would include an assessment of the pupil's articulation abilities and language competencies, fluency, voice quality, and hear-

FIGURE 6.8.

SAMPLE EVALUATION TEAM REPORT

Part A. MULTIFACTORED EVALUATION

STUDENT ___John Doe___ D.O.B. _____ TEACHER _____

SCHOOL _____ GRADE ___4___ DATE OF REPORT _____

I. REASON FOR REFERRAL

John was referred for a multifactored evaluation by the school building's intervention assistance team (IAT) because of continuing academic problems, including difficulty following directions and poor reading comprehension and written expression skills. John has recently begun to exhibit some behavior problems in school and has difficulty sustaining peer relationships.

II. EDUCATIONAL HISTORY

Evaluators _____ (classroom teacher, parents) _____

Date _____

By parent report and teacher comments noted in the student's cumulative report, John has experienced difficulty following directions and completing written assignments since kindergarten. His grades in reading, language arts, and spelling have been average or below average even though he was retained in the first grade and received Chapter I reading services during first and second grade. Both his parents and teachers indicated that John has tried hard and has had a good attitude until recently.

During third grade, John's performance on competency examinations reflected mastery of mathematics objectives at the third grade level and reading and writing objectives at the first grade level. It was noted that his handwriting was legible and neat.

Throughout the years, John's parents have attempted to follow teacher suggestions to help him at home. While John was willing to listen to stories being read to him by his parents, he was reluctant to read out loud to them, especially when his brother was present. His parents admitted to becoming frustrated when trying to help John complete assignments in his language arts and reading workbooks. They have always been puzzled that John could do mathematics so easily but has so much difficulty reading.

Teacher Checklists Initiated for Teacher's Own Use

In September, John's fourth grade teacher observed that he was doing below average work in language arts and content areas. His mathematics skills were at grade level. As a result of this observation, the teacher completed Teacher Checklists for listening comprehension, oral expression, reading comprehension, and written expression to determine what interventions to attempt. On the checklists, the following weaknesses were noted:

John responds to abstract questions with off-topic responses and has trouble following multi-step directions when listening or reading. He also has difficulty answering detail questions about material heard or read. John rarely asks for clarification or assistance. He has limited oral and written vocabulary. John's ability to write grammatical sentences that convey appropriate meaning is poor. He requires additional time to work on written assignments.

Analysis Questions Used by Teacher

Based on these observations, the teacher applied the Teacher Analysis Questions to her classroom instructional approach and identified appropriate Teacher Accommodations to address John's difficulties. The accommodations that seemed to best match both John's needs and the classroom's structure were placed in priority. The following were implemented:

Accommodations Attempted

1. For listening and speaking difficulties,
   a. have John's hearing checked first;
   b. simplify "who-what-when-where" questions to the underlying idea (i.e., where = what place);
   c. make two-step commands pertinent to the environment and use visual cues whenever possible; and
   d. use manipulatives to demonstrate concepts.

FIGURE 6.8. (*Continued*)

2. For reading and writing difficulties,
    a. have John's vision checked first;
    b. have John read action-oriented sentences in games, such as "Simon Says" and treasure hunts;
    c. when reading, use semantic mapping to show story structure;
    d. when writing, teach the use of organizers (e.g., outlining and webbing); and
    e. teach the use of taping orally and then transcribing taped materials.

3. Teach John that "I don't know" is an acceptable answer, if appropriate.

Results of Teacher Accommodations

John's teacher reported that the accommodations were incorporated into the instructional process for all students in the class, rather than applying the accommodations for John only. The end result was that many of the below average and average students in the class seemed to "catch on" to new concepts better than before. John made some improvements in following simple oral instructions and understanding vocabulary words with uncomplicated meanings. However, John's progress was significantly less than other students in the class. While most students learned 20 new concepts over a four-week period, John could use only five new concepts correctly on a consistent basis.

III. HEARING AND VISION STATUS

Initially Suggested as Teacher Accommodations; Then Considered by IAT; Now Used in MFE

Evaluators _____ (school nurse, parents, physical education teacher) _____

Date _____

Hearing Test Results:
John passed his hearing screening at 20dbHL in both ears.

Relationship to Academic Functioning:
John's hearing is normal and appears adequate to hear both teacher instructions and peer discussions in the classroom as well as high- and low-sound frequencies associated with various phonemes.

Vision Test Results:
John also passed the vision screening with 20/20 in both eyes.

Relationship to Academic Functioning:
John's vision is within normal limits and appears adequate to see written work on the chalkboard as well as materials placed on a desk. Left-to-right eye movements were smooth and appeared adequate to track lines of words and sentences in books.

John's parents reported no history of chronic ear or eye infections or injuries. John's physical education teacher indicated that John has adequate vision and hearing to follow directions and perform motor tasks in physical education class.

Results Related to School Performance:
It appears that any difficulties with reading, writing, or following directions are not due to hearing or vision problems. No follow-up in either of these areas is warranted at this time.

IV. EDUCATIONALLY RELEVANT MEDICAL FINDINGS

Considered by IAT; Now Used in MFE

Evaluators _____ (school nurse, parents, physical education teacher) _____

Date _____

John's parents reported that he walked, talked, and reached other developmental milestones at expected time periods. John has had no serious illnesses or injuries. He has a good appetite and sleeps well at night. His energy level is high but typical of other boys his age. John's physical education teacher indicated that John's activity level adjusts appropriately to various demands during physical education class.

Relationship to Academic Functioning:
John appears to be a healthy child who attends school regularly. There do not appear to be any physical or medical factors affecting John's performance in the classroom.

FIGURE 6.8. *(Continued)*

V. COMMUNICATIVE STATUS

Evaluators _____ (speech/language pathologist, classroom teacher, parents)

Date _____

Because only marginal success was attained in helping John improve his classroom performance after several instructional accommodations were made, John's teacher asked that John's case be discussed by the building's IAT. After reviewing the instructional interventions attempted by John's teacher and John's learning response, the IAT requested more information about John's learning response.

Test Results:

1. *Clinical Evaluation of Language Fundamentals-Revised (CELF-R)*

	Standard Score	Discrepancy from IQ
Receptive Language Score:	78	- 2.19
Expressive Language Score:	54	- 3.79
Total Language Score:	66	- 2.99

2. *Test of Written Language-Revised (TOWL-2)*

Written Language Quotient:	70	- 2.73

3. Pragmatic Skills Checklist (see discussion)

4. Language Sample (see discussion)

Parent
Information

When being assessed by the speech/language pathologist, John was cooperative but reluctant to take risks and elaborate in responses. He rarely asked for clarification or repetitions of stimuli and often responded that he "didn't know." Similarly, John's teacher reported that John seldom initiated comments during class discussions, and when called upon, John provided only brief responses. Because John has been reluctant to ask for help, the teacher has reinforced John for admitting when he did not know an answer so that an alternative way of explaining the information could be provided to him. However, John is still reluctant to let the teacher know when such help is needed. John's parents stated that John tends to become a little shy around strangers.

Teacher
Information

John showed adequate ability in processing basic word and sentence structures, but he experienced difficulty with lengthy and more complex sentence forms, especially those with multiple meaning words and passive transformations. Comprehension of abstract language skills, such as idioms and metaphors, was severely limited. John's teacher agreed with these observations and added that John also has difficulty understanding puns made by his peers and jokes that require understanding of a "play on words."

Parent
Information

John had difficulty with multi-step directions presented through the auditory channel alone. Visual cues presented in conjunction with auditory stimuli (e.g., writing the text and page number on the board when giving assignments) improved John's ability to follow directions. John's parents commented that John usually remembers one or two of the things he is asked to do at home, but he never seems to remember all of them.

Classroom
Observation
Related to
Referral
Concern

When observed by the speech/language pathologist in the fourth grade classroom, John failed to carry out written directions on worksheets, often misinterpreting specific constructs used or completing only partial requirements. His teacher indicated that this problem tends to occur three to four times each week.

Relationship to Academic Functioning:

John's expressive language skills were significantly depressed in content, form, and use. He still confused relatively simple constructs, such as verb tense and spatial orientation. John did not produce compound or complex sentences without prompting and could not combine sentences easily, even with a model. He consistently showed little advanced planning of message content and could not sequence events into a coherent whole, making his conversation difficult to follow. In addition, John demonstrated significant word-finding problems in conversation and tended to rely on nonspecific vocabulary ("yellow thing" for "bulldozer") and overuse of fillers ("uhm" and "uh").

Parent and
Teacher
Information

Pragmatically, John was unaware that his responses lacked sufficient information for the listener, and he did not pick up on nonverbal cues that would indicate confusion on the listener's part. Both John's teacher and parents commented that John sometimes has difficulty maintaining friendships because he inadvertently "sticks his foot in his mouth" by blurting out comments, interrupting the conversation of others, or saying things in a way that hurts people's feelings.

FIGURE 6.8. (*Continued*)

Work Sample and Analysis	John's written language difficulties reflected his oral limitations. Analysis of a sample of his classroom writing revealed immature language in both content and form. His sentences tended to ramble and lacked a clear focus or relationship to the main topic. Sentences and words within sentences were poorly sequenced and difficult to follow. Specific vocabulary was used on a limited basis, and grammar and syntax rules were inconsistently applied. It appears that style, spelling, syntax, and semantic skills were extremely limited as John could not construct a meaningful passage. Due to John's extremely limited use of language, particularly in the areas of semantics and abstract language use, a measure of his overall ability and achievement levels was requested.

VI. ABILITY

Requested by IAT	Evaluators _____ (school psychologist) _____ Date _____

Test Results:
Kaufman Assessment Battery for Children (KABC)-Nonverbal Scale (Selection of IQ test based on assessment of vision, hearing, and communicative status)
    Nonverbal Scale IQ = 111

Selection of IQ Test Based on Vision, Hearing, and Communication Assessments	The *KABC-Nonverbal Scale* was administered to assess intellectual functioning. The Nonverbal Scale is intended to provide a reliable measure of overall intellectual functioning for individuals who cannot be assessed validly by the complete Mental Processing Scale because of communication problems. John meets this criterion. The results indicate a nonverbal score of 111, which is within the high average range. There were no significant strengths or weaknesses on the test. John's best areas were Hand Movements and Triangles, with scaled scores of 13. Other scaled scores were Matrix Analogies, 10; Spatial Memory, 11; and Photo Series, 11. On the Hand Movements subtest, John was able to copy precise sequences of movements of the examiner's hand. Success in this area is usually contingent upon a good attention span and concentration. It further measures motoric reproduction of a sequence. On the Triangles subtest, John was able to assemble several identical triangles to match a picture of an abstract design. This task measures mental processing in the visual-motor channel and requires abstract thinking.

Relationship to Academic Functioning:
Based on his performance on the KABC, the results indicate that John has adequate mental ability to learn and achieve in school at least as well as other students his age. John appears capable of achieving fourth grade level outcomes.

VII. ACADEMIC FUNCTIONING

Initiated for MFE	Evaluators _____ (school psychologist, classroom teacher) _____ Date _____

Test Results:
Woodcock-Johnson Test of Achievement-Revised (WJ-R) (Results were computed and compared to others at John's grade level of 4.4.)

Cluster Scores:

	Grade Equivalent	Standard Score	Discrepancy from Norm
Broad Reading	1.9	66	- 2.99
Letter-Word Identification	2.1	74	- 2.46
Passage Comprehension	1.7	67	- 2.83
Broad Mathematics	4.0	95	- .40
Calculation	4.5	102	- .86
Applied Problems	3.3	91	- .13
Broad Written Language	2.1	79	- 2.13
Dictation	2.8	84	- 1.79
Writing Sample	2.0	78	- 2.19

FIGURE 6.8. (Continued)

John was very cooperative during the testing session. He attempted every test item presented to him. Near the end of the testing, John began to yawn and appeared tired.

Mathematics Results:

John's academic strengths appear to be in the mathematics area. John scored highest in the calculation section with a grade equivalent score of 4.5. His next highest score, a grade equivalent of 3.3, was in the applied problems section.

Relationship of Mathematics to Daily Performance:

Following the completion of the mathematics section, John was presented the numerical calculation required to answer the applied problems that he had missed. Under these circumstances, John again was able to correctly solve fourth grade level problems. When asked to explain what made it possible for him to solve the numerical calculation in one situation but not the other, John commented that it was hard for him to find the number problem among all the words. Some of the words made the problem more confusing, and John couldn't figure out what the problem meant.

John's teacher indicated that John did well on most of his mathematics homework assignments and tests as long as they involved computation only. John typically struggles with story problems. His performance tended to improve when either the teacher or another student read the story problem to him in short segments at a time or when he drew pictures or diagrams to depict the story before setting up the calculation.

Reading Results:

On the WJ-R, John experienced the greatest difficulty in the areas of reading and written language, both having developed from a late first grade to an early second grade level.

The most difficult words that John was able to identify when presented individually were "must," "part," and "faster." The next higher level included such words as "knew," "whole," and "shoulder." It appears that John tends to identify single-syllable words or words that contain a smaller word (e.g., cat). He has difficulty identifying words that include initial blends, more than one syllable, double vowel combinations, and silent letters.

On the Passage Comprehension subtest, John was asked to read a short passage and identify a missing key word. John was able to provide appropriate words to complete the sentences in the first few situations. Thereafter, he described rather than labeled an idea, or he provided a word clearly not related to the main idea.

Relationship of Reading to Daily Performance:

John's teacher indicated that these results are typical of John's daily performance. Similarly, John passed all reading pupil performance objectives at the first grade level except recognizing vocabulary, recognizing inflected words, identifying multiple-meaning words, and stating main ideas.

Classroom Observation Focused on Referral Concerns; Relationship of Observation to Academic Functioning

During a 20-minute observation period conducted by the school psychologist, John was seated with four other students in a reading circle. John and one other student had difficulty locating the correct story after receiving directions the first time. Unlike the readings by other students in the group, John's oral reading in the late second grade level book had so many errors that it was difficult for the listener to maintain an understanding of the meaning of the passage. After having completed his reading, John was able to answer one of three comprehension questions. John's teacher indicated that John's reading that day was typical of his performance. As a result, John is reluctant to read aloud during class. John's poor reading skills tend to interfere with his ability to acquire new information in other areas, such as science, health, and social studies.

Written Expression Results:

John's performance on the writing portion of the WJ-R appears to be consistent with information shared by the teacher and speech language pathologist. John's writing skills were developed to the second grade level. His sentence construction was awkward, he tended to omit key words that were essential to conveying sentence meaning, and his sentences were brief. It was interesting, however, that John exhibited slightly higher skills when asked to write a dictated sentence; this task relies more on remembering key ideas than creating and organizing ideas.

Relationship of Written Expression to Daily Performance:

John's teacher reported that the above results are typical of John's daily performance. Tasks such as writing a letter to a friend are difficult and often frustrating. Writing is not a useful learning tool for John. Consequently, taking notes during class renders little benefit to John.

FIGURE 6.8. (Continued)

On the whole, John appears to do better in areas requiring rote memorization (recognizing letters and words, calculating mathematics facts, and writing dictated words or sentences) than he does in areas requiring the development of concepts and understanding (reading comprehension, mathematics-applied problem solving, and conveying ideas in writing).

VIII. MOTOR STATUS

Initiated for MFE

Evaluators _____(school psychologist, classroom teacher, and physical education teacher)

Date _____

Fine Motor Test Results:
Beery Visual Motor Integration Test (Beery VMI)
      Standard Score   10
      Age Equivalent   10 years, 1 month
OSPA Fine Motor Skills Checklist

John uses his left hand for pencil/paper tasks. On the *Beery VMI*, he was very precise in the reproduction of designs. John's fine motor skills were typical of other children his age. According to John's teacher, John appropriately uses classroom supplies, such as scissors, and successfully performs eye-hand coordinated tasks, such as opening doors, sharpening pencils, and drawing lines with a ruler.

Relationship to Academic Functioning:
John's teacher reported that when writing, John forms letters correctly, uses proper spacing, and produces handwriting that is legible and neat. John has the five motor skills necessary to complete academic work and self-help skills in the regular classroom.

Gross Motor Test Results:
OSPA Gross Motor Skills Checklist

Using the *Gross Motor Skills Checklist*, the physical education teacher indicated that John's balance, stamina, and coordination are adequately developed for a child his age. He demonstrates efficient movement of body parts, including those that require eye-hand and eye-foot coordination.

Relationship to Academic Functioning:
John moves about the school grounds and building without difficulty and participates in both school and outside sports activities. In the classroom, he is physically able to participate in activities at his desk, at the chalkboard, or in other areas that may require standing, sitting, or even reclining. John appears physically able to participate in field trips or other activities outside the classroom. Therefore, John's difficulties with academic functioning do not appear to be related to fine or gross motor problems.

IX. SOCIAL-EMOTIONAL STATUS

Initiated for MFE

Evaluators _____(school psycholologist, speech/language pathologist, classroom

teacher, and physical education teacher)

Date _____

Results:
    Devereux Behavior Rating Scale
    OSPA Gross Motor Skills Checklist
    Structured Student Interview

The *Devereux Behavior Rating Scale* was completed by John's classroom teacher. Except for John's academic achievement, all areas assessed were within the normal or expected range as compared to the average child in his grade and his age. Academic achievement was below expectations.

John's classroom teacher and physical education teacher both indicated that John was particularly good at respecting the property of others and following classroom rules. He is responsible and begins tasks when assigned.

Relationship of Social-Emotional Status to Disability

Those behaviors that were below expectations for a typical fourth grader involved cooperating and interacting with peers. Such difficulties may stem from John's underdeveloped pragmatic language skills. According to the speech/language pathologist, John tends to have difficulty demonstrating positive conversational skills, such as turn-taking, listening without interrupting the speaker, using tact, and considering the wishes of the other person.

FIGURE 6.8. *(Continued)*

Interview Structured to Address Referral Concerns

Relationship to Academic Functioning:

John's teacher noticed that John is frequently one of the last students selected by his classmates to participate in team activities whether in the classroom or on the playground. John tends to associate with one peer at a time rather than being involved in a peer group, and he seems to have difficulty sustaining a friendship.

During the structured student interview, John indicated that his greatest difficulty at school involved reading and having to talk in front of the class. The problem that bothered John the most was not having many friends. Both problems were perceived as being pretty serious to him because he wants to earn good grades and be liked by other students.

When asked to describe specific situations in which he experiences difficulty, John stated that when he is called upon to answer questions in class, the other students make fun of him or laugh at him. John said that he sometimes didn't understand why they were laughing. John stated that during physical education class or lunch, some students reminded him that he didn't do the homework assignment or told him he's "just plain dumb" because his answers are "off the wall."

When asked how he felt about these situations and what he had done to make things better, John stated that he felt frustrated and angry every time his teacher gave directions to the class because he never seemed to do the assignment the way the teacher wanted. It didn't seem to matter whether the directions were worksheets or explained during class. At the present time, John feels that there is no use in trying because he will get a bad grade anyway. John indicated that school has always been hard for him and that it seems to be getting worse lately. He said that he would like to get an award just once.

X. IMPLICATIONS FOR INDEPENDENT FUNCTIONING AND EMPLOYABILITY

Purposes of Special Education

At the present time, John only achieves success when given assistance by the teacher or another student. It is important for him to gain the skills that will enable him to complete assignments on his own. Because John's language difficulties seem to affect all areas of language (listening, speaking, reading, and writing), it seems likely that he will experience difficulty maintaining employment after graduation and independence as an adult unless these areas are improved.

XI. TEAM SUMMARY AND INTERPRETATION OF HOW THE MFE RELATES TO ACADEMIC PERFORMANCE IN THE REGULAR CLASSROOM

John demonstrates a severe receptive and expressive language deficit that is affecting his ability to read, write, speak, and listen effectively in school. Although John has high average nonverbal ability, his achievement is far below expected levels except in the areas of mathematics.

With regard to the learning disabilities discrepancy formula, John has discrepancy areas (2.0 deviations below expected performance) in oral expression, written expression, listening comprehension, and reading comprehension. John's difficulty is not due to physical limitations, because his vision, hearing, and motor skills are normal.

Language areas are influencing John's ability to acquire concepts in other content areas that require language skills as a tool for learning.

Part B. MULTIFACTORED EVALUATION TEAM CONCLUSIONS

I. HANDICAP DETERMINATION

The multifactored evaluation team concludes that John has a learning disability in the following specific areas:

X Oral Expression
X Written Expression
X Listening Comprehension
X Basic Reading Skills
X Reading Comprehension
___ Mathematics Calculation
___ Mathematics Reasoning

FIGURE 6.8. (*Continued*)

The multifactored evaluation team also concludes that John has a language handicap that has an adverse effect on his educational performance in the following areas:

X Receptive Oral Language   X Morphology
X Expressive Oral Language   X Syntax
                                      X Semantics
                                      X Pragmatics

General Supporting Data

For each identified area, this determination is based on the following evidence:

1. John has a history (dating back to kindergarten and including retention in first grade) of difficulty with following directions, reading, and writing.

2. John's learning difficulties do not appear to be due to vision, hearing, motor, or medical problems or to other factors related to emotional disturbance, mental retardation, and environmental, cultural, or economic disadvantage.

3. John's age was not a factor that influenced the team's determination.

4. Despite the provision of appropriate accommodations, a severe discrepancy exists between John's ability and his achievement in multiple areas.

5. There is evidence that a severe discrepancy between ability and achievement *is not* correctable without special education services.

6. John indicates that school seems to be getting harder; he expresses feelings of frustration, anger, and futility.

Supporting Data for Each Specific SLD Area

For the sake of brevity only for this *Handbook*, the basis of only two of the five areas identified as a learning disability or language handicap will be discussed and documented below.

Specific Area: READING COMPREHENSION

Source	Evidence
Intervention	John has experienced little improvement in learning despite the provision of Chapter I reading service and teacher accommodations that focused on simplifying directions, reinforcing comprehension of ideas and vocabulary, using story mapping to organize main ideas, and establishing relationships of words to ideas.
Teacher Information	John's reading skills interfere with learning new science and social studies material. John does not like to read in front of the class.
Parent Information	John is reluctant to read in front of his brother. He likes his parents to read to him.

Individualized Tests	Test	Standard Score	Discrepancy from IQ
	WJ-R		
	Broad Reading	66	- 2.99
	Letter-Word Identification	74	- 2.46
	Passage Comprehension	67	- 2.83

John reads with comprehension at the end of the first grade level. He tends to describe key words in passages rather than label them precisely. John tends to identify words that have single consonants and single vowel combinations.

Group Tests	John passed all first grade pupil performance objectives, except vocabulary, inflected nouns, locating main ideas, and multiple-meaning words.
Observation/ Work Samples	While reading aloud in a small reading group, John made frequent reading errors. It was difficult for the listener to understand the meaning of the passage. Afterwards, John was able to answer one of three comprehension questions.

FIGURE 6.8. (Continued)

Specific Area: ORAL EXPRESSION

Source	Evidence
Intervention	John has difficulty explaining ideas even when manipulatives are used to help guide his thoughts.
Teacher Information	John has difficulty carrying on an appropriate conversation with peers because he interrupts others or says things that offend others. John has limited speaking vocabulary and seldom initiates comments during class discussions.
Parent Information	John blurts out comments without taking time to listen to the comments of friends and family. He tends to be shy around strangers.
Student Information	Other students sometimes make fun of John when he answers questions in class. John does not understand why the other students are laughing.

Individualized Tests	Test	Standard Score	Discrepancy from IQ
	CELF-R Expressive Language	54	- 3.79

Observation/ Pragmatic Skills	John was unaware that his responses lacked sufficient information for the listener and did not pick up on nonverbal cues that would indicate confusion on the listener's part.

II. IMPLICATIONS FOR IEP DEVELOPMENT

John needs to acquire the following skills:
1. listening and reading with understanding
2. expressing ideas clearly when speaking and writing
3. demonstrating appropriate conversational skills with peers

III. IMPLICATIONS FOR INSTRUCTION

The following approaches should be attempted:
1. Ask John to write and read his own stories based on his own experience and using his own vocabulary.
2. Check that John can recognize and comprehend words in a sentence before asking him to read.
3. When giving oral instructions, make sure that John is looking at the instructor; ask John to repeat the instructions in his own words. Use visual cues whenever possible to help build meaning.
4. Allow John to participate in role-play activities to practice his pragmatic language and social interaction skills.

The following team members *agree* with the content and conclusions of this report.

Date _____   Chairperson/Title

Signature   Title

_____   _____

_____   _____

_____   _____

_____   _____

_____   _____

The following members *disagree* with one or more points of this report and will provide a separate statement.

_____   _____

_____   _____

This separate statement will be due by _____

Reprinted with the permission of The Ohio Department of Special Education.

154

**Chapter 6:
Case Finding,
Case Selec-
tion, and
Caseload**

ing acuity and perception. there should also be an examination of the peripheral speech mechanism. It is also important to have additional information, which can be obtained through a case history. Such information would include developmental history, family status and social history, medical history, and educational history. A physical examination may be needed as well as a psychological and educational evaluation.

Figure 6-9 provides a listing of components of communicative status that should be evaluated for children with various disabilities (Ohio Statewide Task Force on Language, 1991).

Parental permission is required for the evaluation procedures. The permission should be in writing, and usually a form is utilized for this purpose.

In some cases the school system may not be able to provide some of the diagnostic procedures because of lack of specialized personnel. In this event the school system may arrange to have these procedures carried out by a qualified agency with qualified personnel in the immediate community or nearby. It is the responsibility of the school system to see that the required procedures are carried out. Such referrals are made only after written permission is obtained from parents.

It should be kept in mind that the purpose of the appraisal and diagnostic procedures is to select children who may be placed in the speech, language, and hearing programs in the school. The school clinician must be prepared to describe how the pupil's disability will interfere with his or her ability to profit from classroom instruction.

Steps in Diagnosis. To obtain a clear picture of the child's communication problems, the first procedure is to gather as much pertinent information as possible through a case history and an interview with the parents, the teachers, and if possible, the child. Each informant contributes information vital to the whole picture. The parents can give background information on the development of the child, the teachers may provide needed information on the present status of the child. The teacher should be interviewed to determine the communication requirements for success within the classroom setting and the student's present communication performance on educational and social tasks. A classroom observation as part of the appraisal process will yield valuable information for formulating the diagnosis and developing an intervention plan. Holzhauser-Peters developed the observation checklist for conducting classroom evaluations presented in Figure 6-10 (Holzhauser-Peters and Husemann, 1988).

If provided with guided questions geared toward the child's developmental age and level of understanding, the student may also be able to contribute information which may be of great value to the clinician.

After the background information is obtained, the clinician needs to add to it by describing the problem. This is done by observing the child's performance on appropriate tests that measure the degree of the problem and suggest associated aspects. The clinician must be an astute observer and must be able to record information objectively and without bias. In other words, the clinician must be a good "reporter."

After all the information has been gathered, the clinician makes a diagnosis of the communication problem (or problems). A diagnosis, or an identification

FIGURE 6.9. Suggested components of the evaluation of communicative status for each handicapping condition.

Rules indicates that communicative status is to be evaluated for all handicapping conditions, except visually handicapped. However, because language acquisition is fundamental to the learning process of all students, it is suggested that the communicative status of visually handicapped children be evaluated. Only specific learning disabled delineates the areas to be assessed under communicative status, i.e., oral expression, listening comprehension, and written expression. For the remaining handicaps, evaluation of communicative status is required, but the specific areas are not indicated.

Developmentally Handicapped
- listening comprehension
- oral expression
- written expression
- articulation/phonology
- pragmatic skills survey

Hearing Handicapped
- audiological/auditory tests
- articulation screening/evaluation
- listening comprehension
- oral expression
- written expression
- sign expression
- pragmatic skills survey

Multihandicapped
- listening comprehension
- oral expression
- written expression
- articulation/phonology
- assessment of augmentative potential (if nonverbal)

Orthopedically and/or Other Health Handicapped
- oral/motor examination
- articulation screening/evaluation
- listening comprehension
- oral expression
- written expression
- assessment of augmentative potential (if nonverbal)

Severe Behavior Handicapped
- listening comprehension
- oral expression
- written expression
- articulation/phonology
- pragmatic skills survey

Specific Learning Disabled
- listening comprehension
- oral expression
- language sample
- written expression
- pragmatic skills survey
- observation of classroom language
- articulation screening/evaluation
- meta-linguistic skills assessment
- auditory segmentation skills

Speech Handicapped
- specialized assessments in phonology, articulation, voice, fluency, pragmatics, semantics, syntax, morphology, auditory processing, and memory
- language sample
- observation of language skills in the classroom
- analysis of problem areas in curriculum and school
- teacher-student interviews
- auditory segmentation skills
- written expression

Visually Handicapped
- listening comprehension
- oral expression
- articulation/phonology
- pragmatic skills survey
- assessment of augmentative potential (use of Braille and other devices)

Reprinted with permission of The Ohio Department of Special Education.

156

**Chapter 6:
Case Finding,
Case Selec-
tion, and
Caseload**

FIGURE 6.10. Classroom Observation Checklist for Use by SLP

Student's Name _____ Time of Observation _____

Classroom Teacher _____ Class Observed _____

School _____

1) Presentation of Information
Where does teacher stand to present information?
- ☐ front of room _____
- ☐ side of room _____
- ☐ walks around _____
- ☐ Lecture _____
- ☐ Oral reading by various students in class _____
- ☐ Dittos _____
- ☐ Drill _____
- ☐ Hands-on activities _____
- ☐ other _____

2) Presentation of Assignments/Homework
How are assignments presented?
- ☐ written on board _____
- ☐ verbally presented _____
- ☐ both _____
- ☐ other _____

3) Seating Arrangement
Where Is Student Sitting?
- ☐ front _____ ☐ back _____
- ☐ center of room _____ ☐ by window _____
- ☐ other _____

4) Environment — Overall
- ☐ Relaxed — time to do things at an even pace
- ☐ Fast — pushed for time
- ☐ Noise level _____
    - noisy _____
    - quiet _____
    - moderate _____
- Comments: _____

5) Distractions
- ☐ Is child distracted by other children? _____
    - noise _____
    - other _____
- ☐ Does child distract others?
    - Describe: _____

6) Textbooks
Look at
- ☐ vocabulary _____
- ☐ language complexity _____
- ☐ concepts presented _____
- ☐ concepts needed to understand _____
- ☐ other _____

Textbook format

   ☐ topic headings

   ☐ summary at end of chapter _____

   ☐ other _____

_____

7) How Does This Child Indicate What He Knows?   How Does Teacher Determine Competency Level?

Dittos

   ☐ Are dittos used a great deal?

   ☐ What skills must student possess to complete the dittos?

   ☐ Are dittos black _____

            blue _____

            clear _____

Written Essays/Papers _____

Tests

   Types of tests given

   ☐ ditto _____

   ☐ multiple choice _____

   ☐ fill in blank _____

   ☐ other _____

8) Does student have option of taking test?

   ☐ orally _____

   ☐ written _____

   ☐ both _____

9) Does Child Participate In Class?

   ☐ Raises hand appropriately _____

   ☐ Shouts out _____

   ☐ Does child have time to respond when called upon _____

_____

Does child respond

   ☐ immediately _____

   ☐ need more time to respond _____

   Comments: _____

_____

9) Transition

When class moves from one subject or task to another, how does teacher cue children into transition?

   ☐ physically (with body movements) _____

   ☐ verbally _____

   ☐ bell _____

   ☐ other _____

   ☐ Does student pick up on this cue? _____

10) Child's Organizational Skills

Does child remember?

   ☐ homework assignments _____

   ☐ books needed to take home _____

   ☐ what books and materials to take to next class _____

   ☐ schedule of classes and daily events _____

   Comments: _____

_____

11) Study Skills

Does child know how to study?

   ☐ to remember only important information _____

   ☐ scan chapter first to review headings _____

(*continued*)

158

Chapter 6:
Case Finding,
Case Selec-
tion, and
Caseload

FIGURE 6.10. (Continued)

☐ read chapter summary first _____

☐ get clues by looking at ditto first to determine how to do and then read directions _____

☐ how to take notes _____

☐ how to outline _____

Comments: _____

_____

12) Verbal Organizational Skills

Student:

    ☐ answers simple questions requiring a one word or 1-2 sentence response

    ☐ relates information in an understandable cohesive manner

        ☐ during conversations with adults

        ☐ during conversations with friends

        ☐ during class discussions through

        written assignments _____

        oral presentations _____

    ☐ communicates wants and needs

    ☐ relates the sequence of events in the proper order

    ☐ communicates something that has happened recently _____

        in the distant past _____

        will happen in the future _____

    ☐ relates feelings

    ☐ relates thoughts

    ☐ relates opinions

    Comments: _____

_____

13) Requests For Assistance

When the student has difficulty with a task he

    ☐ requests assistance   ☐ gives up   ☐ other (Describe) _____

_____

14) General

Does child seem to exhibit skills comparable to other children in the class or does the student stand out? Describe how the student "stands out" from the group. Give examples of specific situations when the student "stands out" and also when he "fits in."

_____

_____

_____

_____

Permission to photocopy by *The Clinical Connection,* 109 S. Fairfax Street, Alexandria, VA 22314.

Reprinted with permission of the author (Holzhauser-Peters) and *The Clinical Connection.*

of the problem, is in reality a tentative diagnosis because as a human being grows and changes, the problem changes. A diagnosis is much more than putting a label on a person. It is convenient for professional persons to use diagnostic labels when communicating with one another if all parties concerned understand that the label is not the diagnosis. A diagnosis involves weighing all the evidence, discarding some of it as not being pertinent, and keeping that which merits further investigation.

On the basis of the gathered information, the testing, and the tentative diagnosis, the clinician then determines the prognosis and sets up a long-range plan for the remedial procedures. The long-range plan includes therapy appropriate to the communication problem as well as other strategies and treatment. The school clinician is involved in collaborative team approach with others who are interested in the child's welfare, and these individuals work as a team in establishing an IEP of IFSP. The school clinician is responsible for the appraisal and diagnosis of the communication problem, but the clinician is a team member in the overall appraisal, diagnosis, and treatment of the child.

The clinician uses professional judgment about whether or not to utilize a long case history form or a short one. The clinician should have available tests and forms appropriate for specific problems, including assessment of language and speech, voice, fluency, articulation, and hearing. A form for the oral peripheral mechanism examination should also be available.

Case Selection

After students with communication impairments have been identified and assessed, the clinician faces three difficult tasks. First, the SLP must determine if the student meets the *eligibility criteria* for placement in the program. Second, the *severity of the disorder* needs to be determined. Third, children selected need to be *prioritized* on the caseload. These steps will help the clinician determine the type of service delivery model to be used as well as the frequency and intensity of treatment.

Before eligibility, severity, or priority case selection systems can be put into use, you'll need the endorsement and support of the school administrator responsible for determining policy for the speech, language, and hearing department. The case selection system should be in written form and made available to administrators and educators within the district in order to improve accountability and understanding of the functioning of the program. The understanding of the case selection system and the cooperation of other school personnel would have to be enlisted for the system to function satisfactorily. The principal would be a key factor in the success of such a program. Teachers would also have to be familiar with case selection procedures in order for them to work well. Having a documented system for selecting cases can also be useful in helping parents understand the rationale for recommendations regarding their child's program.

Eligibility Criteria

Clinicians develop eligibility criteria to enable a more definitive means of identifying the population to be served and to provide a more consistent means of applying criteria across the school district (Work, 1989). The eligibility criteria established should be standardized within the school district and appropriate to the population served. Some state departments of education have established eligibility criteria for speech, language, and hearing programs as well as for other special education programs. Where statewide criteria are not available, clinicians often establish criteria for their local districts. Clinicians within a district should work together to determine how they will interpret specific aspects of the eligibility criteria such as terminology and application to certain populations such as adolescents or students who are mentally retarded (Work, 1989). In 1988, the State of Florida, Bureau of Education and Exceptional Students implemented the following eligibility criteria for articulation, language, voice, and fluency disorders:

160 *Eligibility Criteria*

Chapter 6:
Case Finding,
Case Selec-
tion, and
Caseload

A. *Language.* Language disorder is present when:
1. For students below age five (5), there is a significant language delay based on criteria presented in the test or evaluation manual and at least one (1) of the following is met:
    a. There is a significant difference between language performance and other developmental behaviors; or
    b. There is a significant difference between receptive and expressive language abilities
2. For students age five (5) and above, the language scores on standardized tests are more than one (1) standard deviation below the mean for the student's chronological age and at least one (1) of the following is met:
    a. There is a significant difference between language performance and nonverbal performance; or
    b. There is a significant difference between receptive and expressive language scores; or
    c. Two (2) or more, but not all, components of the language system are rated moderately or severely impaired on a language severity rating scale.

B. *Articulation.* An articulation disorder is present when at least one (1) of the following is met:
1. Based on normative data, the frequency of incorrect sound production and the delay of correct sound production are significant; or
2. The error pattern is characteristic of disordered rather than delayed acquisition; or
3. Articulation is rated as moderately or severely impaired on an articulation severity rating scale.

C. *Fluency.* A fluency disorder is present when:
1. Fluency is rated as mildly, moderately, or severely impaired on a fluency severity rating scale; and
2. There are supportive data presented by a primary care giver, a teacher-educator, or the student when appropriate, in addition to a speech-language pathologist, that a disorder exists.

D. *Voice.* A voice disorder is present when:
1. Voice is rated as moderately or severely impaired on a voice severity rating scale; and
2. They are supportive data presented by a primary caregiver, a teacher-educator, or the student when appropriate, in addition to a speech-language pathologist, that a disorder exists.

Priority System of Caseload Selection

Jackson (1986) reported on a priority rating and eligibility system of caseload selection developed by speech-language clinicians in the Akron Public Schools.

The system was implemented to assure continuity and consistency of case selection among the clinicians in the district. It was used to organize the service delivery program according to pupils' needs. It provides a rationale for time allocations, supports accountability, and is adaptable to various scheduling models.

According to Jackson,

> The APS scale (Figure 6-11) allows joint observation of consistent variables by SLPs, teachers, parents, and other professionals without compromising clinical judgment. It assists the clinician in case selection and suggest the intensity of service and the delivery model for the least restrictive alternative in a continuum of service options.

The severity rating scale completed for each student provides a numerical index comprised of information in four categories: (1) standardized test results; (2) eligibility criteria (add points): (3) ineligibility criteria (subtract points); and (4) category or type of disorder (add points). Following is an explanation of each category.

1. *Standardized test results.* Students are provided with a complete multifactored, multidisciplinary test battery. A basic numerical factor is obtained from the results of the evaluation. The student is assigned a numerical value as follows:

Rating	*Category*	*Description*
0 pts.	Normal	Usually those students scoring within one standard deviation from the mean, norm for chronological age, mental age, or grade level.
+3 pts.	Mild	Those students who can understand and be understood by most persons, can use speech and language as an effective communication tool, and have communication skills nearly commensurate with overall ability level. Typically those students who score 1–1.5 standard deviations below the mean, with percentile scores of greater than 36 and standard scores of 70–85.
+5 pts.	Moderate	Those students having difficulty with some aspect of communication. Scores are typically 1.5–2 standard deviations below the norm, 16–35 percentile ranks, and 55–70 standard scores.
+7 pts.	Severe	Those students with severe difficulty understanding or being understood, whose speech/language significantly interferes with communication and educational progress. Scores are usually more than 2 standard deviations below the norm, below the 16th percentile, and below the standard score, with stanine usually 1.

2. *Eligibility Criteria.* Points are added to the student's score if the following eligibility criteria are met:
   a. Articulation stimulability between 20 and 80%.

162

Chapter 6:
Case Finding,
Case Selec-
tion, and
Caseload

b. Organic etiology or difficulty noted in more than one area.

c. Documentation of speech intelligibility using a standardized definition or rating scale. (Example: Speech is defective when it causes the student to be withdrawn or hesitant to speak, causes a social-emotional problem, or interferes with communication.)

d. Documentation of significant educational adverse effect based upon prior documentation by another member of the evaluation team, usually the classroom teacher. Up to three additional points may be added, if SLH pathologist, teacher, and parent all agree there is an adverse effect upon educational performance.

e. Previous enrollment in SLH, but maximum potential has not been reached.

f. Enrollment in special education program with speech-language intervention offered as a related service.

3. *Ineligibility Criteria.* Points are subtracted from the student's score according to specified criteria. This enables the clinician to provide documentation and rationale for reducing services to students. This includes consideration of factors such as prognosis for therapy; comparison of communication skills to mental age or communication characteristics of peers; potential change due to maturation; reaching a plateau in performance or maximum potential; and poor attitude or attendance.

4. *Category or type of problem.* Points are added to the student's score for particular communication impairments.

The total severity index score determines the type of service and suggests the amount of therapy time. A student with 0–5 is within normal limits and therefore ineligible for services. The child with a mild communicative problem (6–10 points) may be served effectively through indirect or direct services. The severe student (18–23 points) usually receives a minimum of one hour of therapy per week, either in individual or small group, or a combination of direct therapy with teacher consultation and integrated classroom techniques.

Using systematized methods such as these enable the clinician to be accountable for the decisions made regarding caseload selection. Ultimately, this type of information is necessary in order to document the importance and effectiveness of the speech-language intervention program. Data generated will help the clinician support discussion of changes in program design and implementation of new service delivery models.

Rating the Severity of the Communication Impairment

The severity of the impairment is an important factor in determining the need for treatment, the appropriate program placement and/or service delivery model, the intensity and frequency of services, and intervention strategies for children with communication disabilities. Unfortunately, there are no uniform

FIGURE 6.11. Akron Public Schools Priority Rating—Eligibility Services Scale.

AKRON PUBLIC SCHOOLS
Office of Special Education

SPEECH, LANGUAGE, HEARING SERVICES—PRIORITY RATING—ELIGIBILITY SERVICES SCALE

Following referral and testing, the student should be rated on the following scale to determine eligibility for services.

(Student Name) Paul Butler

(Birth Date) 7·11·86

Date 9-10-92

Clinician

Grade/Program

I. RESULTS OF STANDARDIZED TESTING/SEVERITY TESTS (add points)

Priority #4 Normal Range	0	
Priority #3 Mild	+3	
Priority #2 Moderate	+5	+5
Priority #1 Severe	+7	

II. ELIGIBILITY CRITERIA (add points)

Artic. Stimuability 20–80%	+1	+1
Organic Etiology—Multiple	+1	
Causes Student to be Withdrawn—Hesitant to Speak; Social-Emotional Problem	+1	+1

(continued)

163

FIGURE 6.11. (Continued)

Criterion	Points	Score
Interferes With Communication	+1	+1
Significant Educational Adverse Effect 0, 1, 2, 3	+0 to 3	+2
Previous Enrollment SLH Has Not Reached Potential	+1	+1
Enrolled Special Educ. Prog.	+1	+1
III. INELIGIBILITY CRITERIA (subtract points)		
Artic./Lang. Appropriate For MA or CA	−1 to −3	
Not Sig. Different/Peers	−1	
Maturity Will Prob. Correct	−1	
Poor Attendance Pattern	−1	−1
Poor Prognosis (Document)	−2	
Maximum Potential Has Been Reached	−0 to −3	
Poor Motivation/Behavior	−1	
Articulation Disorders		
Inconsistent Intelligibility	+1	
Linguistic Code Difference Dialect/Foreign Language	+1	

IV. CATEGORY OF DISORDER
CHECK ONLY ONE CATEGORY
(add points)

1 to 3 Artic. Errors—Inappropriate for age (r, s, l, ʃ)	+2	
Multiple Artic. Errors 4 Consist. Phonemes	+4	+4
Disorders of Voice	+5	
Disorders of Fluency Primary, Secondary	+5	
Language Disorders Aud. Proc. (A) Syntax (Syn) Semantic (S) Pragmatic (P)	+5	
SLH/Cerebral Palsy	+6	
SLH/Hearing Impaired	+7	
SLH-SMI Any Combination of Above Disorders	+7	
TOTAL SEVERITY INDEX		15

V. THERAPY TIME ALLOTTED CHECK ONLY ONE CATEGORY

0–5	Within Normal Standard Deviation
6–8	Mild: Indirect; Monitor; Tutor; Teacher Conference; ½ hour per month

(continued)

FIGURE 6.11. (Continued)

9–11	Mild–Moderate: Direct; Group of 4–5; $\frac{1}{2}$ hour per week						
12–17	Moderate: Direct; Group of 2–3; 1 hour per week	X					
18–23	Severe: Direct; Indiv.; $\frac{1}{2}$ group of two 1–1$\frac{1}{2}$ hours per week Plus $\frac{1}{2}$ individual						
Therapy Administered							
Type-Direct/Indirect							
Date Initiated							
Days/Time/Week							
No. of Sessions							

Reprinted with permission of the author (Jackson).

procedures or guidelines for rating severity which are common to the profession. The Iowa Severity Rating Scales for Speech and Language Impairments (Jeffrey and Freilinger, 1986) were developed to assist clinicians in case selection and decision making. Its design and underlying theoretical construct are representative of the state of the art.

The Iowa Scales are based on a continuum of performance model. Four parameters of communication are considered (e.g., articulation, language, voice, and fluency). Several variables are considered for each of the parameters. Descriptive statements are provided to assist the user in deciding the rating number to assign. For example, the rating scale for articulation considers intelligibility, phonological processes, error types, and phoneme development. The language category considers results of informal assessment measures, impact on educational performance, pragmatic skills, results of formal measures, and other factors. The voice scale rates symptoms, reactions of casual listeners, reactions of significant others, pupil awareness, and the overall effect on communication. The fluency category rates the number of stuttered words per minute and percentage of words stuttered, speech rate, duration, awareness, and secondary characteristics. The Scales are applicable to students of all ages. Some considerations are made for children with disabilities in addition to communication impairments such as mental and developmental disabilities.

The Iowa Scales use a five-point rating scale to identify the place on the continuum which best represents the student's speech and language performance: 0 = adequate speech and language; 1 = adequate speech and language, maturational delays; 2 = speech and language deviation; 3 = speech and language deviation; and 4 = speech and language disorder. The student is rated in each of the four parameters. The total score achieved is then used to describe the nature and severity of the students' communication impairment and to make clinical decisions.

The Iowa Scales do not dismiss clinical judgment. For example, the speech-language clinician would need to consider the following factors:

1. The consistency of the inappropriate communication patterns
2. The pupil's ability to interact verbally with others
3. The effect of the communication problem on school performance
4. The possible impact of the communication problem on the listener
5. The ability of the pupil to communicate well enough to satisfy his or her needs
6. The status of speech and language stimulation in the home
7. The student's response to stimulation of the deficit in speech and language structures
8. The student's chronological age in comparison with the expected age for developing the communication skills which are in deficit or missing

While the Iowa Rating Scales are too extensive to reprint here, a representative sample of the articulation and language sections are provided as a reference in Figures 6-12 and 6-13.

FIGURE 6.12. IOWA'S SEVERITY RATING SCALE FOR ARTICULATION

	0	1	2	3	4
Intelligibility	Conversational speech reflects standard adult patterns.	Conversational speech contains some sound production differences.	Conversational speech is intelligible although noticeably in error.	Conversational speech contains words and phrases which are not intelligible.	Conversational speech is intelligible only with knowledge of the context and familiarity with the pupil and pupil's sound system.
Phonological Processes			Use of articulatory shift processes which are inappropriate for age such as voicing deviations, deaffrication, frontal distortions.	Excessive use (40% or more) of substitution or omission processes which are inappropriate for age, such as velar deviations, stridency deletion and cluster reduction.**	Excessive use (40% or more) of omission processes (such as syllable reduction, prevocalic and postvocalic sound deletion) or unique processes which are inappropriate for age.
Error Types			Sound productions reflect common types of distortions or substitutions of later-developing phonemes.	Sound productions reflect atypical errors.	Sound productions reflect use of limited number of phonemes or phoneme classes.
Phoneme Development		Sound production differences are developmentally appropriate.	Sound productions appear to be developing in normal progression although delayed up to one year.	Sound productions are not developmentally appropriate and are delayed more than one year.*	Sound productions are not developmentally appropriate and are delayed more than one year.
Phoneme Development		Spontaneous development of standard adult phoneme production is expected.	Sound productions may vary with phonetic context indicating that spontaneous phoneme development could occur.	Spontaneous development of standard adult phoneme production is not expected.	Spontaneous development of standard adult phoneme production is not expected.

*A delay in phoneme development of more than one year may warrant a rating of "3" despite no decrease in intelligibility.
**As prevalence of phonological processes increases the resulting decrease in intelligibility would warrant a more severe rating.
Reprinted with permission of the authors (Jeffrey and Freilinger) and Pro-Ed, Inc., Austin, TX.

FIGURE 6.13. IOWA'S SEVERITY RATING SCALE FOR LANGUAGE

	0	1	2	3	4
Informal Assessments	Age appropriate language skills.	Informal assessment indicates an inconsistent difference from normal language behavior.	Informal assessment indicates a language deficit.	Informal assessment indicates a language deficit which usually interferes with communication.	Informal assessment indicates the pupil has limited functional language skills. Communication is an effort.
Educational Note		Educational progress is not affected.	Educational progress may be affected.	Educational progress is usually affected.	Educational progress is extremely difficult.
Pragmatics			The pupil may have some difficulty expressing thoughts and ideas; however, the listener is able to understand the message.	The pupil has difficulty expressing thoughts and ideas. Most of the time the listener is able to interpret essential information.	Conversational rules are violated so that the listener is not able to comprehend the meaning of the intended message.
Other Factors					Language impairment is frequently accompanied by a phonology problem.
Formal Assessments		When administered, standardized diagnostic tests indicate an inconsistent difference from normal language behavior.	When administered, standardized diagnostic tests indicate a language deficit according to one (1) or more of the following measures: a) 1 to 1.5 SD below mean b) LQ or SS of 78–85 c) 7 to 16 percentile d) stanine 3	When administered, standardized diagnostic tests indicate a language deficit according to one (1) or more of the following measures: a) 1.5 to 2 SD below the mean b) LQ or SS of 70–77 c) 3–6 percentile d) stanine 2	When administered, standardized diagnostic tests indicate a language deficit according to one (1) or more of the following measures: a) more than 2 SD below the mean b) LQ or SS at or below 69 c) below 3 percentile d) stanine 1

When psychological test results are available, decisions concerning the appropriate Severity Rating should be made on the basis of a comparison between the pupil's intellectual ability and language assessment results.

Reprinted with permission of the authors (Jeffrey and Freilinger) and Pro-Ed, Inc., Austin, TX.

170   *Dismissal from Therapy*

Chapter 6:
Case Finding,
Case Selec-
tion, and
Caseload

In the process of selecting students for therapy, diagnosing, providing therapeutic intervention, and maintaining students in therapy, sometimes too little attention is paid to dismissal.

The question of when a pupil should be dismissed from therapy may be predicated on (1) when the pupil reaches maximum anticipated performance or (2) when the pupil's communication problem has been completely remediated.

After the pupil has been placed in a therapy program the short- and long-term performance objectives are identified and written in the IEP. The objectives are based on what is identified through testing, observation, conference with parents and teachers, and sometimes discussion with the pupil. In this way it is determined what the pupil needs to learn.

The long-term objectives are what is hoped the student is able to do at the termination of the therapy program. The short-term objectives are the steps through which the student must progress successfully to reach the long-term objectives. This, in effect, means that long-term (or terminal) objectives constitute the exit criteria, or the point at which the student is dismissed from therapy. This is part of the IEP.

Obviously, the nature of the disorder will have a direct bearing on the expected outcome of therapy. For example, a student with cerebral palsy and apraxia of the speech musculature may not be expected to attain "normal" speech patterns, depending on the extent of the involvement. This dismissal point for this pupil may be "adequate" speech. A student with an phonological problem may be potentially able to attain a more complete mastery of the distorted sounds, and the dismissal point for this pupil would be when the student could use the sounds correctly.

The SLP must develop dismissal criteria for each student and terminate therapy when these criteria are met. This means that dismissal from therapy may occur at any time during the school year. Students who have not reached optimum improvement at the end of the school term are carried over into the following term. Students who transfer to another school are referred to the SLP in that school system. Parents should be urged to inform the new school that their child has been in therapy and they wish it to continue. In this situation, the referring clinician secures the proper release forms to transfer the student's therapy records to the new school.

Dismissals need not be absolute. No clinician is wise enough to be able to dismiss a child from therapy with the absolute certainty that the child will never again need it. When a dismissal is made, the child should be scheduled for periodic rechecks to find out if the therapy has held. In a school it is important to have the classroom teacher check this also. It will be necessary to be very specific with the teacher on what to check. The same holds true for parents. A dismissal, then, could be called a *temporary* dismissal.

Sometimes a student may be put on *clinical vacation*. This may occur when the clinician feels that the student has reached a plateau or has been in therapy for a very long time without a break. Before the point at which boredom and apathy set in, the clinician may put the child on a "vacation" from therapy for a designated amount of time. Clinicians have reported that gains in progress have been made when the student was on clinical vacation.

The conditions of a clinical vacation should be carefully explained to the student. I recall one little fellow who, when told he was going to be on clinical vacation, seemed elated. Several days later his mother called to report that he was disappointed when he found that being on clinical vacation did *not* mean he was being sent to Disneyland!

What we are doing as clinicians is trying to make each client his or her own clinician. In other words, we try to bring students to the point where they are able to monitor their own speech, language, or auditory problem to such an extent that they no longer need us. This is sometimes painful for clinicians to do, and at times the student is reluctant to be dismissed from therapy. Both these factors must be objectively viewed by the clinician, and when the optimum levels of performance have been reached by the student, as stated in the long-range goals, the student is ready to be dismissed. The criteria for dismissal are unique to each child and must be carefully established, evaluated, and reevaluated during the course of therapy. If necessary, they must be adjusted or modified in the light of more knowledge about the student.

In addition to providing rating scales for determining selection for the caseload (entrance criteria), it is also important to provide guidelines for determining readiness for program completion (exit criteria). Examples of program completion criteria for articulation and language impairments from the Iowa Scales are as follows:

Program Completion Criteria: Articulation and Language

A pupil's speech and language program should be completed when one or more of the following conditions are present unless professional judgement indicates otherwise.

  I. Terminal I.E.P. speech and language goals and objectives have been met.
 II. Speech and language skills are developmentally appropriate or are no longer academically, socially, personally, or emotionally handicapping. Documentation must be present by one or more of the following: pupil, teachers, parents, Speech and Language Clinician.
III. The pupil has made minimal or no measurable progress after one academic school year of consecutive management strategies. During that time, program modifications and varied approaches have been attempted and a second opinion has been obtained.
 IV. Maximum compensatory skills have been achieved or progress has reached a plateau due to:
   a. cognitive ability level;
   b. structural deviations (e.g. severe malocclusion, repaired cleft lip or palate, physical condition of the vocal mechanism, or other physical deviations or conditions);

172

Chapter 6:
Case Finding,
Case Selec-
tion, and
Caseload

c. neuromotor functioning (e.g. apraxia or dysarthria);

d. hearing impairment.

V. Limited carryover has been documented due to the pupil's lack of physical, mental or emotional ability to self-monitor or generalize in one or more environments.

VI. Lack of progress or inability to retain learned skills due to poor attendance and participation, although program I.E.P. goals and objectives have not been met. Poor attendance and participation records should not stand alone, rather it is the lack of progress or retention which is of primary concern when utilizing this criteria.

Program Completion Criterion Unique to Language:

I. The following criterion is unique to language, but is used in conjunction with any of the above program completion criteria. Adequate language skills achieved as defined by one or more of the following measures:

a. greater than 16 percentile;

b. language quotient or standard score greater than 85;

c. less than one standard deviation below the mean.

Program Completion Criterion Unique to Fluency:

I. 0 to 3 stuttered words per minute or 0 to 3% stuttered words of total words spoken.

a. 130 +/− 20 spoken words per minute

b. Average duration of dysfluency of 0.5 seconds or less

Program Completion Criteria Unique to Voice:

I. The pupil has made minimal or no measurable progress after *six months* of consecutive management strategies. During that time, program modifications and varied approaches have been attempted and a second opinion has been obtained.

II. Current voice production is rated as a 0, 1, or 2 on the voice severity rating. This program completion criterion should only be utilized when pupils have previously been enrolled for voice services with original severity ratings of 3 or 4, but who currently have made progress to the 0, 1, or 2 level of severity. Vocal status is documented by teachers, parents and the speech and language clinician via service or observation logs.

Placement in the Speech-Language Program

The Placement Team

The appropriate placement of the child with disabilities must always be made by a placement team involving, in addition to the child's parents (or surrogate parents), those individuals knowledgeable about the child. The federal law also specifies that the team should include a representative of the local educational agency, the teacher, and if appropriate, the child. Although the law does not state that other individuals are required to be present, good educational practice would suggest that other team members also attend. This list would include those persons who by virtue of their professional backgrounds and the child's unique needs would reasonably be expected to be involved. It might include the principal, psychologist, reading teacher, occupational therapist, physical therapist, vision consultant, and speech-language clinician and audiologist.

The parent need not be the natural parent of the child as long as he or she meets the legal qualifications of the parent surrogate.

The child may be included *whenever appropriate*. Schools may develop their own criteria in regard to appropriateness.

The results of the evaluation and the possible placement options should be available when the placement team meets.

Coordinator of the Placement Team. The representative of the local educational agency usually is the *team captain* and coordinator, and as such arranges for the meeting, presides over the meeting, determines that all necessary persons are present, and acts as spokesperson for the school system. The chairperson presents the necessary information and data or calls on the person responsible for presenting it. The chairperson also has the responsibility of informing the parents of their rights. Setting the tone of the meeting and seeing that all the basic ingredients of the individualized education program are present, and that the procedures are carried out according to state and local guidelines, are also within the responsibilities of the chairperson (Sherr, 1977).

The Teacher As a Team Member. The teacher is the person most responsible for implementing the child's educational program. The teacher in the case of the child with communication handicaps may be the speech-language and hearing clinician or the classroom teacher. The teacher's responsibilities as a team member at the meeting include explaining to the parents the learning objectives, curriculum and various techniques used to meet the annual goals. The teacher will also explain to parents why one particular strategy was used instead of another. In addition, the teacher will answer questions parents might have about events that occur within the classroom. In effect, the teacher is the main emissary between the school and the parents (Sherr, 1977).

Speech-Language Pathologist's Role on the Team. The role of the speech-language clinician on the placement team may vary according to the guidelines and practices of the local education agency. If the child in question has a communication problem, the person providing the language, speech, and hearing services in the school needs to participate in the placement process. Although the placement team has the responsibility of developing an educational program for each pupil, the school clinician will need to provide input into the process of establishing goals, objectives, prognosis, and intervention strategies. The school clinician will also be responsible for reporting to the placement team the results of any diagnostic and assessment testing and may recommend further testing.

174

Chapter 6:
Case Finding,
Case Selec-
tion, and
Caseload

Family As Team Members. Family members can provide insights about the home situation, the impact of the disability on interactions and home activities, and factors which may be contributing to the child's problems. Making family team members gives both family and speech-language pathologists, as well as other members of the team, an opportunity to observe each other's interaction with the student. The family may be team members in the actual diagnosis, treatment, and carrying out of the IEP or IFSP. Furthermore, the more the caregivers are included in these processes, the smoother and the more consistent is the delivery of instruction to the child.

Both family and SLPs gain from the insights of the other, and both will be able to use each other as a source for added ideas. Also, family and SLPs will be able to keep each other informed about the progress of the child.

Reports to caregivers, both oral and written, should be in clear, understandable language and not in professional terminology. Clear explanations of the diagnosis and treatment strategies should be made to caregivers. The SLP should make it plain to caregivers that diagnosis is an ongoing process and that, as the child changes and progresses, the assessment of his or her condition will change.

Speech-language pathologists should avoid labels as much as possible when talking with family. If labels have to be used, it should be made clear to family that they are merely a device for communicating.

The Placement Team's Purpose. The ultimate result of the placement meeting is to develop an IEP or IFSP for the child and to achieve agreement to that plan by the parents and professionals. The plan must be a written document, filed and distributed according to the policies of the state and local education agencies. Policies also regulate who shall have access to the report and how these copies shall be made available. A copy of the report is made available to the parents. All placement team members sign the report.

In most cases the speech-language pathologist is a member of the team if the child displays communication difficulties. If the clinician is not on the team (an unlikely but not impossible situation), a copy of the document should be made available to the clinician.

Ethics and Responsibilities

Our selection of testing procedures and, ultimately, of those students who will or will not receive services in our programs should be guided by our professional ethics and standards of practice. For example, if during the testing session with a child you learn of a need in another area, it is your responsibility to refer that child for services by the appropriate professional. This may mean a medical referral for a physical condition you might observe, the school psychologist for a learning disability you detect, or the guidance counselor for an emotional or social problem. This necessitates looking at the "whole child" not just the speech, language, or hearing behaviors displayed. Children are complex creatures. We cannot diagnose or treat them in isolation. We must report the total picture we observe when we create our description of the child's behaviors and needs (Peterson and Marquardt, 1990).

A Philosophy: The Basis on Which to Build

Knowing who and what you are and where you fit in will provide the basis from which to make many decisions and plans for the program.

Traditionally, the concept of categorical labeling, whereby children with handicaps were diagnosed, tested, and labeled according to the functional area of the handicap, has been the approach to dealing with children in a classroom. This psychological-medical orientation failed to provide information the impact of the communication impairment on educational performance for individual children. To provide better services for children in the school it is necessary to describe the problem in terms of the educational deficits it is imposing on the child. Furthermore, it is important that the classroom teacher as well as the parents understand the connection between the communication handicap and the child's ability to profit from the instruction in the classroom. For example, it is not enough to describe a child as having a hearing impairment and let it go at that. In the school it is necessary to describe how the hearing loss affects the child's ability to hear the teacher's and other children's voices; to monitor his or her own speech, language, and voice; to discriminate among sounds of the language; and to receive information. The effect of the hearing loss on the child's self-image should also be explained.

Speech, language, and hearing clinicians work in many settings. The clinician who chooses to work in an educational setting has the responsibility of removing or alleviating communication barriers that may hinder the child from receiving the instruction offered in the school. The clinician who works in the schools also has the responsibility of evaluating the communication problem and assessing its impact on the learning process. Another responsibility of the school clinician is to serve as a resource person for the classroom teachers and specialized teachers who have children with communication disabilities in their classrooms.

Perhaps it is the term *special education* that has led our thinking astray. It is in reality education for children with special problems. The education of children with disabilities is not something distinct and set apart from education; it is a part of the total school program.

DISCUSSION QUESTIONS AND PROJECTS

1. How would you introduce yourself to a first-grade class you were about to screen for speech-language? How would you explain to them what you were going to do? Role-play this situation in your class.

2. The third-grade teacher sends not only the students who have articulation problems but also all the "problem" readers as well, when you ask for referrals. How would you handle this situation?

3. How would you generate self-referrals on the high-school level?

4. Compose a memorandum to the teachers of Gibbs Elementary School in which you explain the procedures of the speech-language screening you will be conducting there.

176

**Chapter 6:
Case Finding,
Case Selec-
tion, and
Caseload**

5. Is it legal to screen only selected grades when Public Law 94-142 says all handicapped children must be served?

6. Interview a school SLP to find out what speech-language screening tests he or she uses.

7. Survey several SLPs in the schools to find out how they identify students who may have a hearing loss.

8. Invite an educational audiologist to speak to your class on protocols for screening and testing for hearing impairments.

9. Find out what is required in your state in regard to diagnostic procedures for children with communication impairments.

10. Find out how preschool children are identified in your area.

11. Explain those modifications which can be made in your assessment procedures to appropriately test children with the following characteristics or impairments: unable to speak; severe sensory impairment (blind or hearing impaired); unable to move or use hands; or unable to be understood.

12. Develop a library of examples of speech and language disorders.

13. Develop a listing of materials which can be used to present an inservice meeting.

Models of Service
Delivery and Scheduling

Introduction

The roles of the speech-language pathologist and audiologist working in the educational setting have changed greatly in the past few decades. The roles will continue to change as understanding of the needs of children and youth with communication disabilities expands, as the impact of communication impairments on learning becomes more clearly defined, and as methods for delivering services improve. Clinicians still function as specialists who work with children with communication disabilities. However, they are no longer implementing their programs in isolation from the rest of the educational system. Speech-language and audiological services are an integral part of the total educational program for children with disabilities. Clinicians have increased responsibilities for demonstrating how communication disabilities impact upon the learning process. There is a demand to design intervention programs which will increase childrens' potential for benefiting from the educational process.

Public Law 94-142, a legislative landmark, had the greatest impact on the role of the speech-language pathologist and audiologist in education. The law specifies requirements for identifying children with impairments, providing appropriate services based on individual needs, and making available a continuum of service options. Other legislation which followed continued to mandate changes in practices.

In this chapter, we will explore programming alternatives for children and youth with communication disabilities. Emphasis will be placed on explanation of the continuum of service delivery options currently available in school speech-language pathology programs. The chapter also presents definitions of terms that are generally agreed upon and used by professionals in the field. The

178

Chapter 7:
Models of
Service
Delivery and
Scheduling

definitions of communication disorders and an understanding of the continuum of service delivery options are basic tools for the school speech-language pathologist. They may be considered the building blocks of good program development and management. We will also consider scheduling alternatives and variables of importance when scheduling different age or disability groups.

Many of the topics in this chapter have been vigorously debated by speech, language, and hearing professionals, and there is not always agreement on what is the right way or the wrong way to approach and solve these problems. But fortunately, the discussions continue, often generating more research, and eventually common ground is reached. (Read Iglesias, 1985, "The 'Different' Elephant," on how a position paper was developed.)

The Definition of Terms

A good place to start any process is to come to an agreement on the definition of terms. In 1978 the Committee on Language, Speech, and Hearing Services in the Schools (1982) began work on a revision of terminology and submitted the definitions of communicative disorders and variations to the membership of ASHA. The definitions were accepted by the association and disseminated for use by federal, state, and local agencies and others concerned with programs for those with communication impairments. The school pathologist must be able to define and interpret the terminology to parents, teachers, medical personnel, and legislators.

The definitions are as follows:

Definitions:* Communicative Disorders and Variations

I. A COMMUNICATIVE DISORDER is an impairment in the ability to (1) receive and/or process a symbol system, (2) represent concepts or symbol systems, and/or (3) transmit and use symbol systems. The impairment is observed in disorders of hearing, language, and/or speech processes. A communicative disorder may range in severity from mild to profound. It may be developmental or acquired, and individuals may demonstrate one or any combination of the three aspects of communicative disorders. The communicative disorder may result in a primary handicapping condition or it may be secondary to other handicapping conditions.

   A. A SPEECH DISORDER is an impairment of voice, articulation of speech sounds, and/or fluency. These impairments are observed in the transmission and use of the oral symbol system.

      1. A VOICE DISORDER is defined as the absence or abnormal production of vocal quality, pitch, loudness, resonance, and/or duration.

*Prepared by: Committee on Language, Speech, and Hearing Services in the Schools (1982). Efforts to revise these definitions were initiated by ASHA's Language in the Schools Task Force in 1991. They were not yet complete at the time of publication.

*Various definitions and eligibility criteria may exist for determining degree of handicap and disability compensation. The definitions in this document are not intended to address issues of eligibility and compensation.

2. An ARTICULATION DISORDER is defined as the abnormal production of speech sounds.

3. A FLUENCY DISORDER is defined as the abnormal flow of verbal expression, characterized by impaired rate and rhythm which may be accompanied by struggle behavior.

B. A LANGUAGE DISORDER is the impairment or deviant development of comprehension and/or use of a spoken, written, and/or other symbol system. The disorder may involve (1) the form of language (phonologic, morphologic, and syntactic systems), (2) the content of language (semantic system), and/or (3) the function of language in communication (pragmatic system) in any combination.

1. Form of language

   a. PHONOLOGY is the sound system of a language and the linguistic rules that govern the sound combinations.

   b. MORPHOLOGY is the linguistic rule system that governs the structure of words and the construction of word forms from the basic elements of meaning.

   c. SYNTAX is the linguistic rule governing the order and combination of words to form sentences, and the relationships among the elements within a sentence.

2. Content of Language

   a. SEMANTICS is the psycholinguistic system that patterns the content of an utterance, intent and meanings of words and sentences.

3. Function of Language

   a. PRAGMATICS is the sociolinguistic system that patterns the use of language in communication which may be expressed motorically, vocally, or verbally.

C. A HEARING DISORDER is altered auditory sensitivity, acuity, function, processing, and/or damage to the integrity of the physiological auditory system. A hearing disorder may impede the development, comprehension, production, or maintenance of language, speech, and/or interpersonal exchange. Hearing disorders are classified according to difficulties in detection, perception, and/or processing of auditory information.

Hearing-impaired individuals frequently are described as deaf or hard of hearing

1. DEAF is defined as a hearing disorder which impedes an individual's communicative performance to the extent that the primary sensory avenue for communication may be other than the auditory channel.

2. HARD OF HEARING is defined as a hearing disorder whether fluctuating or permanent, which adversely affects an individual's communication performance. The hard of hearing individual

180

Chapter 7:
Models of
Service
Delivery and
Scheduling

relies upon the auditory channel as the primary sensory avenue for speech and language.

II. COMMUNICATIVE VARIATIONS

A. COMMUNICATIVE DIFFERENCE/DIALECT is a variation of a symbol system used by a group of individuals which reflects and is determined by shared regional, social, or cultural/ethnic factors. Variations or alterations in the use of a symbol system may be indicative of primary language interferences. A regional, social, or cultural/ethnic variation of a symbol system should not be considered a disorder of speech or language.

B. AUGMENTATIVE COMMUNICATION is a system used to supplement the communicative skills of individuals for whom speech is temporarily or permanently inadequate to meet communicative needs. Both prosthetic devices and/or nonprosthetic techniques may be designed for individual use as an augmentative communication system.

Classification of Procedures and Communication Disorders

In 1987, the ASHA Executive Board approved *The American Speech-Language-Hearing Association Classification of Speech-Language Pathology and Audiology Procedures and Communication Disorders,* commonly referred to as the ASHA Classification System (ASHACS). This provides a standardized system for coding and indexing procedures and diagnoses commonly used by speech-language pathologists and audiologists. The school speech-language pathologist or audiologist can use the nomenclature and classification system to uniformly describe communication disorders and the procedures being used. The system is especially valuable for clinicians who are interested in analyzing their service programs, generating research data about their caseloads, or developing a computerized information management system. While the actual code numbers used in the system do not correspond to those used by third party reimbursement sources, the terminology used in the ACHACS is widely accepted by payers. The Classification System is presented in Appendix A.

Continuum of Service Delivery Models

Before a comprehensive speech, language, and hearing program is organized by the pathologist, some basis must be established for its implementation. We will call this basis a *model.*

A model is an approximation of the real world and is meant to be used, manipulated, changed, added to, diminished, and expanded. The speech-language pathologist in any school district is the decision maker who must take into account all the information available, and using the model as a guide, construct the program in speech, language, and hearing for that particular community.

[Numerous models for delivering speech-language pathology and audiology services are being practiced across the country. They were designed based on the requirements of the federal and state laws, the needs of the school district, and the insights of professionals. There are variations in service delivery models from school district to school district. Differences may be due to the populations served, funding capabilities, administrative support (or nonsupport), and professional expertise and energy. One of the primary factors in the numbers and types of options available is the availability of staff.]

The laws regulating special education are very clear on one major point. Regardless of the model implemented, the school district should make available a continuum of service delivery options for providing services. The continuum of service delivery options for speech-language pathology may include providing services directly in the regular or special education classroom, implementing a consultation/collaboration model, providing direct services in resource rooms or self-contained classrooms, conducting inservice education programs for others and many more (Dublinske, 1988).

If the continuum of service delivery model is effective, the options will not be mutually exclusive and the clinician will be able to use them individually or in combination to best serve the needs of a particular student. The service delivery option selected should be the most appropriate to meet the child's needs and should be the least restrictive in terms of enabling the child to participate in the activities of the school as much as possible. Consideration should be given to the student's level of functioning and should serve children and youth with communication disabilities ranging from severe disorders to developmental problems. The model needs to be applicable to children of all ages in regular education as well as special education programs. It should also make provisions for providing preventive services to the overall school population.

Organizational models used to deliver services should allow adequate frequency and intensity of help for optimum progress. The program selected should provide students with the best chance for functioning successfully within the school setting and in their future lives. Examples of delivery of service models have been described in the professional literature by Holzhauser-Peters and Husemann (1988); Simon (1987); Dublinske, Minor, Hofmeister, and Taliaferro (1988); Montgomery (1988); and Jones and Healey (1973).

A Statewide Language Task Force sponsored by The Ohio Department of Education, Division of Special Education (1991) devised a comprehensive service delivery model. The model supports four major concepts of service delivery:

1. The importance of recognizing the impact of communication impairments on learning success.

2. The need to create an optimal environment for providing speech-language services.

3. The importance of collaboration and sharing expertise to develop effective program goals, objectives, and intervention strategies for children.

4. The need to integrate speech-language goals, objectives, and techniques into the student's learning experiences.

182

Chapter 7:
Models of
Service
Delivery and
Scheduling

The model is explained in Figure 7-1. There are six service delivery options:

1. inservice;
2. intervention assistance teams;
3. collaboration;
4. pullout intervention;
5. classroom-based intervention; and
6. community-based intervention.

A brief description of each of the service delivery options mentioned above with implementation examples and advantages is provided.

In addition to the options presented in the Ohio model, other options suggested are diagnostic centers, resource rooms, home and hospital services, parent/infant instruction services, and residential programs (Jones and Healey, 1973; Montgomery, 1988).

Some school districts maintain diagnostic centers where thorough diagnostic assessments can be conducted by an interdisciplinary team. Students are enrolled in these programs for only a short period of time. After evaluations are completed, results and recommendations are shared with the parents and school personnel. Resource rooms are part-time classrooms staffed by SLPs. Pupils remain in regular or special education classrooms for the majority of the day. They receive individualized attention in the resource room. Children with moderate and severe disorders are often served through the resource room model.

In the home and/or hospital option, clinicians travel to serve students who are unable to attend school because of confinement to their homes or to a hospital setting. Parent/infant instruction services are often provided to parents with preschool children who have developmental disabilities or who are at risk. The clinician provides guidance and instruction in techniques for assisting infants and preschoolers in developing appropriate communicative behaviors and skills. The services may be provided in the school, a center, the child's home, or other approved facilities. The residential placement option is usually reserved for pupils with severe and profound impairments. Education and specialized services are provided in addition to residential care.

Characteristics of Good Service Delivery Models

According to Flower (1984) the essential characteristics of good service-delivery models fall under five headings: efficacy, coordination, continuity, participation and economy.

1. The first obvious criterion, efficacy, is whether the service makes any difference to the consumer. Screening services can usually be judged in fairly objective terms; however, other services are often more difficult to assess. Evaluation by the clinician and the insights of families, clients, and other

(Text continues on page 190)

FIGURE 7.1. Models of Speech/Language Service Delivery

Service Delivery Models

Public Law 94-142 and *Rules* state that to be eligible for services, a speech/language handicapped student must have a significant deviation from the developmental norm, which has an adverse effect on the student's educational performance. This means that speech/language pathologists, intervention assistance teams, and individualized education program teams must consider the student's level of educational functioning and decide from a continuum of delivery models which model affords the student the best chance for success. At the same time, speech/language pathologists are charged with providing preventive services to the overall school population.

Numerous innovative and effective service delivery models can provide quality service to both the regular and special education populations. A description of the models most frequently employed and examples of their implementation, including advantages, follow.

SPEECH LANGUAGE SERVICE DELIVERY MODELS

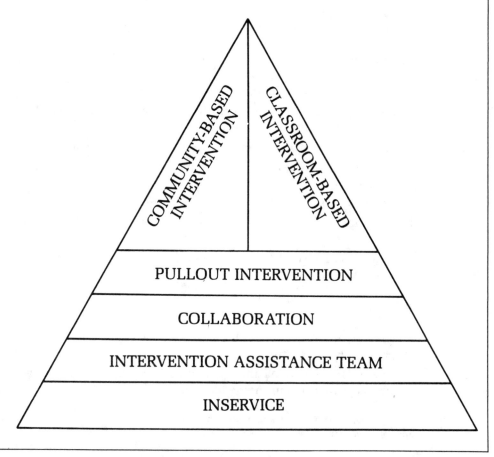

Inservice

The speech/language pathologist interfaces with the regular education program.

"The role of the school speech/language pathologist is in metamorphosis. While change can be threatening, the transformation of the speech/language pathologist from a 'broom-closet' therapist, isolated from the educational mainstream, to a classroom-based communication specialist has the potential of being more professionally rewarding and more relevant to the needs of school-age children."* This quote emphasizes the need for speech/language pathologists to begin spreading the word about language and its impact on educational and social success.

Inservice, both formal and informal, is a functional way to reach teachers and thereby impact the greatest numbers of students without having to provide direct service. Also, speech/language pathologists should attend inservice programs geared toward regular education so they can better understand the relationship between speech/language pathology and classroom instruction.

Implementation Examples

1. Provide information to teachers on topics related to language and learning via five-minute "quick-hits" at faculty meetings, written hand-outs, flyers, and reproducible materials.
2. Share ideas informally with teaches by taking part in the staff "routines" (e.g., informal lunchroom and lounge conversations).
3. Have a loan library of fun and useful materials the teachers may borrow.
4. Involve staff in special speech/language-related activities (e.g., "Better Speech/Hearing Month").
5. Volunteer to participate on curriculum committees, etc.
6. Be aware of curriculum content students are exposed to at various grade levels.
7. Communicate weekly with teachers, offering suggestions they can use with students in speech therapy.

Advantages

1. Greater numbers of students are impacted by the speech/language pathologist's expertise.
2. Referrals for individual therapy may decrease due to increased attention to language concerns in the regular classroom setting.

*Charlann S. Simon, "Out of the Broom Closet and Into the Classroom: The Emerging SLP." *Journal of Child Communication Disorders*, Vol. II. No. 1 (1987), pp. 41–46.

3. The speech/language pathologist can apply langua[ge]
of the classroom curriculum.

4. The speech/language pathologist, by sharing exp[erience]
members, is considered a more integral part of the

Intervention Assistance Tea[m]

The speech/language pathologist participates as a member of a team of professionals on the intervention assistance team (IAT).

The intervention assistance team may include the speech/language pathologist, regular or special education classroom teachers, the principal, various supplementary service personnel (e.g., occupational therapist, physical education specialist), and parents. The team members share observations and formal assessment results regarding the student for the purpose of coordinating the data into unified recommendations for the student. The team may monitor the student from the initial referral through a variety of assessments, interventions, and direct services. As part of the team, the speech/language pathologist has the opportunity to provide information to other team members regarding the sequential steps of language development and the impact and linkage of language with the curriculum and other supplemental services.

Implementation Example

The IAT meets to review information gathered about a student who is performing well below grade level expectations in reading and spelling. The speech/language pathologist helps the team make recommendations regarding intervention strategies for the student.

Advantages

1. Each time the speech/language pathologist is part of an IAT, the other team members learn about language development and intervention strategies. These staff members can then use their knowledge to impact greater numbers of students in the classroom.

2. The speech/language pathologist has the opportunity to educate and collaborate with other school personnel.

3. The speech/language pathologist, in working directly with other professionals, learns to view the student and the student's educational needs from a broader perspective.

Collaboration

The speech/language pathologist collaborates with the teacher and/or parents regarding a specific student, group, or class of students.

The speech/language pathologist observes a class and assembles information about the various levels of language competence among the students. Following analysis of the information, the speech/language pathologist meets with the teacher to share observations and recommendations to enhance the students' language skills and incorporate language development into the curriculum. The speech/language pathologist demonstrates or suggests specific teaching strategies and techniques and may provide supplementary materials to the teacher. Periodic collaboration may continue.

If a student in the class is determined to be handicapped, an IEP is developed, which includes goals and objectives that link the student's language performance with the curriculum. The speech/language pathologist may provide specific suggestions to the teacher so he or she can help the student reach the goals and objectives specified in the IEP.

Implementation Examples — handout

1. Explain or demonstrate specific remediation techniques that the teacher, peer-tutor, or parent volunteer could use to assist the student in carrying over language skills to everyday life. These techniques may include use of computer-enhanced therapy.
2. Provide informal analysis and suggestions for modification of the classroom environment, teacher delivery, or student-learning strategies.
3. Provide "language packets" that may include pictures, word lists, etc., for parents and other volunteers to use with preschool, kindergarten, or high-risk students.
4. Provide language/speech enrichment sessions in the classroom as needed.
5. Provide classroom learning centers for both phonologically-impaired and language-impaired students.

Advantages — overhead / handout

1. Greater numbers of students are impacted by the speech/language pathologist's expertise.
2. All students in a class can benefit from this model, regardless of the category in which they fall: (a) students who have normal language development, (b) students who have language problems but by rule definition are not handicapped, and (c) students who are handicapped by rule definition.
3. The opportunity exists for the teacher and the speech/language pathologist to share techniques; the pathologist learns more about the curriculum, the teacher's style, and classroom routines.
4. A strong language orientation can be established and incorporated into the curriculum.

Pullout Intervention

The speech/language pathologist removes the student from the classroom to provide direct therapy in a separate room.

Pullout intervention has historically been the primary model used by the speech/language pathologist to deliver service in a school setting. This model is sometimes referred to as an itinerant program, providing intermittent direct services. Speech and language services are provided as a supplementary service to regular or special education programs.

Pullout intervention may be aimed at an individual student or a group of students. Criteria for grouping students into a particular session may include age, grade level, type and degree of communication disorder, and functional level. Typically, the students scheduled into a group session exhibit similar communication disorders (e.g., language, articulation, fluency, and voice).

Implementation Examples

1. Traditional Scheduling

Traditional scheduling provides for direct service an average of twice per week to an individual student or group of students. Group size may average from two to four students but may include as many as ten students. The number of sessions per week, length per session, and number of students per session are influenced by the nature and degree of the students' problems and the speech/language pathologist's caseload demands. Creative use of learning centers, computers, and parent volunteers can maximize the benefits of pullout intervention.

2. Intensive Cycle Scheduling (Block Scheduling)

Intensive cycle, or block scheduling, involves servicing a particular site for a concentrated period of time, averaging five to ten weeks, and scheduling students three to five times per week. The block is then alternated with a time block at another school while the initial site is without direct service, or receives minimal direct service, for an equal period. A minimum of two cycles per year is scheduled at each school. Intensive cycle scheduling is less frequently employed than traditional scheduling but is often chosen when travel time between schools is too long.

Advantages

1. Students receive individual direct therapy.
2. Some students may be more willing to give oral responses and engage in group language interaction.
3. Pullout intervention also accommodates articulation, fluency, and voice disorders, especially in the early stages of remediation.
4. Distraction is less of a factor.

Classroom-Based Intervention

The speech/language pathologist provides direct therapy in the classroom setting to one or more students and uses the team approach with the classroom teacher.

The speech/language pathologist conducts classroom activities while the teacher observes and sometimes teams with the pathologist to work with the students. The speech/language pathologist may give the teacher ideas and materials to use in other classroom activities and interactions as a follow-up to the lesson. The speech/language pathologist may previously have conducted individual assessment of some of the students in the class.

Implementation Examples

1. Small Group (Regular or Special Education)

Several students in a class have language problems. The speech/language pathologist services these students through a weekly group activity lesson in the students' classroom. Other students in the class may participate in the lesson. The lesson addresses the students' specific language needs and links language development with the academic or vocational curriculum. IEPs may have been written only for those students who were identified as having a specific language handicap. The teacher observes the lesson and attempts to reinforce the targeted concept/skill during other daily classroom activities and interactions. The speech/language pathologist sometimes provides specific follow-up activities and/or materials. Also, some or all of the identified students may receive individual or group language therapy via pullout intervention.

2. Special Education

Orthopedically Handicapped

The speech/language pathologist and an interdisciplinary team of professionals may serve an orthopedically handicapped student who is learning to use an augmentative communication device by combining collaboration, pullout intervention, and classroom-based intervention.

Multihandicapped Class/Developmentally Handicapped Class

The speech/language pathologist, teacher, and support staff determine the communicative skills necessary for the student to function independently, e.g., in a fast-food restaurant. Objectives, vocabulary exercises, and developmental activities are planned and implemented in the classroom. Pullout intervention may be conducted at any point to emphasize and reinforce the skills.

Developmentally Handicapped Secondary Unit

The speech/language pathologist visits the secondary developmentally handicapped unit weekly or biweekly for a group lesson. The focus may be on the development of pragmatic communication skills that would impact the student's future vocational and social abilities. The teacher and speech/language pathologist work as a team. The teacher then reinforces communication objectives throughout the week.

3. **Junior or Senior High School Class for Credit**

One class period of the student's schedule is devoted to work on language skills. The course might be titled "Communication Skills." During the class period, the speech/language pathologist services several students whose language learning/remediation needs would benefit from this type of scheduling. Course content may include vocabulary development, problem-solving techniques, listening skills, social and conversational speech, question-asking and answering strategies, nonverbal communication skills, study skills related to language, and survival/pragmatic language.

Advantages

1. Greater numbers of students may be served by this method.
2. Nonlanguage handicapped students also may benefit.
3. Service is provided in a more natural environment than is possible in a separate speech therapy room.
4. Examples of language interactions, language modeling, and cueing may enhance the teacher's and the paraprofessional's interaction with students.
5. Language skills are incorporated into the academic curriculum.
6. Enhanced opportunity exists for generalization and carryover of language skills into everyday life.
7. This model is compatible with others.
8. Flexibility of scheduling for the speech/language pathologist is increased.

Community-Based Intervention

The speech/language pathologist collaborates with the special education teacher and other staff members to assist the student with functional speech and language in community sites.

Programs for low-incidence special education students are beginning to emphasize community-based instruction. As part of their school program, severely involved students learn how to function in their own communities. The speech/language pathologist provides direct or indirect services to students on-site in such community settings as restaurants, laundromats, libraries, banks, post offices, etc. The speech/language pathologist helps students with communication skills, monitors their progress, and assists in planning instruction. As a collaborator in a community-based intervention program, the speech/language pathologist assists the teacher, occupational therapist, physical therapist, or other staff members in developing plans and strategies to encourage the growth of the students' functional communication areas.

Implementation Examples

1. Because the school is a community site, development of the student's skills and carryover of those skills into everyday life can be worked on in the school setting. The speech/language pathologist can enlist the support of many resources in the school to aid in remediation of a student's communication skills. Intervention assignment may be given to school personnel—the school secretary, maintenance person, librarian, cafeteria worker, and other teachers and peers—who are often successful in monitoring a student's language skills and in encouraging appropriate adjustments for each site or setting.

2. In community-based sites, the speech/language pathologist analyzes the experience site to identify relevant vocabulary to be learned, develops language concepts relevant to assigned tasks, and guides staff in using directional language most likely to clearly convey instructional messages to students.

Advantages

1. Service is provided in a real-life vocational context.

2. Language objectives are integrated with the student's vocational life objectives.

3. Immediate opportunities are provided for carryover of language skills to everyday life.

4. Language content, form, and use targets can be applied daily.

5. Student motivation is maintained because this method appeals to teenagers.

*This model was developed by the Ohio Statewide Language Task Force. The Ohio Department of Education. Division of Special Education (1991). Reprinted with permission.

professionals all provide information of a subjective nature, but it is frequently difficult to determine whether achievements have, in fact, occurred.

2. Clients with communicative disorders are served by several different professionals. Some of these may provide services that are directly related to the communicative disorder, for example, the learning disabilities specialist working with a child with problems in language acquisition. Other professionals provide services with only peripheral relevance to the communicative disorder, for example, the teacher of a classroom in which a young stutterer is enrolled. Whenever multiple professional services are provided to the same client, the effectiveness of any of those services will often depend on the *coordination* with all other services.

3. Good care depends on the *continuity* of sequential services over a period of several months or sometimes several years. This often requires multiple pro-

fessional services, that is, a total plan for services, with each phase staged and integrated into an uninterrupted sequence toward the ultimate goal.

4. Professional services carried out with little regard for the clients' wishes or little concern for their understanding of what was occurring seriously impair the effectiveness of those services. *Participation* by the client and the family in all decision-making processes ensures the opportunity for excellent services.

5. *Economy* does not only mean spending as little money as possible. It refers also to the conservation of time and energy. The conservation of financial resources, as well as the orderly management of services to avoid waste, and the achievement of efficiency through careful planning constitute the broader definition of economy.

Flower's five criteria will be helpful in assessing service delivery models.

Each school system is unique. The major ingredient in selecting the model to be used is the school speech-language pathologist who must become the information processor and decision maker. The school clinician needs to implement the service delivery options that best fit the organization of the school system, needs of the students, and professionals on staff. There are a number of factors which may influence the number and types of options a school district is able to make available to its students including:

1. The geographic location of the schools, the clinician's "home" office, and the distance and travel time between these locations

2. The availability of working space in each of the schools

3. The type and severity of the communication problems within the schools

4. The number and population of the schools (Would some schools warrant a full-time clinician?)

5. Time allotted for coordination activities, including in-service training; supervision of paraprofessionals or aides; recordkeeping; parent conferences; placement team conferences; and collaborating with classroom teachers, special education personnel, and administrators; administration of diagnostic tests; and so on

6. School policies affecting the transporting of students from school to school to place them in locations where they may receive the appropriate services

7. The level of the school (It is entirely probable that the junior high schools and the senior high schools may have smaller population of students with communication impairments than elementary schools.)

8. The support of the school administration and teaching staff.

Caseload Size and Composition

Caseload size and composition vary from state to state, district to district, and clinician to clinician. The minimum and maximum number of students and types of disabilities which can be served are often mandated by state and local

192

Chapter 7:
Models of
Service
Delivery and
Scheduling

education agencies. More often than not, the numbers of students the SLP is expected to serve are extremely high. This impedes the quality of services and slows down the progress of individual children.

Caseload Composition

The complexity and severity of cases served in public school programs has increased over the past years. For example, studies of caseload composition in 1961 indicated that 81% of most caseloads were made up of children with articulation disorders. In 1981, 47% of the caseloads were comprised of children with articulation disorders and 47% with language disorders. Seventy percent of the cases were classified as being moderate to severe and 43% were multihandicapped (Dublinske, 1988).

Each year, ASHA conducts an Omnibus survey to obtain demographic information about the membership. In 1988, they focused on personnel working in the school setting. Table 7-1 shows the mean percent of clinicians who serve specific types of disorders and the median percent of clients with each disorder. The SLPs' caseloads were largely comprised of children with language disorders (50.2%) and articulation disorders (39.7). The mean monthly caseload size was 55.7 students (Shewan, 1989).

Speech-language pathologists in the Allegheny Pennsylvania Intermediate Unit conducted a study comparing the composition of their caseloads over a seven year time period. Information on 6,500 students was contributed by over 100 clinicians. They documented a shift in their caseload emphasis from 60.8% articulation impaired and 31.7% language disordered in 1981–1982 to 38.3% articulation impaired and 52.8% language disordered in 1987–1988 (Eger et al., 1988). Over the 12-year time period between 1976 and 1988, there was an increase in the percentage of language cases from 13.5% to 49.1%.

TABLE 7.1. MEAN PERCENT CLINICIANS WHO REGULARLY SERVE INDIVIDUALS WITH SPECIFIC DISORDERS AND MEDIAN PERCENT OF CLIENTS WITH EACH DISORDER

Disorder Type	Mean Percent Clinicians Regularly Serving Individuals	Median Percent Clients With Disorder
Articulation	98.6	39.7
Voice	75.5	3.0
Fluency	90.3	4.6
Laryngectomy	2.5	2.0
Dysphagia	18.5	8.0
Childhood Language	99.5	50.2
Aphasia	20.9	5.1
Degenerative Neurological	17.8	4.6
Traumatic Brain Injury	27.4	2.7
Conductive Hearing Loss	60.9	4.6
Sensorineural Hearing Loss	59.7	2.3
Mixed Hearing Loss	32.9	2.4
Central Auditory	42.5	5.1

Source: 1988 Omnibus Survey. Reprinted with the permission of The American Speech-Language-Hearing Association.

The Allegheny clinicians also reported changes in the types of students they were seeing and the types of service delivery models implemented. The population was diverse and included students who were severely and profoundly mentally retarded, severely emotionally disturbed, severely and profoundly hearing impaired, and learning disabled. Speech services were being integrated into the classroom curricula and there was an increase in the use of indirect service delivery services. Clinicians were also involved in early intervention, prevention, and parent training activities.

Guidelines for Determining Caseload Size

The ASHA Committee on Language, Speech, and Hearing Services in the Schools (1984) established guidelines for determining caseload size based on a continuum of service delivery model. The guidelines are not intended to be regulatory or to establish universal minimum standards. Rather, the intent is to provide speech-language pathologists and school administrators with the information they need to cooperatively plan programs. Establishing guidelines provides a basis for determining the appropriate service delivery options to meet the school districts' needs.

The guidelines specify seven program characteristics which need to be considered and four service delivery options from least restrictive to most restrictive. The four service delivery options are:

1. Consultation programs (indirect service);
2. Itinerant programs (intermittent direct services);
3. Resource room programs (intensive direct service); and
4. Self-contained programs (academically integrated direct service).

The seven program characteristics are:

1. cases served;
2. services provided;
3. group size;
4. times per day;
5. times per week;
6. rationale; and
7. caseload maximums.

The model is presented in Table 7-2.

Following is a brief description of each of the seven program characteristics discussed in the guidelines.

Cases Served. Any of the service delivery options can be used to treat students with communication disorders of articulation, language, voice, fluency, or hearing. However, because of factors such as severity, some program options may be more effective than others.

TABLE 7.2. RECOMMENDED CASELOAD SIZE FOR SPEECH-LANGUAGE SERVICES IN THE SCHOOLS

	Consultation Program (Indirect Service)	Itinerant Program (Intermittent Direct Service)	Resource Room Program (Intensive Direct Service)	Self-Contained Program (Academically Integrated Direct Service)
Cases served	— All communicative disorders — All severities (mild to severe)	— All communicative disorders — All severities (mild to severe)	— All communicative disorders particularly language and articulation — All severities	— Primary handicap: communication — Several/multiple disorders particularly language and articulation
Services provided	— Program development, management, coordination — Indirect services	— Program development, management, coordination, evaluation — Direct services — Coordination w/educators	— Program development, management, coordination, evaluation — Direct service/self-study/aide — Coordination w/teacher(s) — Teacher has academic responsibilities	— Program development, management, coordination, evaluation — Direct services plus academic instruction
Group Size	— Individual or Group (indirect service)	— Individual or small group (up to 3 students/session)	— Individual or small group (up to 5 students/session)	— Up to 10 students/speech-language pathologist — Up to 15/speech-language pathologist w/supportive personnel
Time Per Day	— Variable; Possible range — ½ hr. (mild) to 3–4 hrs/day	— ½ to 1 hour/day	— 1 to 3 hours/day	— Full school day
Times Per Week	— 1 to 5 times/week	— 2 to 5 times/week	— 4 to 5 times/week	— Full time placement
Rationale for Caseload Size	— Time necessary by organization — Variable needs	— Complex cases demand lower caseloads — Approximates national average	— Cases require intensive services — Consistent w/regulations	— Consistent w/regulations — Provides for intensive services
Caseload* Maximums	— Up to 15–40 students	— Up to 25–40 students	— Up to 15–25 students	— Up to 15 students w/aide — Up to 10 students w/out aide

Draft prepared by the Committee on Language, Speech, and Hearing Services in the Schools August 1981. Final revision July 1983.

Services Provided. This section of the guidelines specifies that the speech-language pathologist is the primary person responsible for providing services related to program development, management, coordination, and evaluation of communication disorders. It also indicates that service can be provided directly by the speech-language pathologist or indirectly by other individuals involved with the student including teachers, parents, other specialized personnel, or supportive personnel. In cases where the student receives services in a resource room setting or a self-contained classroom, guidelines are provided for selecting the person who will be primarily responsible.

Group Size. Since services are often delivered in a group setting, recommendations are also made for group size ranging from one in an individualized session to a group of 10 to 15 in a self-contained class. Decisions regarding a group versus individualized or combined group/individualized program should be based on student need rather than factors such as administrative direction and time or budget constraints.

Times Per Day and Times Per Week. These categories refer to the amount of actual time (per day and per week) that service is provided to the student. This does not include preparation time, recordkeeping, continuing education activities, school duties, or conferences. As with group size, decisions regarding the length and frequency of intervention should be based on the student's needs and clinical factors rather than budgetary and administrative issues.

Rationale. The caseload size and service delivery option selected should be based on several variables relating to the student and personnel available, and federal, state, and local requirements for serving students with communication disorders. This includes the type and severity of the student's communication impairment, the effect of the communication disorder on academic performance, the relationship of the communication disorder to other handicapped conditions, the stage of development of the communication disorder, the student's history in the speech-language intervention program, amount and type of contact needed to implement intervention strategies, and scheduling constraints. (ASHA, 1984; Eger et al., 1990). Because students' needs are constantly changing, these factors should be re-evaluated and the program adjusted periodically. Consideration needs to be given to the number of children who can be adequately served using a particular service delivery option or combination of options.

Caseload Maximum. Ranges of maximum caseload sizes are specified for each service delivery option. The ranges are dependent on severity of the communication disorder, other student related factors, treatment strategies, number of persons to be involved, and frequency of contact. The maximum caseload size recommended for clinicians using the itinerant or consultative models is approximately 40 students. The number is reduced to 25 for the resource room model and 15 for self-contained classes. Since variations in caseload size and composition are inevitable, it is recommended that each district establish the minimum and maximum number appropriate for its needs.

Other issues that affect the caseload decisions are reimbursement policies, the number of schools served, travel time between schools, and the many additional responsibilities of the school-based clinician, such as conferences, paperwork, and school duties.

Service Coordination

Children with disabilities and their families frequently require a broad range of intervention services. Physical and mental health care are necessary as well as financial assistance and habilitative services. Therapies might include speech-language pathology, aural habilitation, physical therapy, occupational therapy, visual training, counseling, and the like. Numerous professionals representing multiple agencies are charged with delivering the services. As a result, goals, treatment programs, and services are often fragmented and/or duplicated. In addition, complications arise for reimbursement for services because the agencies may each have different funding streams.

To improve the quality of services offered to children and their families, Public Law 99-457 mandated the coordination of services for children. The central question asked is "What help does the family of a child with disabilities need to function well?" Emphasis is placed on collaborative planning and efficient, effective service delivery. To achieve this service coordination, professionals from a variety of disciplines and agencies must strive to understand one another's disciplines. Through this model, the family is involved meaningfully in all aspects of planning, implementing, and monitoring their child's programs.

One of the agencies involved in service delivery for children is the educational system. School clinicians have opportunities to coordinate their services with professionals both inside and outside of the school system. The clinician can contribute to the service coordination process in the following ways:

1. sharing information about the services the school can offer;
2. explaining the child's communication impairments and their impact on the child's ability to function;
3. discussing the speech-language program and educational program planned for the child; and
4. collaborating with other professionals to determine areas of redundancy and ways to facilitate each others' goals.

Scheduling Services

In Chapter 6 systems for case selection were discussed. One aspect dealt with the identification and further diagnosis of individual children who were possible candidates for intervention. Let us now turn our attention to the scheduling of children for services.

In implementing a program based on the continuum of service/delivery concept the SLP would allocate his or her time so that the children in the highest priority category would receive the most attention. As the children progress, their priority ratings change, and they move along the continuum receiving appropriate services until they reach maximum potential and are dismissed from therapy.

This system is based on the needs of the child and meets the letter and the spirit of PL 94-142. Rather than servicing "schools" the SLP is servicing children. Too often administrators expect the SLP's time to be divided equally among schools without regard to the needs of the children. This puts at risk the reputation of the program and may result in lack of support and fewer referrals from teachers, principals, and eventually parents.

Guidelines for the establishment of a case selection priority system were described in Chapter 6. The guidelines are flexible and can be adapted to large, small, or medium-sized school systems. They can also be applied to pupils from preschool through high school.

Length and Frequency of Therapy Sessions

In considering the length and frequency of therapy sessions, the most basic consideration would be the best possible use of the time allotted. This is not much help to the beginning clinician, however, who must decide whether to schedule children for 30-minute sessions or longer. Perhaps the best approach is to take a careful look at the schedule of classes in the school and then have the therapy schedule coincide with the class schedule. This does not necessarily mean that therapy sessions should be the same length as classes, but it would be helpful to both teachers and students if there were some coordination between the two.

Nor does it mean that all the sessions should be planned for the same amount of time. Some sessions may be 20 minutes in length, and some may be 45 minutes. The decision about the amount of time should be made by the clinician on the basis of the child's needs. More time may be needed for group sessions. The child in the generalization stages of therapy may require ten or 15 minutes several times a week. High-school students who may be able to assume more responsibility for themselves may need only one one-hour session per week.

The amount of time needed for each child may change as the child progresses in therapy. Classroom teachers should be informed of the fact that change will occur during the year and that their input would be valuable tin considering any changes in the time.

The key word in planning the amount of time per therapy session is *flexibility* and the criterion is *what is in the best interests of the child*. The responsibility for making good use of the time is the clinician's.

The Itinerant Scheduling Model

Traditionally, speech and language services have been provided on an itinerant basis and have been based on state regulations that define caseload, number of child-contact hours per week, and ratio of clinicians to school populations. By providing more options for delivery of services instead of relying solely on the itinerant model, more children who need help can be reached. This does not

198

Chapter 7:
Models of
Service
Delivery and
Scheduling

imply that the itinerant model is not a good model when it is used in the appropriate circumstances; however, it does mean the speech-language pathology and audiology professions must break the habit of thinking of it as the only option.

Many of the children with severe communication disorders, as well as those with mild to moderate deviations, will be in regular classrooms with speech, language, and hearing services provided by the school clinician on an itinerant basis. The itinerant model has been used from the time it was suggested in 1910 by Ella Flagg Young, who felt that it protected the young teacher from "depression of spirit and low physical conditions resulting from confinement in one room for several successive hours while working with abnormal conditions." Not until recent years, with the advent of mandatory legislation, more sophisticated tools of identification, evaluation and program management, larger numbers of children needing services, and the recognized need for an interdisciplinary approach, have other systems of scheduling been developed.

The itinerant model may be effective in situations where schools are within a few miles of each other or where school populations and caseloads are low. It may also provide continuous therapy for children who need more frequent intervention over a longer period of time, such as children with fluency problems, hearing problems, and problems resulting from such conditions as cleft palate and cerebral palsy.

The itinerant (or traditional) model may take several forms. The school clinician may serve one, two, or three schools, working with a small group of children (two to five) or individual children on an intermittent basis of twice a week. An example of this schedule follows:

	Monday	Tuesday	Wednesday	Thursday	Friday
AM	School A	School C	Coordination	School A	School C
			and Consultation		
PM	School B	School C	Day	School B	School C

Intermittent therapy may also be provided by a clinician based in a single building. This would be appropriate for a school with a large population and a large number of pupils with communication problems.

Another possible option in a school system with two or more SLPs would be to assign the clinicians on the basis of their areas of specialization. In a variation of this model in a large school system, part of the staff might be on an itinerant schedule while several clinicians would serve as "specialists," matching their strengths to the students' needs.

Intensive Cycle Scheduling

Another model of scheduling services is the intensive cycle, sometimes called the block system. In this model the child is seen four or five times a week for a concentrated block of time, usually four to six weeks.

MacLearie and Gross (1966) reported on an experimental program in intensive cycle scheduling in the Ohio communities of Brecksville, Cleveland, Dayton, and East Cleveland city schools and the Crawford County schools. The

research was carried on over a period of four years, and the results were reported both subjectively and objectively. The Ohio study indicated the following
advantages of the plan:

1. A greater number of children could be enrolled during the school year.
2. A larger percentage of children were dismissed from therapy as having obtained maximum improvement.
3. The length of time children with articulatory problems were enrolled in
   speech therapy was reduced.
4. Although not statistically significant, the Brecksville study gave some indications that a greater carryover of improvement occurred.
5. Closer relationships between the therapist and school personnel and parents
   was noted because of the greater acceptance of the therapist as a specific part
   of a particular school's staff.
6. Students appeared to sustain interest in therapy over a longer period of time.
7. Less time was needed in reviewing a lesson since daily therapy sessions occurred.

Participants in the study made the following suggestions concerning the
length and nature of intensive cycle scheduling:

1. The first block scheduled should be longer to account for screening and
   program organization.
2. Sessions should be a minimum of four weeks in duration.
3. A minimum of two cycles, and preferably three to four each year, are needed
   for best results.

Problems related to intensive cycle scheduling follow:

1. Some problems of a psychogenic nature may need more frequent contacts on
   a regularly scheduled basis.
2. Administrative problems and reactions to students leaving a classroom on a
   daily basis may be a problem if the intensive cycle program is not carefully
   explained to the school staff.
3. Monopolization of a shared room for therapy services may cause scheduling
   problems.

One of the anticipated problems was the reaction of the classroom teachers
to having children leave their classroom on a daily basis. In the Brecksville study,
it was reported that of the 35 teachers responding, 30 felt that the intensive cycle
method fitted better with other aspects of their daily program. Two stated they
had no opinion, and three preferred the itinerant method.

Results of the study in Cleveland (MacLearie & Gross, 1966) indicated that
regardless of the scheduling method used, the group receiving the intensive
program first had a greater average gain than the group receiving therapy on an

200

Chapter 7:
Models of
Service
Delivery and
Scheduling

intermittent basis first. The implication seemed to be that an optimum program may be therapy on an intensive basis first and on an intermittent basis next as the child's communication improves.

Objective Evaluation

a. A breakdown of the articulation caseload by grades indicated that best results were obtained in grades four, five, and six in terms of number and percent of pupils corrected

b. The groups which responded least were made up of seventh and eighth graders

c. Intensive cycle scheduling seemed to be less effective with problems involving organic impairments such as cerebral palsy, cleft palate, and brain injury

d. Intensive scheduling provided the opportunity for a greater number to receive speech therapy and for a greater percent of improvement

e. Experimentation with length of blocks revealed that the eight-week blocks enrolled more pupils than did the eighteen-week blocks. However, the eight-week block schools were first-year schools. The previous study showed that first-year school enrolled more pupils than did those using intensive therapy for the second time. The correction rate of total caseloads was similar in each school

f. The limitation of four buildings per therapist was thought to

   1) Provide an on-going program of once a week therapy for selected children between blocks on the intensive cycle plan

   2) Permit scheduling of selected children as needed.

Subjective Evaluation

The project directors felt that intensive cycle scheduling tended to:

a. Provide better integration of speech therapy with the total school program

b. Result in more consistent oral practice at home and more sustained interest

c. Permit more frequent contacts between therapists and school personnel

d. Minimize the effect of pupil absence on speech progress

e. Shorten time allotted to speech screening

f. Result in fewer problems in scheduling therapy classes for upper elementary children as they could be seen at times which best suited their program

g. Stimulate more frequent conferences with parents and teachers

h. Permit the enrollment of a larger number of children with speech problems without detracting from the quality of the work accomplished

i. Provide a higher rate of correction.

The Combination of Models for Scheduling

Another option for scheduling services would be a combination of models, for example, a combination of the itinerant model with the intensive cycle scheduling system. In this option an intensive program (with children receiving therapy on a daily basis) might be followed by a scheduling model of intermittent therapy. This plan would insure compliance with PL 94-142 in that children needing therapy over a longer period of time would not be dropped because the intensive cycle terminated. Obviously, this would be easier to arrange if there were more than one SLP on the staff, if communication aides were available, if the program were carefully coordinated, and if the clinicians and the school administrators all agreed on the program.

Scheduling Groups of Children

Although some therapy in the public schools is carried on in individual therapy sessions, a great deal of it is also done in group sessions.

Initially, the clinician is faced with the task of deciding which children should be placed in a group. The answer would depend on the needs of the child at any given stage of therapy. Some children may need an intensive approach to master some skills, and this may best be accomplished by working alone with the clinician. Later that same child may be ready to use these skills in a social situation, and a group experience would best fit this need.

The makeup of the group is an important factor in planning for optimal therapy results. Some clinicians find it more productive to work with a group of children who have similar problems, whereas for other clinicians the homogeneity of problems is not as important as grouping children of the same age level.

On the junior and senior high-school levels it may be more productive to have students with fluency problems in a group. On the other hand, some students with stuttering problems may not be ready for a group situation until after a series of individual therapy sessions.

In deciding when children should be put in a group and which group they should join, several things need to be considered. First, there are no right or wrong ways of grouping children. Groups must be flexible and must meet the needs of each child enrolled. Second, grouping is done to control the factors that enhance learning. Third, groups should not become static. As children learn and as needs change the composition of the group should change. Fourth, groups should be structured but not rigid. A structure assists learning, and if learning is not taking place there is no purpose for the existence of the group. Fifth, the size of the group should depend on its major purposes; however, a group of more than five or six students to one instructor tends to lose its tutorial effect (Stimson, 1979).

Often, several children from a single classroom need to be scheduled for therapy. Depending on their disabilities and needs, they may or may not be able to be accommodated in the same group and scheduled for the same therapy time. The teacher's input in scheduling is essential so consideration can be given

202

**Chapter 7:
Models of
Service
Delivery and
Scheduling**

to subjects the children will miss and disruptions which will occur as they enter and leave the classroom.

Students with speech, language, or hearing disorders should not be put in therapy groups simply to accommodate more students in the SLP's caseload. The rationale for placing a student in a group should depend on the needs of the student and the purpose of the group.

Scheduling in Junior and Senior High Schools

Some special considerations need to be taken into account in scheduling junior and senior high-school students. Because of the inflexibility of the classes and the study programs on those levels, the Task Force on Traditional Scheduling Procedures in Schools (1973) recommended these alternatives: (1) the clinician discuss scheduling with the school principal before the beginning of the school year, (2) consideration be given to regularly scheduled speech and language classes with credit as part of the academic curriculum for those pupils in need of such services, (3) a rotation system be developed so students do not miss the same class each time, (4) scheduling during the regular academic year be omitted completely and intensive services be provided during the six-week summer period, or (5) additional staff be employed to serve only these students.

Receiving grades and academic credit for participating in the speech-language intervention program often motivates junior high and high school students. The credit is usually one-quarter or one-half as much as a regular course and enrollment may be repeated. Clinicians wishing to use this model must work with administrators, teachers, and counselors to determine where the course best fits in the school curriculum. Some districts offer a course of this nature as an elective in the language arts area, others consider it a personal enhancement class. Students who might qualify for the program can be identified by reviewing caseloads from elementary programs in the district or through referral and screening programs.

There must be a defined course content, objectives, learning activities, and grading criteria commensurate with other courses on the schedule. For example, students can be objectively evaluated on factors such as attendance, level of involvement and participation in class activities, completion of assignments, and efforts made toward reaching identified targets and goals. The course can be listed as an elective course option in the student's school handbook and scheduling can be done through the school computer along with all other academic scheduling. If the scheduling system is refined, groups of students with similar communication disabilities can be formed.

Organizing the program in this manner makes it more acceptable to students who may be sensitive about their speech or language difficulties. It also promotes interaction of students with similar concerns. This enables practice of functional speech and language skills. Another advantage to this scheduling plan is that students begin the year with the speech-language therapy program as *a part of* their schedule rather than an addition to it.

Flexibility in Scheduling

The therapy program has many facets, many ramifications, and requires much from the school SLP. Decisions must be made, and they will not always be the right decisions. Speech-language pathologists are conscientious and intelligent people, but they are not infallible. They usually learn from their mistakes and often from the mistakes of others. The beginning clinician might be wise to avoid getting locked into a course of action that later, because of circumstances, might not be the best one. This can occur on the intervention level and on the organizational and management level. For example, if the clinician determines that the client is not responding to a particular approach in therapy, the clinician changes the procedures. On the organizational level if the SLP has "sold" the school administration on the idea that the itinerant service delivery model is the only feasible one, the SLP may have difficulty if it becomes apparent in the future that other service delivery models should be utilized. Allowing for some flexibility will enable the school clinician to maintain a viable program.

Nonscheduled Service Time: Coordination Time

In addition to the time spent in conducting therapy sessions and diagnostic activities, the clinician has many other duties to perform. Some time must be set aside during the week to carry out activities necessary to the overall program. In some states this is referred to as *coordination time*. It may be a half day or a full day. Usually it is a block of time set aside on a regular basis in the week's schedule. Some school clinicians set aside a block of time during each day for this purpose.

Some of the activities carried on during coordination time are parent conferences; staffing of cases; staff conferences; in-service training; correspondence; maintaining records and reports; classroom demonstration lessons for speech and language development and improvement programs; consulting with the school nurse, psychologist, guidance counselor, reading teacher, and others; and other activities important to conducting an effective program. In some geographical areas school clinicians employed in different school systems get together for professional meetings and to assist each other in screening, in-service training programs, and other professional matters. This can be especially effective where there may be only one clinician in a school district or where the opportunity for getting together may be limited by distance and time.

Because of the myriad of activities carried on during coordination time, it is highly desirable for the clinician to keep the school administrators informed of what is done during this time. Some clinicians use a monthly report form on which they record their activities during the nonscheduled service time. Periodically they send the reports to the school administrators.

Sometimes misunderstandings arise between the classroom teacher and the school clinician when the teacher sees the clinician leave the building during coordination day to carry out duties elsewhere. If the SLP informs the teachers and the principal of his or her activities during that time, criticism and skepticism are allayed and there is a better understanding of the program.

Summer Programs

One way in which many school clinicians have extended their services is to offer a summer program. There may be several reasons for carrying out a summer program: to provide more intensive therapy for children who need it, to provide services of an intensive nature to children with such problems as stuttering or communication problems associated with physical disabilities, and to offer a preventive program of therapy along with a parental guidance program.

School clinicians have provided summer programs for a number of years. Some of the programs have been financed by the local education system, and some have been underwritten by foundations, grants, or a local service club. In some cases, the program has been a joint effort of both the school system and a voluntary organization. In this sort of program, usually the building, facilities, supplies, and so on have been furnished by the school, whereas the clinician's salary has been paid by the community group.

The clinician in charge of the program will need to establish criteria for accepting children and will need to carry out the necessary diagnostic procedures. Often only a limited number of children can be accepted, depending on the number of staff members available.

Summer programs are usually well received in a community, and once started are often repeated during subsequent summers.

DISCUSSION QUESTIONS AND PROJECTS

1. Why is it important to have definitions of communicative disorders that are uniform and agreed on by professionals in the field?

2. You are the school SLP. How would you utilize the service delivery options model in explaining your program to a meeting of elementary teachers in a specific school?

3. Can you give examples of the various service delivery options in your community?

4. Interview some SLPs presently working in the various service delivery options.

5. Using Flower's list of essential characteristics of good service-delivery models, devise a list of questions under each of the five headings. The purpose of the questions would be to evaluate the service delivery models found in a typical school.

6. List professionals who might be in attendance and topics which would likely be discussed during a meeting to coordinate services for the following chil-

dren: an infant born with Down syndrome, a preschool child with cerebral palsy, a 13-year-old boy who sustained a traumatic brain injury.

7. Using an itinerant scheduling model, schedule the following children in School A, School B, and School C:

School A, 8:30 A.M.—3:00 P.M., 19 students
Kindergarten: 3 language/articulation
Grade 1: 2 articulation, 1 primary stutterer
Grade 2: 1 voice, 1 foreign language, 2 articulation
Grade 3: 2 voice, 1 stutterer, 2 articulation
Grade 4: 1 aural rehabilitation
Grade 5: 1 voice
Grade 6: 1 articulation, 1 stutterer

School B, 8:15 A.M.—2:30 P.M., 30 students
Grade 1: 3 language, 1 severe articulation, 1 hearing impaired
Grade 2: 3 articulation
Grade 3: 3 voice, 1 cleft palate, 3 articulation
Grade 4: 4 articulation, 1 stutterer
Grade 5: 2 hearing impaired, 1 stutterer, 1 voice
Grade 6: 2 articulation, 1 voice, 3 language

School C, 8:30 A.M.,—3:15 P.M., 28 students
Kindergarten: 4 language/articulation
Grade 1: 3 severe articulation, 5 articulation
Grade 2: 2 articulation, 1 language
Grade 3: 1 foreign language, 1 voice, 1 stutterer
Grade 4: 1 cerebral palsy, 1 hearing impaired, 1 articulation
Grade 5: 1 foreign language, 1 stutterer, 2 articulation
Grade 6: 1 foreign language, 2 hearing impaired

8. Interview a school SLP about the type of scheduling models being used.

9. Would you schedule children during recess? Art Class? Physical education? Reading? Social Studies? Explain.

10. Does the severity of the problem have any influence on the time of day you would schedule a student?

CHAPTER 8

Intervention: Planning, Implementing, Evaluating

Introduction

The school clinician spends most of the working day involved in actually performing therapy. The type of intervention used will be the decision of the clinician and will be appropriate to the age of the child as well as the type of problem. It is not necessary at this time, nor would there be space in this chapter, to discuss the various treatment approaches and philosophies. Suffice it to say that the school clinician should not only be well versed in the remediation approaches used in the past but also aware of current developments in treatment approaches. There are a number of approaches available to the clinician, and the choice will depend on what best serves the child. Beginning school clinicians will reflect on what they learned in academic courses as well as in practicum courses. They will gain additional information and practice during student teaching. In this chapter we will discuss planning, implementing, and evaluating intervention services.

Planning Individualized Programs

Effective intervention begins with the planning process. A planning conference is held. At that time, the clinician works with the student's parents, a representative of the school district, the student's teacher, and other appropriate professionals to plan the intervention program. During the conference, decisions made are based on data gathered during the multi-factored assessment. The nature and degree of special education programming and intervention is determined. The mode for service delivery is selected, and the goals, objectives, and procedures for intervention are identified. The SLP and/or audiologist should come to the meeting prepared to discuss the nature of the student's communication impairment, its impact on educational performance, and recommendations for treatment. In cases where only speech, language, or hearing problems are the primary concern, fewer individuals may be involved in the planning. An Individualized Education Program (IEP) is developed for school age children. The Individualized Family Service Plan (IFSP) is used for preschoolers.

Individualized Education Program

An IEP must be developed for each school-age student identified as having a disability and needing special education placement or support services. The IEP should include a description of the student's current educational level and a plan of future goals. Earlbaum (1990) states that the IEP should provide "a cohesive picture of where the child has been, where the child is, and where the child is going." Section 121.a 346 of PL 94-142 regulations specifies the following content in the IEP:

1. A statement of the child's present levels of educational performance

2. A statement of annual goals, including short-term and related services to be provided to the child and long-term instructional objectives

3. A statement of the specific special education and the extent to which the child will be able to participate in regular educational programs

4. The projected dates for initiation of services and the anticipated duration of the services

5. Appropriate objective criteria and evaluation procedures for determining, on at least an annual basis, whether the short-term instructional objectives are being achieved

The IEP must be specific for each child who receives either special education or related services or both. A single IEP is written for a child enrolled in special education and receiving both special education and related services. The related service may be in speech, language, or audiology. Presumably, the SLP and/or the audiologist is present at the planning meeting and contributes to the planning. When the SLP or audiologist provides the related service and the child is not enrolled in any other special education program, the IEP is written by that professional, with appropriate input from parents, teachers, or administrators.

When out-of-school services are purchased by the local board of education for a specific child, the IEP is written by the school personnel involved and contains the information regarding the nature of the service provided. The out-of-school professional is often asked to contribute to the preparation of the IEP.

Each of the major components necessary for the IEP is described in the following paragraphs (Dublinske, 1978). The components conform to the IEP requirements contained in Public Law 94-142. Many alternatives exist to develop the IEP and comply with the law. The suggested components are designed to

208

Chapter 8:
Intervention:
Planning,
Implement-
ing, Evalu-
ating

provide speech-language pathologists and audiologists with decision-making information that can be used, if necessary, to improve program and case management procedures. A sample IEP is found in Figure 8.1. The content included in the sample IEP shows how the information might appear on an IEP. Many IEPs will be more complex and detailed than the sample IEP. Terminology may vary from district to district.

I. *Identification/Development Information*

This section contains demographic information related to the child and information on IEP development and implementation activities. Components included in this section may vary depending on information required by the local education agency.

The "case coordinator" could be a staff person assigned to coordinate case assignments within the agency, or the person with primary responsibility for implementing the IEP.

If the IEP has to be approved by an immediate supervisor, this person can sign off in an "approved by" space.

The "IEP initial placement date" indicates the date services will be initiated. The "last MFE date" indicates the date services included in the IEP will end. Since IEPs have to be reviewed on an annual basis, the duration of services indicated between the entry and exit date is typically one year.

The time between the entry and exit dates constitutes the "service year." Space is provided to indicate the "follow-up/review dates." The IEP can be reviewed as often as necessary but must be reviewed at least annually. The review can take place anytime during the service year.

The "persons developing the IEP" must include as a minimum the parent, teacher, and person qualified to provide or supervise special education and related services.

II. *Assessment Information*

Informal and formal "assessment procedures" used to determine the child's eligibility for special education should be included. No child can be placed in special education based on a single assessment procedure. "Results" of the assessments should be described and interpreted in a manner that facilitates understanding by other persons viewing the IEP. Complete names of assessment instruments should be used. The "date" of assessment and the name and title of the "examiner" also should be included.

III. *Special Education and Related Services Needed*

This section must indicate all of the special education and related services the child needs to receive an appropriate education. Statements should include information on the specific placement alternative the child needs and the frequency service will be provided.

The percentage of time the child will spend in each special education and related service program and regular education program must be indicated. The percentage can be computed by determining the total number of educational hours available during the year and dividing the number into the number of hours spent in the various special and regular education programs.

IV. *Placement Justification*

If the IEP is used as a placement document, the parents' signatures must be secured to indicate they approve of the child's special education placement. As a placement document, the IEP should include a summary statement indicating the placement recommended and the rationale for the placement.

V. *Current Levels of Performance*

From the assessment information collected, data-based statements of performance must be developed. These statements indicate the performance level for specific tasks or behaviors. Preferably, each statement will include a numerical reference to the child's performance level. Performance levels can be indicated for such areas as language, speech, hearing, or any other breakdown appropriate for the child or the informational needs of the LEA.

VI. *Need Statements*

Need statements show the direction of change that is to occur as the present level of performance is modified. Need statements indicate that a behavior is going to increase or decrease.

VII. *Annual Goals*

Goals indicate the projected level of performance for the child as a result of receiving the special education and related services indicated in the IEP. Goals should include the components when, what, and criterion and should be numbered, 1, 2, 3. . . .

VIII. *Short-term Instructional Objectives*

"Area" refers to the specific performance area to which the instructional objective relates, for example, language or articulation.

"Instructional Objectives" indicate the specific behaviors that will be acquired as the child moves toward accomplishment of the annual goal. Each annual goal may have a number of instructional objectives depending on the intermediate steps needed to accomplish the goal. Each objective should include the components when, who, to whom, what, criterion, and evaluation.

IX. *Recommendations*

Primary or unique methods and materials that are needed to complete the instructional objectives are included under "recommendations." Recommendations should include the following components: what, how many, and how often.

X. *Status Report*

Including a "status report" section provides a method for reporting progress made in accomplishing objectives. On the date the instructional objective is to be accomplished, or on any other regularly scheduled review date, the evaluation component in the instructional objective can be executed. Progress the child has made in completing the objective can be indicated by using a status code. The "mastery codes" allow staff to indicate the amount of progress made by the child in those instances when 100% of the indicated criterion has not been met.

"Revision" made in any objective or "comments" on why the objective was not completed should be included to provide information that can be used in developing future IEPs.

Creating IEPs for a large caseload can be a very time-consuming task. Some clinicians have made the job more efficient by using computers and word processors. They select intervention goals from a data bank of goals and objectives. Appendix B provides an example of one such data bank developed by school clinicians in Stark County and Cincinnati, Ohio (1991). Wilson, Lanza, and Evans (1991) created a comprehensive resource containing functional IEP goals and

FIGURE 8.1. Summit County Public Schools

SUMMIT COUNTY PUBLIC SCHOOLS
Individualized Education Program

Richards _____
Local School District

☐ Initial Placement
☐ Periodic Review
☐ Amendment - Exit

Initial Placement Date: 9-15-92
Next Scheduled Review _____
Last MFE Date _____

IDENTIFYING INFORMATION:

Name Bill Prinzo   D.O.B. 7-11-83   C.A. 9.3   School Year 1992   Grade 4   Building Wayne

Parent/Guardian Norman and Shirley Prinzo

Address 301 Warren Ave   City Wilkins   Zip 12345   SS.# 410-68-5304

Phone 528-8524   District of Residence Richards

Recommended District/Agency _____

SPECIAL EDUCATION PROGRAM AND RATIONALE: Individual/small

group instruction for speech – language and collaboration with teachers

IEP AMENDMENT (Check as appropriate)

☐ Change Placement
☐ Same Placement but Change in Goals/Objectives Times. etc.
☐ Change of Related Service.
☐ Change of Participation in Regular Education.
☐ Discontinue Special Education Program and Services   If checked, indicate below the appropriate reason:

☐ Does not meet eligibility requirements
☐ Full time placement in Regular Education is considered to be the most appropriate placement.
☐ Student will follow Regular Education course of study
☐ Student has withdrawn.
☐ Student has graduated.

PLACEMENT AND RELATED SERVICES Check (✓) Needs

	Date Initiated	Anticipated Duration
☐ Regular Class		
☐ Supplemental Services		
☑ Individual/Small Group Instr.	9-15-92	6-5-93
☐ Special Class/Learning Center		
☐ School in Separate Facility*		
☐ Home Instruction*		
☑ Speech/Language	9-15-92	6-5-93
☐ Occupational Therapy (OT)		
☐ Transportation (TR)		
☐ Work-Study/Vocational (WS)		
☐ Physical Therapy (PT)		
☐ Other		

*PLACEMENT IN SEPARATE FACILITY (Complete if Applicable)   (BE SPECIFIC)

It is necessary to educate this student in a separate facility because: _____

_____

IEP WAS DEVELOPED BY THE FOLLOWING CONFERENCE PARTICIPANTS

Parent/Guardian: Norman & Shirley Prinzo   Date 9-15-92

Teacher: Brian Williams   Date 9-15-92

Speech-Lang Therapist: Sarah Retzer   Date 9-15-92

Psychologist: Mari Halkovich   Date 9-15-92

Other: James Broccio (teacher)   Date 9-15-92

District Rep: Brian Neidet   Date 9-15-92

Chairperson: Sarah Retzer   Date 9-15-92

AGREEMENT AND PLACEMENT: *I HAVE REVIEWED THIS IEP AND:*

✓ Agree with the program and placement recommendations.
___ Do not agree with the program and/or placement recommendations.
___ I waive my right to receive notification of placement by certified mail.
___ State and Federal Rules and Regulations mandate that every handicapped child be re-evaluated at least every three years. This is to notify you that your child will be provided that mandated re-evaluation prior to your child's next Annual Review.
___ I have received the due process information and been informed of the continuum of program options.

CIRCLE DEGREE OF PARTICIPATION IN REGULAR PROGRAM

(All Regular Classes)   Selected Regular Subjects   Non-Academic Activities

COMMENTS: If any, list regular subjects or activities.

_____
_____
_____
_____

Parent/Guardian Signature _____ Date _____

Superintendent/Designee _____ Date _____

SCSE 106 R 9/91

Reprinted with permission of The Summit County Board of Education, Akron, Ohio.

STUDENT: _____Bill Prinzo_____

Area of Instruction: Communication Skills   **Test Administered:** 1) Clinical Evaluation of Language Functions (CELF–R) **Score:** 66   –2.99

Summary of current performance: Adequate hearing vision & motor skills   2) Test of Written Language   70   –2.73
to complete instructions; difficulty following multiple-step instructions
presented verbally or in writing; improves if teacher gains attention to – and   3) Pragmatic Skills Checklist   Below expectations for age
uses strategies such as gestures, lists, varied voice patterns.   4) Language Sample   Below expectations for age

Annual Goals	Short-term Objectives	Criteria & Evaluation Procedures	Periodic Review	
To improve skills for listening and understanding classroom instructions presented orally and in writing	1) To maintain attention to teacher while instructions are delivered during reading, spelling and math.	(1-7) Teacher observation and checklist		
	2) To state instructions to a peer or the teacher to confirm understanding	(4,6) Periodic review of written work to determine improvement		
	3) To increase the number and complexity of instructions followed from sequences of 2-4.			
	4) To accurately perform tasks during classroom reading, spelling and math activities according to teacher's instructions	Criteria for all objectives: 3 out of 4 instances as measured during classroom activities		
	5) To identify written instructions by underlining or high lighting them on worksheets and in text books			
	6) To follow instructions of increasing complexity using a variety of language forms ("instead", "before", "after", "if", "but")			
	7) To use compensatory strategies when needed – ask peer or teacher for assistance			

* * * MASTERY CODES: M=Mastery   PM=Partial Mastery   NM=Non Mastery   or   percentages *** * ***

SCSE 106z R

(continued)

FIGURE 8.1. (Continued)

SUMMIT COUNTY PUBLIC SCHOOLS   Page __3__ of ____   I E P

STUDENT: ___Bill Prinzo___

Area of Instruction: ___Communication Skills___   Test Administered _____   See page 2   Score: ____
Summary of current performance:
Difficulty maintaining communication with others in small group and social situations; does not initiate conversation, take turns appropriately, or listen attentively.

Annual Goals	Short-term Objectives and Criteria	Criteria & Evaluation Procedures	Periodic Review
To demonstrate appropriate use of pragmatic strategies for social interaction and informal classroom activities.	1) To plan and organize thoughts prior to expressing them	(1-7) Guided teacher observation during informal and small group activities (once per week)	
	2) To develop awareness of conversation partners' nonverbal behaviors indicating a communication breakdown	(1-7) Completion of Teacher checklist (once per week)	
	3) To talk at appropriate times during informal conversations with peers	(8) SLP observe and complete checklist	
	4) To share information with peers during small group activities	(5) Language sample during structured activity (once per month) – SLP	
	5) To describe objectives or events to peers using appropriate semantics	(1-8) Readminister the Pragmatic check-list (once every 3 month)	
	6) To respond to topics discussed by peers with questions or comments.		
	7) To reduce inappropriate interruptions	Criteria for all objectives: 3 out of 4 instances as measured during classroom situations.	
	8) During a 5 minute conversation, maintain the topic and provide sufficient information for listeners to complete a task described.		

*** MASTERY CODES: M=Mastery   PM=Partial Mastery   NM=Non Mastery   or   percentages   ***

SCSE 106r R

212

objectives that are appropriate for children ages birth to 18. The resource, The IEP Companion, is available through LinguiSystems, Inc., 3100 4th Avenue, P.O. Box 747, East Moline, IL 61244.

Individualized Family Service Plan

Public Law 99-457 provides guidelines for serving the needs of infants and toddlers presenting developmental delays. The law requires that the services be multi-disciplinary and that service delivery plans reflect coordination of services among local agencies. Provision of services to the child's family is an integral component of the law. Federal regulations state that a systematic service plan be developed. This is referred to as the Individualized Family Service Plan (IFSP). The plan must span one year with a six-month review, specify outcomes for the child and family, and name a service coordinator from the profession most relevant to the child's or family's needs (1992). Collaboration is reinforced as a service delivery model for this population.

With the exception of services provided to the family and the emphasis on the child's health-related needs, several components in the IFSP are similar to those of the IEP. A meeting is held with the family and professionals who can provide services to the child. The goal of the meeting is to establish a plan for achieving the desired outcomes. Gillette and Robinson (1992) describe a process for developing an IFSP. They include a sample meeting agenda, time schedule for discussing pertinent topics, and sample planning forms. Prior to the meeting, the coordinator should gather pertinent background information about the child and family to facilitate greater understanding of the needs and possible ways to meet the needs.

The IFSP format can be used to focus the attention of meeting attendees and guide the discussion. A sample format is included in Figure 8-2. The components of the IFSP are similar to the IEP. The topics listed below should be addressed in writing and face to face during discussions:

1. Introductions and background information including identifying information about the child, family, and disciplines/agencies represented

2. An overview of current medical, health and rehabilitation services being provided to the child

3. A summary of the child's current health, development and family functioning including the child's strengths and needs and the family's strengths and needs in relation to the child

4. The child's health outcome, providers, and methods of service delivery including determining who will be the providers, the location, duration, frequency, and intensity of each service

5. The child's development outcome, providers, and methods; again determining professional providers, service schedules (numbers of contacts, length of contacts, and location of service), family involvement and measures of child development to be used

214

Chapter 8:
Intervention:
Planning,
Implement-
ing, Evalu-
ating

6. The family's life outcome, providers and methods; determining services which may be needed in the following areas: support, child care, education, family life planning, financial resources, and community resources

7. As the meeting draws to a close, a service coordinator should be identified.

FIGURE 8.2. Sample Individualized Family Service Plan

Date: Feb. 24, 1992	
Name: John Ondick	
Birthdate: Jan. 1, 1991	Corrected Birthdate: Feb. 5, 1991
Age: 13 Months	Corrected Age: 12 Months
Parents/Guardian: John & Mary Ondick	Relationship to Child (please circle)
Address: 1010 Sunset	biological parent, foster parent,
City: Home City	residential facility
State: Ohio 10101	Referred by: Children's Hospital
Phone: 222-2222	Referral Date: Jan. 5, 1991
County: Home County	Next review date: Aug. 24, 1991
School district/residence: Home City	

I. CHILD'S CURRENT SERVICES

Primary Physician: Dr. Mosnott
Nursing: Sharon Short, R.N., County Services
Early Intervention: Nancy Hill, Teacher; Annette Manning, Speech; (County) Trevor
  Blosser, Physical Therapy; Cheryl Pelland, Occupational Therapy
Human Services: Respite Services; Family Resources; Nutritional Funds
Other: Denise Wray, Summer Occupational Therapy; Dr. DePompei, Neonatology
  Follow-up Clinic; Dr. Jackson, Surgery; Dr. McCarthy, Opthamology; Dr.
  Butler, Cardiology; Dr. Ryan, Genetics; Dr. Renick, Neurosurgery
Case Manager: Nancy Hill, Teacher

II. SUMMARY OF CHILD/FAMILY CURRENT STATUS

Child Health (Past History, Current Status):

Differences from last plan: (1) shunt revision: 10/91; (2) hernia repair: scheduled for
  4/3/92; (3) chailasia scan 2/5/91 - mild reflux
Immunizations: DPT: 4/91; OPV: 4/91, 7/91; MMR: HIB:
Flu shot: 1/26/92
Nutrition: 2/6/92, videofluoroscopy - swallowing mechanism intact
Hearing: 1/26/92, hearing evaluation - behavioral - intact hearing
Vision: follow-up scheduled for 3/17/92
Technology Dependence: None

Child Development (Assessment, Date, Findings):
(Battelle 1/26/92 Age Equivalents)

Movement: 5 months
Communication: Receptive - 5 months; Expressive - 2 months
Understanding: 5 months
Social: 6 months

(continued)

FIGURE 8.2. (Continued)

Living Skills: 2 months
Other: INFANIB. Abnormal muscle tone - low

Family Functioning:

Financial Resources: Provider (Name, Address, Phone)
Insurance: HMO; 1212 Trail Rd., Home City, OH 10101
Public Assistance: (Medicaid, SSI): SSI for 2 older children
Other: (MCMH, Model 50, Family Resources): for nutritional supplement
    allowance
Transportation: added additional family car
Child Care: none
Respite Care: grandmother and county respite
Support Systems (family, church, counseling, etc.): extended family, many friends
Child's Strengths: enjoys moving and touching people and objects; smiles
Child's Needs: needs to improve eating habits and make weight gains; development
    in all areas delayed

**III. OUTCOMES - CHILD HEALTH, CHILD DEVELOPMENT, FAMILY
FUNCTIONING**

    A. Outcome: John will continue toward best possible health in terms of:

    (1) Eating and Growth (Methods and Providers):
        (a) Measure and chart weight, length, head circumference weekly.
            (Provider - county nurse)
        (b) Review measurements above monthly. (Provider - pediatrician)
        (c) Continue to feed John with nutritionally supplemented formula.
            (Provider - mother)
        (d) Regularly follow and revise oral motor skills program. (Provider - mother
            and county)
    (2) Breathing and Hearing Patterns
        (a) Review vital signa monthly. (Provider - family and pediatrician)
        (b) Attend scheduled cardiology appointments. (Provider - family and
            pediatrician)
    (3) Neurological Status
        (a) Monitor fontanelle and shunt site
        (b) Observe for signs of shunt malfunction
        (c) Attend hearing, vision, and neurosurgery appointments. (Provider for a,b,
            and c - family and neurosurgeon)
    (4) Routine Health Care
        (a) Schedule and attend appointments for follow-up of health status and
            immunizations. (Provider - family and pediatrician)

    B. Outcome: John will continue toward his best possible development integrating
the following skill areas: movement, understanding, communication, socialization,
self help.

    (1) Attend classes 2 times a week for 2 1/2 hours to address the 5 skill areas above
        and to plan home interventions and teach family skills.

(continued)

216

Chapter 8:
Intervention:
Planning,
Implement-
ing, Evalu-
ating

FIGURE 8.2. (*Continued*)

(2) Work towards self-help in feeding following plan under health.
(3) Attend evaluation at orthopedic clinic to determine best intervention and
   appropriate equipment for Mark's low tone.
(Provider for 1,2, and 3 - county, parent-infant program, teacher, speech,
 occupational and physical therapists, and family)

C. Outcome: The family will continue to meet John's needs with their choice of
health, developmental and social services.

(1) Continue to provide allowance for nutritional supplement. (Provider - county)
(2) Continue to take advantage of county and family for respite. (Provider - family)
(3) Explore financing through county's family resources for any equipment
   recommended. (Provider - family)

Planning and Evaluating the Lesson

There are considerations the school SLP needs to make when planning instructional objectives for individual lesson plans. First to be considered are the goals
for that particular lesson. What does the clinician hope to have the student
accomplish? Are the clinician's aims reasonable? Is the student aware of the
goals for that lesson? Has he or she helped formulate them? Do the clinician
and student agree on the goals? Will these goals bring them closer to the final
goal?

Along with the specific goals for éach therapy session, the clinician and
student must be in agreement on the general, or long-range, goals. In other
words, what is to be finally accomplished in the way of improvement of communication? In formulating the long-range goals, the physical, emotional, intel-
they produce only frustration and disappointment for both the clinician and the
student.

The next thing needed in the lesson plan is the list of materials. If the list
contains curricular materials, the subject, text, page numbers, and worksheets
should be listed. The list should be so complete that a person unfamiliar with the
session would be able to assemble the materials from the list. A complete listing
of materials will provide a ready future source of reference not only for the
beginning clinician but for the experienced therapist as well.

Following the list of materials, the lesson plan would then go on to the steps
or the procedures in the lesson. These can be listed in order of use and include
the estimated time for each. This would be particularly helpful to the beginning
clinician, who has not yet been able to judge accurately the amount of time
needed for each step. It is a common occurrence for the novice to complete all
the activities of the lesson in half the time allotted or else to complete only the
first few steps in the entire amount of time. It should be a comfort to the

beginning clinician to know that with continued experience comes a more accurate judgment of the passage of time during a therapy session.

The steps in the lesson should be based on the child's needs, the general and specific goals of therapy, and the evaluated results of the previous lesson. The clinician may wish to consult with the parents concerning home assignments or with the classroom teacher on generalization.

The clinician must have justification for listing the steps in a particular order; otherwise the therapy session becomes a hodgepodge of activities unrelated to the goals. On the other hand, the order of activities must not become so sacred that it cannot be changed. I recall one professor's lecture to a class in which she said, "I expect each student teacher to teach from a lesson plan, complete with goals, materials, estimated time for each activity, and the activities listed in order of presentation. But if I come into the room and find the student teacher teaching the right activity at the right time according to the clock and the lesson plan, I'll know there's something wrong with the lesson."

Her point, of course, is that any lesson plan, no matter how carefully thought out, should be abandoned or rearranged to suit the needs of the student. If Jimmy comes to speech class and proudly announces that he has a new baby sister, or if Susie wants to show off her new shoes, or if the first snow of the season has fallen during the night, all these things are much too important for the clinician to ignore and not utilize in the therapy session.

By using meaningful activities, curricular materials, and real-life situations, generalization becomes much less of a problem. The clinician doesn't fall into the trap of playing endless, meaningless games with the student.

In most schools, classroom teachers are required to submit lesson plans each week to the principal or curriculum supervisor. This is done for two reasons. One, if the teacher becomes ill, a substitute teacher can take over the class. Two, the teacher's plans can be monitored to make sure that curricular objectives are being met. Speech-language pathologists also need to keep their lesson plans current and have them available for review if asked.

Developing individualized lesson plans for large numbers of children can be a time-consuming and complex task for school clinicians. Experienced SLPs often evolve unique systems for preparing their lesson plans. Pascu-Godwin (1991) devised a comprehensive lesson planning procedure and form illustrated in Figure 8-3. She uses abbreviations, numbers, and codes to record therapy objectives and procedures for each child on the caseload. Her system enables planning for many children individually or in groups.

Motivation

Much has been written about motivation, and probably much more has been said. Everyone seems to be in agreement that motivation is necessary to produce good and lasting results in therapy. It is not uncommon to hear clinicians express the wish that they could motivate their client. This would imply that motivating is something one does to another person.

However, motivation is something that is within the person, driving him or her from inside. It is not realistic to think that clinicians are able to motivate

FIGURE 8.3. LESSON PLANS FOR COMMUNICATIVE DISORDERS

SCHOOL: _Smith School_   SPEECH-LANGUAGE CLINICIAN: _Vicky Pascu-Godwin_
DAY(S): _Mon. and Thurs._   TIME: _11:30 - 12:00 noon_   SCHOOL YEAR: _1991-92_
DELIVERY MODE: 1) PULL OUT, 2) CLASSROOM COLLABORATION, 3) TEACHER
           CONSULTATION, 4) COMMUNITY-BASED INTERVENTION

STUDENT	LESSON PLAN GOALS IN ACCORDANCE WITH IEP	DELIVERY MODE	ANNUAL REVIEW	ROOM
1.) Jennifer Midcap	↑ Receptive Language Skills ↑ Expressive Language Skills ↑ Pragmatic / Social Language Skills	1, 3	10-15-91	Kdg. 1
2.) Robert Williams [ESL]	↑ Expressive Language Skills ↑ Pragmatic / Social Language Skills	1, 3	5-30-92	Kdg. 1
3.) Rema Metcalf [H.I.]	↑ Receptive Language Skills ↑ Expressive Language Skills ↑ Pragmatic /Social Language Skills	1, 3	5-23-92	Kdg. 2

(↑) = To increase   (↓) To decrease

1. Attendance: A=Absent, E=Excused, T=Tardy, NS=No School; 2. Folder (if circled, folder not returned); 3. Homework due (if circled, assignment not returned on time); 4. Evaluation: M=Mastery, PM=Partial Mastery, NM=Non Mastery, %s

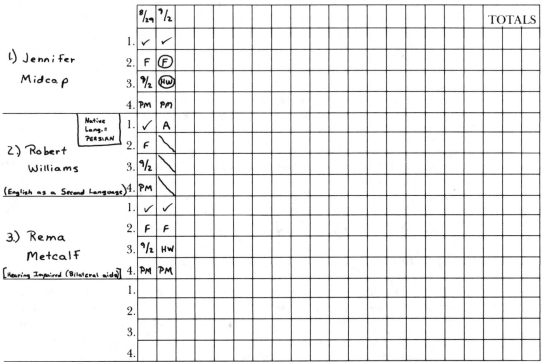

		8/29	9/2												TOTALS
1.) Jennifer Midcap	1.	✓	✓												
	2.	F	(F)												
	3.	9/2	(HW)												
	4.	PM	PM												
2.) Robert Williams (English as a Second Language) [Native Lang.= PERSIAN]	1.	✓	A												
	2.	F													
	3.	9/2													
	4.	PM													
3.) Rema Metcalf [Hearing Impaired (Bilateral aids)]	1.	✓	✓												
	2.	F	F												
	3.	9/2	HW												
	4.	PM	PM												
	1.														
	2.														
	3.														
	4.														

Developed by Vicki Pascu-Godwin.
Consultants: Patty Fry, Maureen Helt, Luan Korosa

(continued)

FIGURE 8.3. (Continued)

OBJECTIVES:	DATE		WEEK OF							
	8/29	9/2	9-9	9-16	9-23	9-30	10-7	10-14	10-21	10-28
I. Receptive Language Skills										
A. ↑ auditory identification of sounds	1,3									
B. ↑ auditory discrimination of sounds/words	1,3	1,3								
C. ↑ auditory memory for 2–3 step direction	1,3	1,3								
D. ↑ complex directions										
E. ↑ sentence recall		1,3								
F. ↑ details from paragraphs recall										
G. ↑ synonyms/antonyms/homonyms										
H. ↑ listening comprehension										
I. ↑ association/categorization										
J. ↑ wh/yes–no questions										
K. ↑ basic concepts development:										
L. ↑ figurative/literal/implied reasoning										
M. ↑ vocabulary										
N. ↑ logical thinking/reasoning										
O. ↑ grammar comprehension of words/sentences										
II. Expressive Language Skills										
A. ↑ morphology										
B. ↑ word recall/confrontational naming	✔	✔								
C. ↑ syntax	✔	✔								
D. ↑ interrogative form	✔	✔								
E. ↑ vocabulary	✔	✔								
F. ↑ describe words/define words	✔	✔								
G. ↑ word finding/closure		✔								
H. ↑ length of utterance		✔								
I. ↑ sentence recall										
J. ↑ sentence production for meaning										
K. ↑ unscramble sentences										
L. ↑ story production										
M. ↑ antonyms, synonyms, homonyms										
N. ↑ semantic absurdities										
O. ↑ associations/verbal reasoning/analogies										
P. ↑ sequencing										
III. Pragmatic/Social Language Skills										
A. ↑ eye contact/attention span	✔	✔								
B. ↑ use of appropriate gestures/facial expres.	✔	✔								
C. ↑ topic initiation, maint., and change	✔	✔								
D. ↑ ability to give directions	✔	✔								
E. ↑ appropriate social interchange	✔	✔								
F. ↑ perseveration										
III. Articulation Skills (Phonology)										
A. ↑ oral motor control aned coordination										
B. ↑ self-monitoring of speech										
C. ↑ auditory discrimination										
D. ↑ isolation/placement										
E. ↑ syllables										
F. ↑ initial word position										
G. ↑ final word position										
H. ↑ medial word position										
I. ↑ phrases										

(continued)

FIGURE 8.3. (Continued)

OBJECTIVES:	DATE										WEEK OF										
J. ↑ sentences																					
K. ↑ reading																					
L. ↑ conversational speech																					
V. *Fluency Skills* A. ↑ obtain baseline																					
B. ↑ fluent speech (↓ repetitions, ↓ hesitations, ↓ prolongations)																					
C. ↑ relaxation/desensitization																					
D. ↑ or ↓ rate of speech																					
E. ↑ stabilize, maintain, generalize fluency																					
VI. *Voice Skills* A. ↑ identify behaviors affecting voice																					
B. ↑ educate NORMAL vs. ABNORMAL function																					
C. ↑ improve vocal quality, pitch, intensity, nasality, range																					
D. ↑ vocal misuse and abuse																					
E. ↑ stabilize, maintain, generalize vocal behavior																					
MATERIALS/ACTIVITIES (See description on activities) NS (Non-Seasonal) S (Seasonal)	2,4,5	1,5,6																			
PROCEDURES: As stated in activity																					
listen	✔	✔																			
read		✔																			
say	✔	✔																			
write																					
motor																					
cue																					
look at	✔	✔																			

*This page flips over and represents ONE SEMESTER OF PLANNING. Only two of these pages are necessary for an entire year of planning per individual group.

MATERIALS/ACTIVITIES FOR LESSON PLANS

NS = NON-SEASONAL	S = SEASONAL
Tchr. Ther; Stud; Parent—Consultation/ Testing Duties mandated by State Standards 1. Blue Book p.p. 87–91	+R = Pumpkins, Ghosts SPEECH-TAC-TOE upon completion of artic., lang., fluency, etc. skill
Hearing screening, evaluation and/or 2. impedance audiometry	+R Spook Spots in conjuction with artic., lang., fluency, etc.... skill.
3. Articulation charting	Paper Bag Owl - Experience-Based Language Activity - follow directions as stated on activity card.
"Open Court": Alphabet / Word / Picture Chart "This is a **ball**, and it begins with **B**. 4. Capital **B**, Lower case b (say sound) b-b-b."	
(Add motions) Rhyme, Rhythm, Repetition - WHOLE LANGUAGE - Alligator Pie, Alligator Pie. If I don't get some I think I'm going to cry. Take away the green grass. Take away the sky, 5. but don't take away my Alligator Pie.	

(continued)

FIGURE 8.3. (Continued)

NS = NON-SEASONAL	S = SEASONAL
6. Barrier Board "SPEECH OFFICES" – To define and describe curriculum – related vocabulary using Alphabet/ Picture flash cards to match card in speech office. Take turns, listen, follow directions.	
7.	Turkey Trot – WH interrogatives
8.	Trim the Turkey – Rhyme Time
9.	Thanksgiving Popcorn Bingo – /r/
10.	" " " /s, z/
11.	" " " /L/
12.	" " " /θ, ǯ/
13.	
14.	
15.	Gingerbread Matching
16.	Snowman / Christmas Stocking SPEECH-TAC-TOE
17.	

clients. Rather, the recipients of our services will make a change in communication behavior only if personal values and attitudes impel them to do so.

The use of games, precision therapy, negative reinforcement, positive reinforcement, rewards, punishment, shaping behavior, and so on provides incentives, inducements, and spurs, which may bring about changes in behavior. If the inner drive, or the motivation, is absent, however, there may be regression or lack of what is commonly referred to as *carryover* or *generalization;* or there may be no change in behavior.

Although the clinician is highly anxious to change the child's speech be-

222

**Chapter 8:
Intervention:
Planning,
Implement-
ing, Evalu-
ating**

havior, it does not necessarily follow that the child will share that feeling. In some cases the child may be highly motivated to hang onto an immature speech and language pattern because it may be a way of coping with other members of the family. Or a child may enjoy the attention of the therapist so much that the child does not wish to improve and end the therapy sessions.

What are the implications for the clinician in regard to motivation in students? Raph (1960) suggested that there must be a shift of focus from a teacher-centered orientation of motivation to an understanding of the attitudes and values present in the child's motivation for learning. She has suggested that it would be desirable for the clinician to have some background in developmental psychology, some sensitivity to the nuances of the therapeutic relationship, and a willingness to learn as much as possible about an individual child's emotional functioning. She also suggested that understanding the feelings of the child may be as important as any diagnostic information that is gathered.

Evaluation of the Lesson

Following each session, the clinician should evaluate the effectiveness of the lesson. What should the evaluation include? In order to decide, let us look at the goals. Did this lesson accomplish the specific goals set forth in the lesson plan? Did the techniques employed bring about the desired results, or could the same results be accomplished by simpler, more direct methods? Did the student understand why he or she was doing certain things? In other words, did this lesson make sense to the student? Did it include an opportunity for generalization? For practice? For review?

Did this lesson have any relationship to the student's specific needs? Were the techniques and materials adapted to the appropriate age level, sex, interests, level of understanding? Paradoxically, it is possible for a lesson to be well taught and interesting to the student yet still not have any bearing on the communication problem and its eventual solution!

Was the clinician able to establish good rapport with the student? Was the clinician genuinely interested in both the student and the lesson? Did the clinician talk too much, or too little? Did both clinician and student seem to feel at ease? Was the clinician in charge of the lesson or did the student take over?

All of these questions need to be answered concerning every lesson. Too often the criteria for a therapy session are based on whether or not the student enjoyed it and whether or not good rapport existed between the student and the clinician. Although both are important, there is much more to a successful lesson. Careful preparation and careful evaluation of therapy sessions, both group and individual, are essential ingredients of good therapy.

The most effective clinicians we have observed have kept a running log of therapy, usually written immediately after each session. This is in addition to the lesson plan.

Lesson plans may serve still another purpose. When progress reports, case closure summaries, periodic evaluation reports, and letters are required, the lesson plan may serve as a source of referral and an evaluation of progress of therapy, and it could facilitate the writing of letters and reports.

Making Speech-Language Intervention Relevant to the Students' Educational Needs

School is a communication-based environment. Therefore, students who exhibit communication impairments are at risk for academic failure. Success in the school setting depends on the ability to communicate effectively in classroom and social situations where functional communication skills are necessary. For example, children must respond appropriately when asked questions. They must understand the meaning of vocabulary words and concepts unique to numerous subject areas. They are expected to interact socially with adults and peers. In order to gain information, they must be able to formulate questions and use appropriate phonology, syntax, semantics, and pragmatics so they can be understood by others. They have to understand relationships between sounds and symbols. It is essential for them to follow written and verbal instructions; organize thoughts in verbal and written expression; and comprehend large amounts of information presented by the teacher.

The school speech-language clinician can increase students' potential for success by making the intervention program relevant to students' academic needs. There are two ways this can be accomplished. One, the clinician can incorporate objectives and materials from the classroom into the therapy program. Two, the teacher can reinforce communication skills during classroom activities. Both of these methods require collaboration between the classroom teacher and speech-language clinician.

The creative clinician need only to look to the classroom to obtain materials and resources for the intervention program. Textbooks, workbooks, and teaching kits provide materials and activities which are age appropriate, interesting, and motivating to children. By developing speech-language therapy goals around the curriculum, the clinician can increase the student's chances of using appropriate communication skills while responding in the classroom. Following are examples of therapy goals based on curricular objectives and communication needs:

1. To appropriately respond to questions *from the end of the social studies chapter.*
2. To correctly produce target phonemes *taken from the student's weekly spelling list.*
3. To generate and combine sentences *about life's events to create an autobiography.*
4. To verbally recall details *from a story assigned in reading group.*
5. To verbally describe (in sequence) four steps to *a science experiment.*
6. To correctly explain *the rules to a sport being taught in gym class.*
7. To comprehend mathematical concepts *stressed in math class.*
8. To produce syntactically correct sentences *using the weekly vocabulary list from language arts class.*
9. To use appropriate pragmatic skills *during a small group craft activity.*
10. To use fluent speech to practice a *book report for English class.*

224

**Chapter 8:
Intervention:
Planning,
Implement-
ing, Evalu-
ating**

School clinicians must have a good understanding of the structure, scope, and sequence of the school curriculum followed for each grade and subject area in their school district. All school districts have manuals available describing these components and the competencies students are expected to gain as they progress through school. The manuals may be referred to by a number of names including "scope and sequence," "course of study," "school curricula," or "competency guidelines." The wise clinician will obtain a copy of the school curriculum from the curriculum director in the school district and make efforts to coordinate the speech-language program with the curriculum. An example of the scope and sequence for a Language Arts curriculum is provided in Appendix C to show you how valuable these materials can be for program planning.

It is helpful to provide teachers with specific suggestions for creating a "communication positive" climate in their classroom. This can be done by jointly arranging classroom materials, space, and activities so that communication exchanges will occur. With guidance from the SLP, teachers can learn to use several interactive communication strategies to elicit correct speech-language production, reinforce children's attempts to practice what they are learning in the therapy program, and facilitate correct productions when communication errors are observed. Several communication strategies teachers can implement are presented in Chapter 9. Fujiki and Brinton (1984) have provided some valuable suggestions on how the SLP can work with the classroom teacher on supplementing language therapy in the classroom. The teacher should:

1. Create a climate of emotional acceptance in the classroom that emphasizes communication

2. Become an attentive listener

3. Avoid complexity in conversation by using shorter utterances, avoiding ambiguous words, using direct requests, and adjusting the degree of conceptual difficulty and abstractedness of words

4. Use extra stress on important words

5. Utilize context as an aid to comprehension

6. Utilize specific techniques for talking with children

7. Encourage the child to make an unintelligible message more intelligible, while at the same time not allowing the child to become too frustrated

Considerations for Special Populations

Since the early 1970s the role of the SLP in the schools has moved into new areas. Much of the terminology has changed, research has added new dimensions, and service delivery methods are becoming more flexible and diverse. In the early days programs known as "speech improvement" were designed to help preschool and early primary children improve speaking and listening "habits." These programs also focused on pupils learning English as a second language and the eradication of substandard usage of the English language.

Interestingly enough, programs for special populations today have their roots in the concerns of the early practitioners. The prevention of speech, language, and hearing problems in infants and preschool children; the communication difficulties of bilingual and nonstandard speakers of English; and language disorders in children and adolescents all constitute areas of interest and concern for today's clinician.

There are many options for the delivery of educational services, which may include self-contained special classrooms, part-time resource rooms, or full-time integrated classes with monitoring or support services. The individual needs of the children determine the amount and type of supplemental services required. The speech-language clinician may be working with teachers of children who are developmentally delayed, emotionally disturbed, hearing impaired, or learning disabled. The children in these modules may also require the help of the reading teacher, academic tutor, psychologist, and others. This means that the school clinician will be working not only with the child's classroom teacher but also with other specialists as well as with the parents of the child.

In working with personnel in the other specialized fields, it is important to keep in mind that the instruction should be child-oriented. The specialists involved work as a team, and each team member has specific responsibilities that are known to themselves and other team members.

For example, in a program described by Parker (1972) in which the speech-language clinician was on a learning center team, the other full-time members included a special education teacher of children, a reading specialist, and a special learning disabilities teacher. Part-time members included a psychologist, a social worker, a hearing consultant, two tutors, a vocational rehabilitation counselor, and a school counselor. According to Parker, the team members did not teach content area subjects, but they did assist classroom teachers in developing and acquiring more diversified methods and materials. The team identified those students requiring team services; diagnosed the students' learning strengths and weaknesses; prescribed behavioral goals according to the students' needs; prescribed plans to carry out these goals; managed the prescribed plans; and evaluated the students' progress, prescribed plans, and methods.

The literature in the field of communication disorders provides professionals with extensive discussion of approaches for treating children with communication impairments. It is not the intent of this book to suggest specific methodologies. However, there are considerations which need to be made for special populations.

Culturally and Linguistically Diverse Populations

The issue of providing speech, language, and audiological services to children whose native language is not English or who speak different dialects has been a topic of intense discussion among professionals. Census figures in 1990 indicated that approximately 26% of the U.S. population is nonwhite. The number and proportion of minorities is increasing. It is projected that by the year 2000, 40% of the school population will be from ethnically diverse backgrounds.

Much of the intervention process is dependent upon the relationship established between the individual with a communication difference or impairment

226

Chapter 8:
Intervention:
Planning,
Implement-
ing, Evalu-
ating

and the clinician. Therefore, the relationship is affected when the client and clinician speak different languages or come from different cultural backgrounds. Clinicians need to have an understanding of the various cultures they will encounter in their communities. Acceptance of speech-language services may be affected by cultural variables such as traditions, customs, values, beliefs, and practices. It is important to know about the speech, language, and behavioral characteristics associated with specific cultures. It is essential to have knowledge of the unique aspects of a language in order to assess or remediate the phonemic, syntactic, morphological, semantic, lexical, or pragmatic characteristics. The clinician should become aware of specific assessment materials and treatment strategies known to be effective for particular ethnic populations. Caution must be taken to avoid making generalizations and formulating erroneous expectations. Terrell and Hale (1992) suggest that it is necessary for clinicians to modify intervention paradigms to incorporate alternate strategies and culturally distinct styles of learning.

With so much blending occuring in the world, it is hoped that future professionals demonstrate a high degree of cultural sensitivity. Clinicians can increase their awareness of the cultures they serve by gathering the following information about the ethnic groups in their communities (Hanson, Lynch, and Wayman, 1990):

—The countries of origin, languages spoken, and numbers of individuals from the ethnic group living in the community;

—The social organization of the ethnic group and resources available within the community;

—The prevailing belief system within the community including the values, ceremonies, and symbols important to that culture;

—The history of the ethnic group and current events directly and indirectly affecting the culture;

—The methods used by the members of the community to gain access to social services; and

—The attitudes of the group toward seeking assistance.

Various degrees of English proficiency may be observed in speakers from minority populations including those who are bilingual English proficient, limited English proficient, and limited in both English and their native language. Assessment and intervention should be conducted in the student's primary language for those who are limited in English.

According to Freeman (1977), "Dialectal differences cannot be construed as speech or language disorders. They are deviations from Standard American English which are based on the rules of the dialect, not on the speaker's ability to understand or speak. They reflect the internalization of the language rules of a primary culture or subculture."

In discussing the bilingual population in the schools, Work (1982) stated, "To consider these children speech-language disordered would be improper. Their difficulty with English is not due to a language disorder but to a language difference. Differences may be found in the linguistic structure, the phonological system, and the inflectional use of voice. Differences also exist in the cultural background at verbal and nonverbal levels."

There is little doubt that speech, language, and hearing deviations and disorders do exist among minority populations, including Hispanics, blacks, Asians (including Pacific Islanders), and American Indians (including Alaskan natives). In identifying communication disorders and deviations in minority populations, the SLP must be careful not to confuse a dialect with a communication disorder. According to a paper drafted by the Committee on the Status of Racial Minorities (1985), "It is apparent that the assessment and remediation of many aspects of speech, language, and hearing minority language speakers require specific background and skills. This is not only logical and sound clinical practice, but it is the consensus set forth by federal mandates. . . ." The report further indicated that state regulations are being developed to acknowledge the need for specific competencies to serve minority language populations. In California, for example, school districts are being encouraged by the education agency to require resource specialists, speech-language pathologists, and school psychologists to pass a state-administered oral and written examination on Hispanic culture, the Spanish language, and assessment methodology before they conduct assessments for Spanish-speaking children with limited English proficiency.

Harris (1985) discussed the importance of the clinician's investing time and effort to learn about the culture of the population that he or she serves. Harris, who was codirector of the Native American Research and Training Center, University of Arizona, stated,

> To appropriately measure and evaluate the English performance of minority language children on measures of speech and language, the examiner must be familiar with the behavioral characteristics of that group as they relate to language learning and language use. The level to which the particular child employs the traditional linguistic/cultural practices of his ethnic/minority group must be determined in order to assess his performance in an appropriate manner.

For example, requesting an Apache child to answer incessant questions, especially to answer in English, may put the child into a cultural conflict in which his or her resulting behavior (silence) may not be indicative of potential or knowledge but rather of cultural integrity.

This is not to say that school SLPs should not evaluate and provide services to children who have limited English proficiency and who have speech, language, or hearing handicaps. Interim strategies may be employed, such as utilizing interpreters or translators; establishing interdisciplinary teams, including a bilingual professional (for example, special education teacher or psychologist); or establishing cooperatives among school districts to hire an itinerant or consultant bilingual SLP or audiologist (Committee on the Status of Racial Minorities, 1985).

In regard to social dialects (black English, standard English, Appalachian English, southern English, New York dialect, Spanish-influenced English), it is the position of the American Speech-Language-Hearing Association (1983) that

228

**Chapter 8:
Intervention:
Planning,
Implement-
ing, Evalu-
ating**

. . . no dialectal variety of English is a disorder or a pathological form of speech or language . . . (however) it is indeed possible for dialect speakers to have linguistic disorders within the dialect. An essential step toward making accurate assessments of communicative disorders is to distinguish between those aspects of linguistic variation that represent the diversity of the English language from those that represent speech, language and hearing disorders.

Public Law 94-142 does not permit federal funds to be designated for services that are elective or for children who are not handicapped.

Attention Deficit and Central Auditory Processing Disorders

In order to benefit fully from the classroom situation, children have to be able to hear the teacher's message and understand what it means. Children who exhibit problems related to attention deficit and central auditory processing disorders are at risk for failure due to their inability to effectively process the information presented to them. They may have difficulty discriminating sounds, attending to spoken messages, making associations, recalling sequences of information, and processing the information they hear. Determining the existence of problems related to an auditory processing disorder is a complex task. There are several assessment and diagnostic tools which can be used to assess auditory processing skills. The educational audiologist and speech-language pathologist should be key members of the evaluation and planning team for this student.

The SLP can stress the importance of listening skills for the learning situation. In addition to providing direct instruction, clinicians can provide teachers with valuable information about techniques they can use to help students with these problems function more effectively in the classroom. Clark (1980) recommends that teachers use the following strategies for increasing listener potential: gain the student's attention, reduce distractions, provide preferential seating, monitor speaking delivery style, provide instructional transitions, block out auditory distractions, use visual and written teaching aids, avoid auditory exhaustion, check the student's concentration and comprehension, encourage participation, and provide support and reinforcement during learning activities.

Severe Communication Disabilities

There are approximately two million Americans who demonstrate severe communication disabilities. The federal laws have mandated the provision of services to children with severe and profound disabilities and has acknowledged that they may be educated to the extent that their limitations allow.

There is wide variation in the degree of disabilites demonstrated and capabilities of children who are impaired. Therefore, SLPs, teachers, and other school personnel must evaluate each child and plan an intervention program specific to that child's strengths and needs.

Some children with severe mental retardation or developmental delays do not begin to use words until the age of five or six, whereas others may learn to communicate by pointing and gesturing. Others with severe and profound deficits may never learn to communicate meaningfully. Early intervention, parent education, and interdisciplinary collaboration are important factors in a program for children with severe and profound mental retardation and developmental disabilities.

Some students have neuromuscular, neurological, or physical disabilities which are so severe that they are unable to use speech as a primary method of communication. They may even be unable to use standard augmentative communication techniques such as gestures, facial expressions, and writing. The disabilities may be the result of congenital conditions, acquired disabilities, or progressive neurological diseases. These students may have been diagnosed as having cerebral palsy, multiple sclerosis, oral or facial deformities, developmental verbal apraxia, autism, or dysarthria. They may also have central processing disorders or severe expressive aphasia. Children who acquire traumatic brain injuries or spinal cord injuries may have reduced communication skills. Many students who are unable to communicate verbally or vocally have normal or near normal receptive language abilities and normal nonverbal intelligence.

To treat children such as these, the SLP works closely with the family, regular and special education teachers, physical and occupational therapists, psychologists, and health professionals.

The National Joint Committee for the Communicative Needs of Persons with Severe Disabilities developed a number of recommendations for serving individuals with severe disabilities. The Committee was comprised of professionals representing a wide variety of disciplines including speech-language pathologists, special educators, occupational therapists, and physical therapists. Their recommendations included several principle tenets clinicians might use to guide their decision making for facilitating and enhancing communication among persons with severe disabilities: (a) communication is a social behavior; (b) effective communicative acts can be produced in a variety of modes; (c) appropriate communicative functions are those that are useful in enabling individuals with disabilities to participate productively in interactions with other people; (d) effective intervention must also include efforts to modify the physical and social elements of environments in ways that ensure that these environments will invite, accept, and respond to the communicative acts of persons with severe disabilities; (e) effective intervention must fully utilize the naturally occurring interactive contexts (e.g., educational, living, leisure, and work) that are experienced by persons with severe disabilities; and (f) service delivery must involve family members or guardians and professional and paraprofessional personnel (National Joint Committee for the Communicative Needs of Persons with Severe Disabilities, 1992).

Intervention goals generally emphasize development of self-help skills and social and adaptive behavior. It is important to select activities which are representative of common situations which may occur in the pupil's experiences.

The speech and language services provided depend on the needs of each child. Vanderheiden and Yoder (1986) list numerous responsibilities SLPs may undertake when treating persons with severe expressive communication disorders:

230

**Chapter 8:
Intervention:
Planning,
Implement-
ing, Evalu-
ating**

- Assessing, describing, documenting, and evaluating the communication needs;
- Evaluating and assisting in the selection communication aids and techniques;
- Developing speech and vocal communication to the fullest extent possible;
- Evaluating and selecting the symbols for use with the selected techniques;
- Developing and evaluating the effectiveness of intervention procedures to teach skills and strategies necessary to utilize augmentative communication in an optimal manner;
- Integrating assessment and program procedures with family members and other professional team members;
- Training persons who interact with the individual; and
- Coordinating augmentative communication services.

The speech and language services provided depend on the diagnosis of each child. The most advantageous method or methods of communication are determined and may include gestural systems if appropriate, symbol systems, and orthographic or pictorial systems. Depending on the mode of communication selected, the process may include augmentative communication devices such as communication boards, computerized devices, speech output devices, synthetic voice instruments, word processors, and other electronic and mechanical apparatus.

An intervention method found to be successful with clients who have no effective means of communicating is *facilitated communication* (Biklen, 1992). The client types in order to communicate with others. It has been used successfully with autistic individuals as well as people who have neuromotor difficulties such as apraxia. Biklen describes the basic elements of the procedure as follows: the client selects the letters and words to type but is given physical support by another individual (referred to as the facilitator); initial training methods elicit messages from the client which are predictable by using names, matching exercises, and cloze procedures; the facilitator helps the client maintain focus on the activity by providing reminders and guidance if extraneous actions occur; the client is treated as competent and provided with emotional support and encouragement rather than testing to determine competence levels; specific efforts are undertaken to help the client generalize the skills beyond one or two familiar facilitators; and as the student becomes more independent over time, the physical support provided by the facilitator is faded over time.

Autism

Autism is a neurological disability that interferes with the normal development of effective reasoning, social interaction, and communication skills. Some refer to autism as "the ultimate learning disability." Persons with autism experience difficulty understanding what they see, hear, and sense. They are unable to communicate effectively with others and relate to the world outside of the self (Autism Society of Ohio, 1992).

Public Law 101-476 required that school districts take steps to identify and serve students with autism. Because communication skills are so greatly affected by this disability, the SLP plays an important role in assessing and planning intervention for students with autism. Clinicians should be familiar with the characteristics of autism and accepted procedures for evaluating students. Several characteristics associated with this devastating disability are: severe delays in development of communication skills and understanding of social relationships; inability to recognize and respond to the behavior and communication of others; problems with judgement and recognition of simple cause and effect; inconsistent response (oversensitivity or undersensitivity) to sensations of touch, sight, and sound; variable patterns of intellectual functioning (individuals may show high level skills in one domain and contrastingly low performance in another); and restriction of activities and interests including repetition of body movements and routines. Many of these characteristics are symptomatic of other severe disabilities. Therefore, it is important that the diagnosis of autism be made by a team of health care and special education professionals who are familiar with the characteristics of autism.

Development of treatment strategies for this group of individuals is still in its infancy. Although the literature about intervention is growing rapidly, a definitive set of answers regarding the most effective methodologies has not yet been generated. Some general suggestions are to develop functional communication and learning goals to encourage safety and independence, use intervention techniques that emphasize development of pragmatic language skills, work within a highly structured format, stress generalization of skills to various situations outside of the therapy or classroom context, use augmentative communication strategies, and incorporate the family into treatment planning and implementation.

Hearing Impairments

Management of hearing loss should be overseen by the educational audiologist. Most school districts do not employ audiologists. They must rely on services provided on a shared or contractual basis. In the absence of a staff audiologist, the speech-language pathologist has greater understanding of hearing loss than any other professionals in the school setting. There are several aspects of care for these children for which the SLP may be responsible including making medical and audiological referrals when indicated, facilitating acquisition and use of assistive listening strategies and devices, developing teachers' awareness and understanding of hearing loss, making recommendations for general education programming, developing speech and language skills, and monitoring the student's hearing aids.

It is important for educators and parents to understand the problems children will experience if their hearing is impaired. Even mild hearing loss can greatly impact upon school success. Flexer (1991) states that "all hearing losses involve educational issues and some also involve medical issues." In the absence of the educational audiologist, the SLP is the most appropriate person for conveying this information to others.

Flexer, Wray, and Ireland (1989) suggest that speech-language pathologists

232

Chapter 8:
Intervention:
Planning,
Implement-
ing, Evalu-
ating

need to be aware of three areas which are critical to classroom success for children with hearing impairments: hearing and the impact of hearing loss on classroom performance; the use of sound enhancement technology for habilitation and environmental access for persons who are hearing impaired; and, the use of educational management strategies which emphasize hearing rather than minimize it. They offer the following list of hearing-oriented topics to assist the speech-language pathologist in delivering adequate services and answering pertinent questions posed by teachers who have children who are hearing impaired in their classrooms:

I. Hearing
— Classrooms are auditory-verbal environments with "listening" serving as the basis for classroom performance.
— Hearing loss occurs along a broad continuum ranging from a mild hearing loss to profoundly hearing-impaired; not as two discrete groupings of normally hearing or deaf. In fact, about 92% to 94% of hearing-impaired persons are functionally hard-of-hearing and not deaf.
— Hearing loss, whether mild or profound in nature, negatively impacts on verbal language, reading, writing, and academic performance.
— Speech may be audible to someone with a hearing loss, but not necessarily intelligible enough to hear one word as distinct from another.

II. FM Equipment
— Persons with hearing losses need the signal of choice to be 10 times more intense than background sounds in order for speech to be intelligible; an impossible classroom listening situation.
— Appropriately fit sound enhancement equipment, typically FM units (in addition to wearable hearing aids), are necessary for any hearing-impaired child with any degree of hearing loss to function in a mainstreamed classroom because this equipment improves the Signal-to-Noise ratio.
— FM equipment must be fit by an audiologist who is mindful of:
  a. The acoustic characteristics of the equipment;
  b. Methods of coupling equipment to personal hearing aids;
  c. Psycho-social issues of visual deviance;
  d. Multiple equipment settings to allow flexibility in various listening environments.
— FM equipment must be functioning and teachers must be comfortable with its use, or it is of no value.
— The Ling 5 Sound Test is one method by which the classroom teacher can screen equipment function.

III. Educational Management Strategies Which Focus on Hearing
— Auditory Skills training and development should be implemented during all therapy and classroom activities.
— "Listen," as a cue word used by all staff, can alert the hearing-impaired child to upcoming instructions.

— Teachers are encouraged to repeat or rephrase comments from other students in the classroom.
— Pre and Post tutoring programs can provide necessary redundancy of instructional information.

Anderson (1991) provides a summary of the relationship of the degree of long term hearing loss to the psychosocial and educational needs of children (see Table 8-1). She describes problems and barriers that may be encountered and recommends educational strategies for treating children with varying hearing losses. She suggests that special education programming may be appropriate to meet the needs of individuals with any and all degrees of hearing loss. When making educational decisions, the special education placement team should consider the full range of service delivery options. This would include integrating the child into the regular education classroom and providing teacher inservice and supportive services. With adequate training and comprehensive support services, the regular education classroom teacher can have increased awareness of the impact of hearing impairment on a student's classroom function, and learn to adequately meet the student's needs.

In some school districts, SLPs take responsibility for teaching students with hearing impairments to communicate. The Listen Foundation (1991) describes five approaches which are frequently used.

1. The *auditory-verbal* method teaches children to use their residual hearing to learn spoken language. Integration into the hearing world is stressed. Appropriately fitted hearing aids and assistive listening devices are essential.

2. The *auditory-oral* approach is similar. It also uses aided hearing. Intervention is usually presented individually or in small groups and also teaches lip reading.

3. The *oral* approach introduces hearing during specific auditory lessons, and places emphasis on lip reading and written communication.

4. *Total communication* provides the child with a variety of communication methods simultaneously including signs, fingerspelling, lip reading, speech, and use of residual hearing.

5. *Manualism* does not consider spoken language as a necessary component for communication. It considers sign language as the natural language of all deaf persons.

Parents should be provided with a clear explanation of all of these methods and invited to participate in the selection of a teaching method. Of course, before the SLP undertakes implementing a particular method, he or she should understand the philosophical basis and implementation techniques.

Children with hearing impairments should be monitored by an audiologist to ensure that they see a physician when necessary and that they are properly fitted for hearing aids and assistive listening devices. Lesner (1991) recommends that the SLP maintain records on the students' hearing aids (Figure 8-4). She also

TABLE 8.1. RELATIONSHIP OF DEGREE OF LONG-TERM HEARING LOSS TO PSYCHOSOCIAL IMPACT AND EDUCATIONAL NEEDS

Degree of Hearing Loss Based on Modified Pure Tone Average (500–4000 HZ)	Possible Effect of Hearing Loss on the Understanding of Language & Speech	Possible Psychosocial Impact of Hearing Loss	Potential Educational Needs and Programs
Normal Hearing −10–+15 dB HL	Children have better hearing sensitivity than the accepted normal range for adults. A child with hearing sensitivity in the −10 to +15 dB range will detect the complete speech signal even at soft conversation levels. However, good hearing does not guarantee good ability to discriminate speech in the presence of background noise.		
Minimal (borderline) 16–25 dB HL	May have difficulty hearing faint or distant speech. At 15 dB student can miss up to 10% of speech signal when teacher is at a distance greater than 3 feet and when the classroom is noisy, especially in the elementary grades when verbal instruction predominates.	May be unaware of subtle conversational cues which could cause child to be viewed as inappropriate or awkward. May miss portions of fast-paced peer interactions which could begin to have an impact on socialization and self concept. May have immature behavior. Child may be more fatigued than classmates due to listening effort needed.	May benefit from mild gain/low MPO hearing aid or personal FM system dependent on loss configuration. Would benefit from soundfield amplification if classroom is noisy and/or reverberant. Favorable seating. May need attention to vocabulary or speech, especially with recurrent otitis media history. Appropriate medical management necessary for conductive losses. Teacher requires inservice on impact of hearing loss on language development and learning.
Mild 26–40 dB HL	At 30 dB can miss 25–40% of speech signal. The degree of difficulty experienced in school will depend upon the noise	Barriers beginning to build with negative impact on self esteem as child is accused of "hearing when he or she wants to,"	Will benefit from a hearing aid and use of a personal FM or soundfield FM system in the classroom. Needs favorable

Degree of Hearing Loss	Possible Impact on Understanding of Language and Speech	Possible Psychosocial Impact of Hearing Loss	Potential Educational Needs and Programs
	...level in classroom, distance from teacher and the configuration of the hearing loss. Without amplification the child with 35–40 dB loss may miss at least 50% of class discussions, especially when voices are faint or speaker is not in line of vision. Will miss consonants, especially when a high frequency hearing loss is present.	"daydreaming," or "not paying attention." Child begins to lose ability for selective hearing, and has increasing difficulty suppressing background noise which makes the learning environment stressful. Child is more fatigued than classmates due to listening effort needed.	seating and lighting. Refer to special education for language evaluation and educational follow-up. Needs auditory skill building. May need attention to vocabulary and language development, articulation or speechreading and/or special support in reading. May need help with self esteem. Teacher inservice required.
Moderate 41–55 dB HL	Understands conversational speech at a distance of 3–5 feet (face-to-face) only if structure and vocabulary controlled. Without amplification the amount of speech signal missed can be 50% to 75% with 40 dB loss and 80% to 100% with 50 dB loss. Is likely to have delayed or defective syntax, limited vocabulary, imperfect speech production and an atonal voice quality.	Often with this degree of hearing loss, communication is significantly affected, and socialization with peers with normal hearing becomes increasingly difficult. With full time use of hearing aids/FM systems child may be judged as a less competent learner. There is an increasing impact on self-esteem.	Refer to special education for language evaluation and for educational follow-up. Amplification is essential (hearing aids and FM system). Special education support may be needed, especially for primary children. Attention to oral language development, reading and written language. Auditory skill development and speech therapy usually needed. Teacher inservice required.
Moderate to Severe 56–70 dB HL	Without amplification, conversation must be very loud to be understood. A 55 dB loss can cause child to miss up to 100% of speech information. Will have marked difficulty in school situations requiring verbal communication in both one-to-one and group situations. Delayed language,	Full time use of hearing aids/FM systems may result in child being judged by both peers and adults as a less competent learner, resulting in poorer self concept, social maturity and contributing to a sense of rejection. Inservice to address these attitudes may be helpful.	Full time use of amplification is essential. Will need resource teacher or special class depending on magnitude of language delay. May require special help in all language skills, language based academic subjects, vocabulary, grammar, pragmatics as well as reading and writing. Probably needs

(continued)

TABLE 8.1. (Continued)

Degree of Hearing Loss Based on Modified Pure Tone Average (500–4000 HZ)	Possible Effect of Hearing Loss on the Understanding of Language & Speech	Possible Psychosocial Impact of Hearing Loss	Potential Educational Needs and Programs
	syntax, reduced speech intelligibility and atonal voice quality likely.		assistance to expand experiential language base. Inservice of mainstream teachers required.
Severe 71–90 dB HL	Without amplification may hear loud voices about one foot from ear. When amplified optimally, children with hearing ability of 90 dB or better should be able to identify environmental sounds and detect all the sounds of speech. If loss is of prelingual onset, oral language and speech may not develop spontaneously or will be severely delayed. If hearing loss is of recent onset speech is likely to deteriorate with quality becoming atonal.	Child may prefer other children with hearing impairments as friends and playmates. This may further isolate the child from the mainstream, however, these peer relationships may foster improved self concept and a sense of cultural identity.	May need full-time special aural/oral program with emphasis on all auditory language skills, speechreading, concept development and speech. As loss approaches 80–90 dB, may benefit from a Total Communication approach, especially in the early language learning years. Individual hearing aid/personal FM system essential. Need to monitor effectiveness of communication modality. Participation in regular classes as much as beneficial to student. Inservice of mainstream teachers essential.
Profound 91 dB HL or more	Aware of vibrations more than tonal pattern. Many rely on vision rather than hearing as primary avenue for communication and learning. Detection of speech sounds	Depending on auditory/oral competence, peer use of sign language, parental attitude, etc., child may or may not increasingly prefer association with the deaf culture.	May need special program for deaf children with emphasis on all language skills and academic areas. Program needs specialized supervision and comprehensive support

...dependent upon loss configuration and use of amplification. Speech and language will not develop spontaneously and is likely to deteriorate rapidly if hearing loss is of recent onset.			...services. Early use of amplification likely to help if part of an intensive training program. May be cochlear implant or vibrotactile aid condidate. Requires continual appraisal of needs in regard to communication and learning mode. Part-time in regular classes as much as beneficial to student.
Unilateral One normal hearing ear and one ear with at least a permanent mild hearing loss	May have difficulty hearing faint or distant speech. Usually has difficulty localizing sounds and voices. Unilateral listener will have greater difficulty understanding speech when environment is noisy and/or reverberant. Difficulty detecting or understanding soft speech from side of bad ear, especially in a group discussion.	Child may be accused of selective hearing due to discrepancies in speech understanding in quiet versus noise. Child will be more fatigued in classroom setting due to greater effort needed to listen. May appear inattentive or frustrated. Behavior problems sometimes evident.	May benefit from personal FM or soundfield FM system in classroom. CROS hearing aid may be of benefit in quiet settings. Needs favorable seating and lighting. Student is at risk for educational difficulties. Educational monitoring warranted with support services provided as soon as difficulties appear. Teacher inservice is beneficial.

Note: All children with hearing loss require periodic audiologic evaluation, rigorous monitoring of amplification and regular monitoring of communication skills. All children with hearing loss (especially conductive) need appropriate medical attention in conjunction with educational programming.

REFERENCES

Olsen, W. O., Hawkins, D. B., VanTassell, D. J. (1987). Representatives of the Longterm Spectrum of Speech. *Ear & Hearing*, Supplement 8, pp. 100–108.

Mueller, H. G. & Killion, M. C. (1990). An easy method for calculating the articulation index. *The Hearing Journal*, 43, 9, pp. 14–22.

Hasenstab, M. S. (1987). *Language Learning and Otitis Media*, College Hill Press, Boston, MA.

Developed by Karen L. Anderson, Ed.S & Noel D. Matkin, Ph.D (1991).

Adapted from: Bernero, R. J. & Bothwell, H. (1966). Relationship of Hearing Impairment to Educational Needs. Illinois Department of Public Health & Office of Superintendent of Public Instruction.

Peer Review by Members of the Educational Audiology Association, Winter 1991.

*Reprinted with permission of authors and *Seminars in Hearing*.

238

Chapter 8:
Intervention:
Planning,
Implement-
ing, Evalu-·
ating

FIGURE 8.4. HEARING AID DATA SHEET

STUDENT: _____   Date: _____

SCHOOL: _____

Hearing Aid Information	*Right Ear*	*Left Ear*
Make/Model	_____	_____
Serial Number	_____	_____
Date of Manufacture	_____	_____
Battery Size	_____	_____
Battery Type	_____	_____
Volume Control Setting	_____	_____
Tone Control Setting	_____	_____
Output Control Setting	_____	_____
Compression Control Setting	_____	_____

OTHER:

*Developed by Sharon A. Lesner, The University of Akron. Reprinted with permission.

developed a protocol SLPs can follow to determine if students' hearing aids are functioning properly (Figure 8-5).

Traumatic Brain Injury

Each year, over one million American children and youths sustain a traumatic brain injury (TBI) as a result of motor vehicle accidents, falls, sports injuries, and abuse. Years ago, many of these children would have died. However, due to decreased emergency response time and improved medical treatment, lives are now being saved. Approximately 165,000 of the children injured will have to be hospitalized and 16,000 to 20,000 will suffer from severe or moderate symptoms as a result of their injuries (Savage, 1991).

Traumatic brain injury may affect children's capabilities in a broad number of areas including physical, cognitive, communicative, behavioral, and social

FIGURE 8.5. PROTOCOL FOR HEARING AID CHECKS

Visual Inspection
1. Clean case with no cracks
2. Clean microphone opening
3. Volume control moves smoothly
4. No signs of moisture in the tubing or earhook
5. Earhook securely attached to hearing aid
6. No breaks or cracks in earhook
7. Tubing securely attached to hearing aid
8. Tubing is not yellowed, hardened, brittle, or broken
9. MTO switch set correctly
10. Volume control set correctly
11. Tone control set correctly
12. Well fitting earmold
13. Earmold condition satisfactory (not cracked or chipped)
14. Clean earmold bore

Battery Check
1. Battery positioned correctly
2. Clean, non-corroded battery contacts
3. Battery appropriately charged (1.1 volts+)

Listening check while you listen with a hearing aid stethoscope
1. Sufficient output
2. No tinny, muffled, or raspy output
3. No scratchy or crackling sound when volume control is moved
4. No hum or buzz
5. No intermittent sound when case is rotated
6. Quality of the "Five Sound Test"

Listening check while the student listens
1. Lack of feedback when the hearing aid is in the student's ear
2. All sounds of the "Five Sound Test" are detected

*Developed by Sharon A. Lesner, The University of Akron. Reprinted with permission.

skills. While many problems exist with this population following injury, the cognitive-communicative impairments experienced appear to be the main barriers to successful reintegration into home, school, and community.

As an SLP you will be one of the most valuable members on the planning team for this student. Blosser and DePompei (1992) recommend the following assessment strategies prior to planning a treatment program for students with TBI:

1. conduct an environmental assessment to determine communicative situations which might pose difficulty for the student;

2. determine the communication needs required to meet classroom objectives and daily classroom requirements; and

3. analyze the communication behaviors of key persons with whom the student will be interacting.

240

**Chapter 8:
Intervention:
Planning,
Implement-
ing, Evalu-
ating**

Based on the information gathered, they suggest that the SLP work with the student's family and teachers to restructure the environment and modify communicative interactions in order to strengthen communications skills. Recuperation from TBI may be ongoing for years. Students' behaviors may change drastically in that time period. Consequently, more frequent evaluations and revisions of the IEP are required.

The chart in Table 8-2 illustrates a few representative examples of the deficits students with TBI may exhibit, the resulting behaviors teachers might observe in the classroom situation, and the cognitive-communicative intervention strategies which would be effective for developing communicative skills

TABLE 8.2. COGNITIVE-COMMUNICATIVE IMPAIRMENTS, REPRESENTATIVE CLASSROOM BEHAVIORS, AND RECOMMENDED COGNITIVE-COMMUNICATIVE INTERVENTION STRATEGIES
(Blosser and DePompei, 1992)

Cognitive-Communicative Impairments	Behavior	Cognitive-Communicative Strategy
Word retrieval errors.	Answers contain a high use of "this," "that," "those things," "whatchamacallits." Difficulty providing answers on fill-in-the-blank tests.	WORD RECALL: Teach the student association skills and to give definitions of words he can not recall. Teach memory strategies (rehearsal, association, visualizations, etc. . . .).
Verbal problem solving ability is reduced.	In algebra class, the student may arrive at a correct answer but not be able to recite the steps followed to solve the problem.	PROBLEM SOLVING: Teach inductive and deductive reasoning at appropriate age levels.
Poor reasoning skills.	After behaving inappropriately, the student is unable to discuss actions with teacher.	REASONING: Privately (not during classroom situations or in front of peers) ask the student to explain answers and provide reasons.
Reduced ability to use abstractness in conversation (ambiguity, satire, inferences, drawing conclusions).	Says things that classmates interpret as satirical, funny, or bizarre although they were not intended to be that way.	SEMANTICS: Teach the student common phrases used for satire, idioms, puns, etc. . . .
Delayed responses.	When called upon to give the answer, the student will not answer immediately, appearing not to know the answer.	PROCESSING: Allow extra time for the student to discuss and explain. Avoid asking too many questions.
Unable to describe events in appropriate detail and sequence.	When relating an experience, details are out of order, confused, or overlapping.	SEQUENCING: Teach sequencing skills. Direct the context of the student's responses.
Inadequate labelling or vocabulary to convey clear messages.	Inappropriately labels tools in industrial arts class.	SEMANTICS: Teach the student vocabulary associated with specific areas and classroom activities.

(Blosser and DePompei, 1992). Information such as this can be helpful when collaborating with teachers and parents or planning the IEP.

Reading and Writing Disabilities

Many of the same children who exhibit communication impairments also demonstrate reading and writing difficulties. It is important, therefore, for SLPs to understand the relationship between oral and written language. Current research supports using a whole language approach to develop spoken as well as written language skills (Norris and Damico, 1990). This approach is based on the philosophy that language learning should be an integrated process involving interactive and naturalistic intervention practices. Emphasis is placed upon teaching language and reading skills using real conversational contexts and situations.

The components of language and reading are not fragmented into separate components (such as phonology, morphology, syntax, semantics, and pragmatics). Rather, communication is presented as a whole process to be used to understand and transmit meaning. Clinicians who are experienced in using the whole language approach suggest that the SLP work closely with the classroom teacher to plan meaningful learning activities, provide realistic and functional opportunities for facilitating communication, and encourage the student to actively participate during the learning activities. The whole language approach is applicable to all children who demonstrate language disabilities.

Gruenewald and Pollak (1973) described the clinician's role in helping primary classroom teachers develop strategies for teaching the auditory skills necessary in learning to read. They suggested that the clinician utilize knowledge of auditory processes in diagnosing and analyzing auditory skills such as listening attention, identification and localization, discrimination, auditory sequencing and memory, and auditory association and closure. According to Gruenewald and Pollak the appraisal of reading readiness is often weighted heavily toward visual discrimination tasks or the combination of visual and auditory tasks, to the exclusion of auditory learning tasks.

Gruenewald and Pollak stated that although speech clinicians are generally not trained to teach reading as a process, they are trained in the auditory aspects of speech and language development and must not isolate themselves from the total learning process:

> We are suggesting that the clinician use knowledge of auditory processes to assist the primary teacher in diagnosing needs and implementing group and individual programs in the developmental aspects of reading. Our unique contribution to the educational team can be the analysis of speech, language, and auditory learning upon which further symbolic and academic skills are built.

Following is a diagnostic outline showing auditory activities involved in reading readiness (starred items). The outline was developed by Gruenewald and

242

**Chapter 8:
Intervention:
Planning,
Implement-
ing, Evalu-
ating**
Pollak, along with the developmental reading specialist in the Madison, Wisconsin, public schools to provide a framework for the classroom teacher in assessing reading readiness skills (starred items indicate auditory activities):

1. Some components of reading readiness assessment
   A. Following directions
      *(1) Attending behavior (visual and auditory contact)
      *(2) Language of instruction (comprehension of task)
      (3) Performance of task (at what level?—motor, perceptual, conceptual, verbal)
   *B. Language
      (1) Nonverbal
      (2) Social
      (3) Comprehension (nonverbal-verbal)
      (4) Verbal (structure and content)
      (5) Conceptual parameters (classification and relationship)
   *C. Auditory behavior
      (1) Listening behavior
      (2) Recognition, identification, and localization of sound
      (3) Discrimination
         a. Concept: same-different
         b. Nonverbal: sound, pitch, rhythm
         c. Verbal: letter sounds, words
      (4) Auditory memory and sequencing (nonverbal and verbal)
      (5) Auditory association
      (6) Auditory closure
   D. Visual behavior
      (1) Visual reception
      (2) Visual recognition and identification
      (3) Visual discrimination
      (4) Visual memory and sequencing
      (5) Visual association
      (6) Visual closure
   E. Motor behavior
      (1) Gross motor performance
      (2) Fine (visual-motor)
         a. Hand-eye functioning
         b. Eye focus

c. Tracking

d. Midline structure

Wray and Watson-Florence (1984) suggested that SLPs demonstrate activities and strategies for classroom teachers to improve reading proficiency in the classroom. These strategies are based on a language theory paradigm and are in concert with the daily curriculum. In this type of model the SLP shares information on the "language-reading connection" with the teacher, and together they plan the structuring and achieving of goals for the language-delayed child at risk for reading development.

According to Wray and Watson-Florence,

> Guidelines are provided to aid the speech-language pathologist in creating an integrated communication curriculum to be used to teach reading skills. Activities designed to improve oral language development and usage will be related to exercises stressing reading development and usage. To avoid fragmented learning experiences, the child's language program in areas such as writing, spelling, reading, speech and auditory training will be coordinated and based on overall language acquisition. These ideas will be based on the assumption that demonstration for the teacher will initially take place with the speech-language consultant gradually assisting the teacher to independently implement these ideas in the daily curriculum.

Language Procedures to Facilitate Reading Skills

Wray and Watson-Florence suggest activities that:

Stress discrimination among speech sounds to teach grapheme/phoneme correspondence

Teach listeners to discriminate various stress patterns across words

Teach auditory awareness of where one word stops and another begins

Develop semantic awareness of word labels and functions

De-emphasize accuracy and encourage rhythm and melody during oral reading

Acknowledge the child's dialect

Write stories composed by the children using their language patterns

Have adults read various types of materials to children

Involve the children as active participants in meaningful language/reading activities

Demonstrate how stories are typically organized

Demonstrate how to ask questions to obtain additional information

Introduce vocabulary concepts systematically using grouping techniques

Stress comprehension skills

Select vocabulary and reading material from the child's basal reader making certain the reading level is easy

244

**Chapter 8:
Intervention:
Planning,
Implement-
ing, Evalu-
ating**

Apply compare/contrast techniques to language instruction

Present the reading words in the context of a phrase using a modifier or verb, not in isolation

Reading is one of the most important skills taught in the school. Classroom teachers in the primary and early elementary grades are responsible for teaching reading, and the reading specialist in the school system is responsible for helping the child with a reading problem. Sometimes this is done directly with the child and sometimes it is accomplished indirectly through the teacher.

Classroom teachers often use quick screening instruments to place students at appropriate reading levels. Children having reading difficulties are referred for a thorough reading analysis, which may be done by the reading specialist.

The speech clinician and the reading specialist should strive to learn one another's professional terminology. Often they are talking about the same things but using different terms.

The reading specialist and the SLP have much in common and much to offer one another. A close working relationship between them is an important aspect of the speech, language, and hearing program.

Maltreated Children

An unfortunate condition that seems to be more widespread is that of the battered or neglected child, who may also have communication problems. The maltreatment of children usually falls into one or more four general areas:

1. Physical abuse
2. Neglect
3. Emotional maltreatment
4. Sexual abuse

Some forms of abuse and neglect are easily recognized, such as beatings that leave facial bruises or being repeatedly locked out of the home for long periods of time. The more subtle forms of abuse may include verbal abuse, poor supervision, or overly strict discipline. What is the school clinician's role in regard to abused and neglected children? First, the SLP should be alert to the signs of abuse. It is important to keep in mind that abuse occurs among the rich and well educated as well as the impoverished. The next step is to report your suspicions to the principal, backed up with as much evidence as possible. Your suspicions may be wrong, but you may also be saving a life.

Children who are maltreated often exhibit learning disabilities. They show symptoms such as distractability, inappropriate behaviors, poor memory skills, and inattentiveness. These symptoms are often blamed on the emotional distress the child may be experiencing due to the abuse. When symptoms such as these are noticed, the child should be referred for a multi-factored evaluation, including speech-language and hearing testing. The behaviors may actually be related to brain damage caused by physical abuse.

Vocational High School and Secondary Transitional Programs

The interest in preparing adolescents in high schools and vocational high schools for jobs in the outside world provides a unique challenge to SLPs and audiologists. It is not known at this time how many school SLPs serve in vocational schools but the number is probably quite small. By the same token, it is not known how many adolescents with speech, language, and hearing problems are in vocational schools.

A vocational high school is usually jointly operated by a group of existing school districts. In some cases, if the school district is a large one both in numbers and in size, the vocational high school may serve only one school district. Students often retain membership in the "home" school district but may attend classes at the vocational school for all or part of the school day.

The curriculum of the vocational high school may include basic academic classes such as English, American history, and government. It would also contain classes related to the students' vocational choices and laboratory classes during which the theory and training are applied to actual job projects. The students upon graduation receive a diploma from the home school and a vocational certificate from the vocational school.

Because the purpose of a vocational school is to prepare a student for a specific vocation, the needs and the motivations of students in this kind of setting differ from those of students in the regular high school.

Awareness of the psychology of this age group is important to the school clinician. A strong desire to be accepted by peers and not to be different from them sometimes underlies a resistance to therapy. A good working relationship with the vocational instructor can do much to encourage students enrolled in therapy to maintain good attendance.

Regardless of how severe the communication deficit may be, it is of secondary importance to the student at this age level. The intervention program should be based on the student's personal and vocational vocabulary. Remedial sessions can be developed around such topics as hairdressing, automobiles, getting a job, and other subjects of interest.

In addition to a remedial program, a speech-improvement program may fulfill the needs of many of the students. For example, students preparing for their rotation assignments as assistants to area dentists can be introduced to the following topics: (1) selecting correct word choices, (2) eliminating slang, (3) speaking clearly with the appropriate volume and rate, and (4) eliminating syntactical errors.

Programs may also include in-service training programs for both students and staff members. Topics for vocational instructors include information on speech, language, and hearing problems and the recognition of them. In-service topics for students include speech, language, and hearing behavior in the young child for the students enrolled in the child-care program as well as the effects of prolonged and sudden loud noise on students working in shop areas, such as auto mechanics, industrial, carpentry, and agricultural shop areas.

Clinicians may initiate a hearing-conservation program. Staff members and students involved in noisy laboratory and shop classes should be made aware of

246

Chapter 8:
Intervention:
Planning,
Implement-
ing, Evalu-
ating

the ramifications of noise pollution and the effects on the hearing of the persons involved. The clinician may arrange for decibel readings to be conducted in the suspected loud-noise areas. Measures may be taken to make ear protectors available in the school supply store for students and instructors.

High schools may also have transitional programs. In this type of program the student moves from school to the work force, with activities focused on exploring employment opportunities, assessing vocational potentials, vocational training, and job placement. For students in the secondary transitional programs who have communication handicaps or limited communication skills, the services of the SLP and/or audiologist are utilized. The programs are carried out by the school staff, often with the cooperation of potential employers.

Working with Groups of Children

In a sense all therapy is group therapy. A dyadic group (group of two) in speech, language, and hearing consists of the clinician and the student. Therapy groups in the schools consist of the clinician and from two to five students, or in special instances, more students. The purpose of a therapy group is to help the client in such a way that in the future he or she becomes independent of the relationship. The clinician is in a leadership role whether he or she utilizes a nondirective approach or a direct approach. The clinician is a facilitator who is aware of the feelings, values, and tensions of the participants. The clinician may play the role of an impartial judge in the event of friction. He or she keeps the group members moving toward the completion of the tasks at hand.

Beasley (1951) described the advantages of structuring a group therapy session around the development of social skills. She maintained that practice and drill on speech patterns did not give children a way of using them readily in social and interpersonal situations.

Backus (1952) viewed the role of the therapist as one who creates the kind of environment in which the client becomes able to change. She maintained that a group situation provides a greater possibility for this than does a two-person relationship. She also felt that the group situation has a wider availability of "tools" (social situations) than does the one-to-one encounter.

Care must be taken that your group therapy doesn't become individual therapy with one child speaking and the other children in the group simply listening, watching, and waiting for their turn. Passive participation has no therapeutic value. In groups structured like this, group interaction is limited if it exists at all.

Leith (1984) describes a much more interactive and effective model of group interaction. Referred to as "the shaping group," each student is actively involved in the activity. The children elicit responses from one another and provide the modeling, corrections, and feedback. They learn to judge other group members' productions as correct or incorrect and apply the reinforcement. In this model, there is constant interaction and learning is an ongoing process.

There is no rule that says all therapy sessions must take place around a table. Working in front of a mirror, a flannel board, or a chalkboard will help group members to become better participants. It has been said that learning is movement. If this is true, the clinician who sits on a chair without ever moving, and the children who remain in their places during the entire session day after day, may not be making the best possible use of the therapy time.

Counseling

Counseling is an important factor in a holistic approach to therapy. The SLP in the school system counsels both students and parents in communication problems. Some of the counseling is geared toward the prevention of problems. For example, the SLP may give a talk to the families on the nature of speech, language, and hearing problems or the development of speech and language in infants and children. Or the counseling may be directly with the student, entailing self-perception, acceptance of the problem, understanding of the problem, relationship to peers, information about the specific disorder, reluctance to talk, and feelings about the problem.

The school clinician should be alert to any signs that would indicate that the student may require psychological or psychiatric treatment. Even the faintest doubt about seeking further professional help should be pursued.

Many school clinicians have found that fears and apprehensions surrounding many types of speech disorders are based on misinformation or no information. Much of the anxiety for both students and their parents can be alleviated by factual and general information.

The student's negative feelings about the problem may also be allayed by the attitude of the clinician, who says, not only by words but also by actions, "I'm here to help you; we can work on this together."

Although SLPs are not trained as counselors, there is no question about their knowledge of their professional field and the fact that they have been doing counseling. Without counseling, therapy alone would be ineffective. Recognizing that there are some children whose emotional problems may go beyond the communication problem, the school SLP seeks consultation and possible referrals of such children to other agencies and services specifically designed to deal with them.

Two of the most helpful books for those seeking more information on counseling for speech, language, and hearing problems are *Counseling the Communicatively Disordered and Their Families* by David M. Luterman (Pro-Ed., 1991) and *The Psychology of Communication Disorders in Individuals and Their Families* by Walter J. Rollin (Prentice Hall, 1987).

The Prevention of Communication Problems

The Committee on the Prevention of Speech, Language, and Hearing Problems of ASHA (June 1982), views the responsibility of the profession to include not only the treatment but also the prevention of communicative disorders. Included in one of the areas of prevention is the early detection and treatment of young children. Public Law 99-457 mandates assistance to preschool chil-

248

Chapter 8:
Intervention:
Planning,
Implement-
ing, Evalu-
ating

dren, ages birth to five. As discussed previously, services may be provided by a number of disciplines and should be coordinated. Family involvement is essential.

What does this mean to the school SLP? Essentially, it means that if you are employed as a school clinician in a state that includes in its laws the detection and treatment of young children, the responsibility of servicing these children will be with the local health care or education agencies. Because of financial restraints few school systems have this type of program; however, the detection and treatment of young children with disabilities are often being provided by local community voluntary agencies and by private agencies and health care programs.

The school SLP has a stake in encouraging and assisting these agencies in early detection and remediation. The earlier that handicapping conditions are identified, the better chance there is of remediation. And eventually fewer of these children will turn up in the caseload of the school clinician. Communication deviations that go untreated may develop into communication disorders and cause these children difficulties with the acquisition of such academic skills as reading, spelling, writing, and mathematics.

The SLP may intervene by providing information about speech and language development, environmental factors that influence development, and techniques to facilitate and stimulate speech and language development. Talks to groups of parents, early childhood educators such as day-care workers, preschool and nursery school teachers, members of the health professions, elementary school teachers and administrators, student groups, community organizations, and other professional groups, will help individuals understand how they may prevent and ameliorate speech, hearing, and language problems in children. Information may also be disseminated through newspaper articles, radio and television appearances, and other media. In a school or preschool the SLP may also provide demonstration lessons for the teachers.

Other Facets of a Successful Program

Letter and Report Writing. The ability to express ideas on paper as well as verbally is essential for the speech-language clinician. Some persons seem to be born with this knack, whereas others have to learn it. In any event, the techniques of writing professional reports and letters can be learned.

Often, professional letter and report writing is highly stylized and follows a definite pattern. In addition, the basic essentials of good writing must be observed. First, the writing must be clear and concise. Simpler terms are much better than complex ones, and the simplest and easiest way of saying something is usually the best. The professional vocabulary must be adequate and the terminology must be appropriate.

The beginner who is learning the skill of professional writing should keep in mind the person to whom the report is being written. This person may be another clinician, the teacher, the family doctor, or the parents. Appropriate word choices should be made in keeping with the understanding of the potential reader of the report. Avoid professional jargon when writing to parents and do not assume they know the meanings of technical words. Remember that you are one human being writing to another human being; try not to sound like an institution writing to a human being. Put yourself in place of a parent who receives a letter from the school clinician stating, "Periodically during therapeutic intervention the speech-language pathologist will attempt to assess Billy's receptive language abilities by the administration of norm-referenced and criterion-referenced tests to determine his linguistic status in relation to his peers." Why not say, "During the time Billy is enrolled in therapy I will give him several tests to help us find out how well he is progressing."

Following are several different types of reports that the school SLP may write during a professional career:

The Daily Log. The daily log is written for the clinician's own information. It may be nothing more than a simple jotting down of notes following each therapy session. These notes may indicate the child's reaction to the therapy, any progress made on that particular day, and suggestions and ideas the clinician may want to include in the next therapy session.

The Progress Report. The progress report covers a span of time, for example, a period of one month, two months, six weeks, six months, or a year. It may be written for the clinician's own information or at the request of the person responsible for the management of the students in that particular setting. The progress report could include such information as the specific dates of the therapy, the number of therapy sessions, the name of the clinician, an evaluation of the progress, a listing of the therapy goals and a statement concerning whether or not they are accomplished, the methods of therapy, and the overall results of the treatment to date. In a school the progress report may be written for the teacher's use and should be specific about what was done in therapy and what would be recommended for the teacher to follow up on. Progress reports are usually filed in the child's cumulative folder, and if the child moves from one school to another the reports may follow to the new school. Progress reports may also be sent to parents. The clinician must be sure the terminology is geared to the parents' understanding.

Final Reports. Final reports or closure reports may follow a checklist format or narrative style or a combination of the two. The factual information included in the closure summary may include name, date of birth, type of problem, date of the latest service, name of the clinician and the supervisor, date when student was first seen, starting date of the therapy, and the date of recheck and results of recheck. Information about the therapy and the number of sessions may also be included, as well as whether the therapy was in group or individual sessions. A rating of the progress during the time covered by the report could also be included. The rating may be on a continuum, such as "no progress, very slight, slight, moderate, good, excellent." Clarification of these categories should also be included.

Under the mandate of PL 94-142, final progress summaries are required, and in some school systems both progress summaries and final reports are required. The reports would contain information to help determine whether or not the student had achieved the short-term instructional objectives. The contents of the final reports are shared with the parents and, in some cases, with the

250

**Chapter 8:
Intervention:
Planning,
Implement-
ing, Evalu-
ating**

student. The reports must be as accurate as humanly possible and written so that they will not be misconstrued.

If other services were utilized during this time it would be necessary to include a reference to them and, if available, a summary. Such services would include psychological, social, remedial reading, medical, vocational, educational, and psychiatric. In some cases it might be necessary to attach a copy of the report. The report should indicate whether the service was obtained within the school system or in a community agency.

General Information. In writing professional reports the school clinician should keep in mind that opinions, rationalizations, hunches, and unsubstantiated ideas should not be included unless they are labeled as such. They may be included under *clinical impressions* or a similar category. As long as they are labeled it is permissible to include them.

Report writing, as the name implies, means a reporting of the facts without any editorializing by the writer. The reader of the report must be allowed to draw his or her own conclusions from the facts submitted.

DISCUSSION QUESTIONS AND PROJECTS

1. Collect samples of Individualized Education Programs and Individualized Family Service Intervention Plans used in various school systems. Compare and contrast IEPs and IFSPs. How are they alike? How are they different?

2. If you are working with a client in your university based clinic, develop an IEP or IFSP for that client.

3. Prepare a lesson plan for 2 of the students listed below. Be sure to show how you will incorporate information and materials from the school curriculum into your plan. Each speech-language goal should be related to some aspect of the classroom or a school subject. Students: an eight year old girl from Vietnam with limited English proficiency; a 3-year old child with cerebral palsy; a fifth grader with severe dysfluency; a third grader with a language-learning disability that affects reading comprehension; a five year old with delayed articulation; a high school junior with cognitive-communicative impairments as a result of a TBI.

4. Describe steps you could take to motivate a student who is not interested in participating in your therapy program any longer.

5. With a fellow classmate, enact a discussion you might carry on with a class-room teacher to explain a student's communication impairment, the impact of the impairment on the learning process, and recommendations of how the two of you might work collaboratively to facilitate generalization of communication skills within the classroom. Role play your discussion for your classmates (one person assume the role of classroom teacher, one of SLP).

6. Using Flexer, Wray, and Ireland's outline prepare an inservice presentation for the teachers of a child with a moderate hearing loss.

7. Plan a therapy lesson for a group of fourth grade students with multiple articulation problems. Base your lesson on a social studies unit.

8. What behavioral signs would alert you to the possibility that a child is being physically abused? What steps are required of educators in your state if they discover abuse?

9. Plan a presentation for high school students who have had children. What might you tell them to encourage them to help their children develop appropriate communication skills?

10. Develop a lesson plan for a group of vocational education students who are studying cosmotology and/or auto mechanics. Build a vocabulary list. Prepare a list of recommendations for them for preparing for a job interview.

11. Read Terrell and Hale's (1991) article about serving multicultural populations. Discuss the learning styles they describe. Survey your classmates to determine the existence of various learning styles.

12. Gather information about at least one ethnic group served in your university's clinic. Use Hanson, Lynch, and Wayman's suggestions as a guide for the type of information to seek.

CHAPTER 9

Working with Others: Collaboration and Consultation

Introduction

In Chapter Seven, we looked at a collaborative/consultative model of service delivery and intervention. This model reinforces the importance of working closely with other individuals who are involved in the lives, education, and rehabilitation of school children. To implement this model effectively, it is important to understand the roles and responsibilities of family members, administrators, teaching personnel, and non-teaching staff who interact directly with the speech-language pathologist in order to help children with communication impairments. In other words, what can we expect from various individuals and what can they expect from us?

The school SLP works not only with school-based personnel but also with staff from community health and rehabilitation facilities. In fact, federal legislation (Public Law 99-457) mandates that schools and community agencies work closely together to provide services to children with disabilities and their families. In some cases, services are purchased from agencies outside of the school district if they are not available in the local education agency.

Parents and/or guardians are encouraged to take leading roles in the planning of speech, language, and hearing services for their children. Although interactions with parents are not new for school clinicians, the importance cannot be emphasized enough. It is helpful to understand problems which interfere with interactions with families and strategies for forming meaningful relationships with them.

The school speech-language pathologist is also a consultant to the community and a source of information on speech, language, and hearing disorders and services.

The roles of the director of special education, elementary and secondary supervisors, superintendent, assistant superintendents, and board of education have already been discussed in Chapter Three. In this chapter, we will examine the roles, responsibilities, and working relationships we can establish with other individuals who are involved with school children.

The Importance of Collaborating and Consulting with Others

In each situation and environment a child enters, there are demands for communication. Therefore, it is important for individuals with whom children interact to learn the importance of communication for success, to recognize communication delays and disorders, and to play important roles in facilitating speech-language development and modification if problems exist.

The service delivery options presented in Chapter Seven have, as a major component, collaborative-consultative services. In this service delivery model, the clinician, family members, and other professionals work together as a team to develop plans and strategies for helping children with communication impairments. They may also join forces to prevent communication problems from occurring. The child is the central focus of planning and problem solving and each team member brings to the situation their own unique expertise and contributions.

Idol (1986) defines collaborative-consultation as "an interactive process that enables teams of people with diverse expertise to generate creative solutions to mutually defined problems. The outcome is enhanced and altered from the original solutions that any team member would produce independently."

As the collaborative-consultative model has been more frequently applied, communication disorders professionals have begun to expand the purposes for which it can be applied (Hoskins, 1991; Wiig, Secord, & Wiig, 1990; Montgomery, 1990; Eger, 1990). The collaborative-consultative model can be used to:

- Determine the severity of the communication impairment;
- Assess the impact a communication impairment has on the student's academic and social performance;
- Define a student's communicative needs for various educational and social situations;
- Observe a student's communicative abilities under specific circumstances;
- Develop strategies for stabilizing the new skills the student is learning in therapy; and
- Monitor the student's progress after dismissal from a direct service program.

Several professionals (Nelson, 1990; Wiig, Secord, and Wiig, 1990; Marvin, 1990; Damico & Nye, 1990) have described the role of the speech-language pathologist as a collaborative-consultant for children with various communication disorders. To be successful in this role, the SLP must have a solid theoretical

254

**Chapter 9:
Working with
Others:
Collaboration
and
Consultation**

foundation in communication development and disorders; must be able to identify childrens' strengths and needs; must be able to develop prescriptive techniques for problems related to phonology, syntax, semantics, pragmatics; must
understand the school curriculum and learning process; and should be able to
relate these aspects of communication to oral and written language.

The essentials of programs that are successful involve cooperation, communication and joint planning and programming. Professionals focus on how
they can best combine their talents, expertise, and schedules to facilitate a comprehensive program for children.

Intervention Assistance Teams

To promote collaborative planning, many school systems have organized *Intervention Assistance Teams.* The teams are generally comprised of the child's teacher,
a school administrator such as the principal, the school psychologist, a special
education teacher, and other professionals who have knowledge of the child's
skills and needs. This includes the speech-language pathologist and audiologist.
Together, team members and the child's parents make decisions regarding assessment procedures needed and intervention strategies to be used. Specific
responsibilities are assigned and timetables for implementing procedures and
evaluating progress are established.

To implement an intervention assistance team, the following questions
must be addressed: Which children will be served by the team? Who will participate on the team? How will it operate? How will the team's effectiveness be
evaluated? To be most effective, team members must be prepared for the job
they are to do. Goals and expectations of what can be accomplished must be
realistic. It is wise to keep minutes of team meetings. These can then be used to
document assistance as well as to serve as a guide for implementing recommendations in the months following the meeting.

Attitudes

The functions of the school SLP are ideally carried out as an equal member of
the educational team. To provide the best possible treatment for pupils with
communication impairments, the school speech-language pathologist must work
cooperatively with students' families and with other professionals in the education community. Sometimes, this involves providing information and support.
Oftentimes, it means receiving information and support. But most often, it
entails both.

The attitudes others have toward the speech-language-hearing program
are crucial to its success. Equally important are the attitudes SLPs display in
relation to working cooperatively with other individuals to improve students'
communication skills. In most situations, the reactions and quality of cooperation of individuals are determined by what the situation signifies to them. People
possess varying degrees of difference in their understanding and attitude toward
children with communication difficulties and toward the services of the speech-

language-hearing pathologist. There may be a lack of clarity about the roles and responsibilities of the SLP leading to confusion and misinterpretation. This confusion may limit the effectiveness with which the SLP can function in school districts or individual school buildings. A concerted effort must be made to ensure that parents and other professionals are informed of and clearly recognize the functions of the speech-language pathologist within the school setting.

Several researchers have conducted studies on the attitudes of classroom teachers, special educators, and school principals toward speech, language, and hearing programs in the schools (Blosser and DePompei, 1984; Phelps and Koenigsknecht, 1977; Shrewsbury, Lass and Joseph, 1985). Their results have shown that while educators may be favorable toward the speech-language-hearing program, they may not have good understanding of the nature of some types of communication disorders, the impact of communication impairments on academic performance, the functions of the SLP, and how to create favorable conditions for reinforcing speech and language skills or facilitating change and carryover.

There are many school clinicians who are doing a good job of collaborating and consulting with other individuals to build support and understanding of their school therapy programs. Their interactions lead to more comprehensive and effective services for students. Successful clinicians generally have good communication and interaction with parents and school professionals.

The Principal

A key person in the speech, language, and hearing program is the building principal. This individual's attitude toward speech, language, and hearing can make or break a program. Without the understanding and cooperation of the principal it would be extremely difficult to carry out an effective program. The principal is the administrator of the building, and in a sense, the school SLP is responsible to that person while in that building. The school SLP is a member of staff of that particular building in the same way that other teachers are staff members.

What can the school clinician expect from the principal? First, the principal is legally and educationally responsible for each child enrolled in the school. Therefore, it is important for the principal and speech-language clinician to work closely together to ensure that quality services can be delivered.

The principal is often the representative of the local education agency in the development of individualized education programs (IEPs) for children and may serve as the coordinator of the placement team.

The principal is responsible for arranging for adequate working space and facilitating the procurement of equipment and supplies. The principal acquaints the clinician with the policies, rules, regulations, and all procedures in that school.

The principal may help the SLP in integrating the speech, language, and hearing program into the total school program. In some situations, the principal may assist the clinician in scheduling the screening programs and in setting up the schedule for children to be seen in therapy.

256

Chapter 9:
Working with
Others:
Collaboration
and
Consultation

The principal can be expected to visit the therapy sessions and observe. Indeed, a wise clinician will invite the principal to observe therapy sessions and will encourage questions.

The interpretation of the program to other members of the school staff, the parents, and the community is ongoing, and much may be done by the principal. In addition, the principal may arrange opportunities for the clinician to interpret the program to the staff and the parents as well as professional and lay groups in the community. The principal is the liaison between the school and the community and between the school clinician and the school staff. When a parent, a classroom teacher, or a member of the community has a question regarding the speech, language, and hearing program, that person will ask the principal, who may answer the query or refer it to the school SLP. Clinicians may not always be immediately available for questions that come to the school because on that particular day they may be scheduled at another school. When this occurs, the principal will be the one to handle the questions.

A study by Blosser and DePompei (1984) indicated that speech-language pathology may not be a well-understood profession by school administrators. According to Blosser and DePompei,

> The findings appear to indicate that principals continue to view the speech-language pathologist in the traditional role. There was inconsistency in the title given to the speech-language pathologist. Principals agreed the SLPs work with children with articulation, voice, fluency and language disorders; but did not agree that they work with children with learning disabilities or identify hearing loss. Most agreed that SLPs continue to conduct therapy one to one or in small groups.
>
> Several principals indicated that SLPs do share information about their programs with them and participate in selected building level activities. A majority of the principals responded that they agreed correction of communication disorders is important. Few principals agreed that SLPs currently play a role in teaching language skills in the classroom. While 89% of the principals indicated that they understood the role of the SLP, only 37% reported they had had academic exposure to the SLP's role. This may indicate that there is limited discussion of the speech-language pathology profession in the academic preparation of administrators.
>
> In relation to recent discussions in the literature regarding changes in the role of the school speech-language pathologist, the findings of this survey demonstrate that principals do not currently support modifications of the traditional role. Principals indicated they would prefer that the SLP have more direct contact with children with communication disorders, parents, teachers, and the principals themselves. They also appear to understand those factors which interfere with the provision of more direct contact such as paperwork, the evaluation process, and the high numbers of children requiring services in contrast to the low number of SLPs available.

Considering that over 45% of the profession is employed within the school setting, these results are disturbing. It will be difficult to institute changes while school administrators continue to be content with the status quo.

The principals were asked to respond to the following three open-ended questions:

a. What changes would you as a principal like to see in the speech-language therapy program?

b. What changes do you feel your teachers would like to see in the speech-language therapy program?

c. Do you feel there are problems with the way the speech-language therapy program is currently operated? If yes, what are they?

The responses fell into the following categories:

1. Desired Changes: Principals indicated they would prefer more direct contact; increased services at the high school level; more parent contact; and more work with the severely and multiply handicapped. Many stated that they feel SLPs should begin their programs earlier in the year and end them later. Many noted that SLPs take too long to test and do too much testing in relation to teaching. Several remarked that SLPs don't adhere to the same accountability for their time as other teachers do and are not available when needed.

2. Teacher Contact: The majority of respondents indicated they feel their teachers would like the SLP to be more informative about their program and work more closely with teachers and other special educators. They indicated that teachers don't feel SLPs function as a part of the educational team. They would like SLPs to become more involved in school activities. Many stated that they would like to see the SLP provide in-service for the teaching staff regarding when and how to make referrals, the therapy program, and developmental norms for communication skills.

3. Problems: Principals indicated that problems which interfere with the speech-language therapy program include: the paperwork necessary for due process; high caseloads; too many building assignments; and conflicting schedules.

It was interesting to note, however, that the principals rated the SLP's individual qualities high: 91% of the principals rated them high in flexibility, 85% in organization, and 74% in creativity. Approximately two-thirds (65%) agreed that the SLP in their school demonstrates leadership.

The principal can smooth the way for school clinicians in many situations. Perhaps one of the most important is in helping the clinician gain acceptance of the program by the school staff and the parents. The attitude of the principal may be reflected by the teachers, and the attitudes of the children may stem from the way teachers perceive the program. Because of a myriad of duties and heavy administrative responsibilities, principals cannot be expected to know everything about the therapy program, but a willing and cooperative principal with a positive attitude is excellent insurance for a good speech, language, and hearing program.

On the other side of the coin, the school clinician has some important

258

Chapter 9:
Working with
Others:
Collaboration
and
Consultation

responsibilities to the principal. Providing information about the program to the principal is one of the most important factors in maintaining a good relationship.

The clinician will want to confer with the principal regarding major aspects of the screening, assessment, and intervention program. For example, the clinician should provide information to the principal on screening policies and procedures, grades and numbers of children to be screened, plans and time scheduled for follow-up testing, criteria for case selection, scheduling policies and procedures, and plans for developing intervention goals jointly with parents and teachers. The principal needs to know the children on the active caseload, the children dismissed from therapy, and the children being monitored indirectly. It is helpful to identify children by name, age, grade, communication problems, room number, and teacher and to provide a brief statement of progress.

It is advisable to furnish the principal with written reports both periodically and systematically. Some information is valuable if submitted on a monthly basis; other information can be submitted semi-annually or annually. Any plans for inservice programs for teachers and group meetings with parents and local professionals should be discussed with the principal prior to inception. Written reports or correspondence pertaining to a child in that school should be shown to and approved by the principal prior to sending them to parents or other professional personnel. Reporting information to the principal in this manner will help keep your program activities visible and it will keep the principal aware of the important role you play in the school.

If the clinician is itinerant, more than one building and more than one principal will be involved; therefore, the clinician needs to know the policies and procedures in each school. Because clinicians often work in several buildings and with several principals at one time, it is good practice to keep all the principals informed in a general way about the programs in the other schools. This practice serves to keep the principals well informed about the total program in the school system, facilitates cooperation and coordination among schools, and helps keep the clinician's workload well balanced. Care should be taken not to share private information from one building to the next and never gossip about colleagues.

The Classroom Teacher

In the speech-language pathologist's role as a collaborator and consultant to the classroom teacher, several areas should be considered:

• the strengths and needs of the student with the communication handicap;
• the academic and social demands placed upon him or her in the classroom;
• the student's interaction with peers; and
• the teacher's interest in and capability for collaborating.

This means that the SLP must understand the education process in addition to having competency in the communication disorders profession. It also means that the SLP must know what is going on in the classroom as well as making sure that the classroom teacher understands the speech, language, and hearing program and the role of the speech-language pathologist.

In most school systems there is an administrator for curriculum development. With assistance from teachers, principals, directors of special services, or other administrators, this person is responsible for the selection of textbooks and instructional supplies and materials. The business of educators is the selection of what will be taught, at what level, and in what sequence. That which is taught is the *curriculum*. The curriculum is organized by teachers into *instructional units*, each made up of lesson plans, constituting how the curriculum is taught (Rebore, 1984).

One of the ways in which the speech and language program can be integrated into the curriculum is for the SLP to have input into the curriculum committee, either as a member or in an advisory capacity. In this way the pathologist can be perceived by the rest of the staff as someone who does more than correct frontal lisps. As a communication specialist the pathologist can provide information on pragmatics, communication in the classroom, how to help the children follow directions, how to encourage children to ask questions, and how teachers can become better communicators in the classroom. The pathologist can offer suggestions on how the teaching of improved communication skills can be integrated into language arts, social studies, science, art, physical education, math, reading, spelling, and writing.

The integration of the speech, language, and hearing program into the curriculum is a basic factor. It is essential that the classroom teacher understand the program, but it is equally important that the speech clinician understand what is going on in the classroom. It is not enough to give lip service to the idea of integrating the program into the educational framework; it must be put into practice.

How can this be accomplished? The answer is not a simple one, but let us first consider some of the things the school pathologist can expect of the classroom teacher; then let us look at some of the expectations of the classroom teacher in regard to the clinician.

The school SLP can expect the teacher to provide a classroom environment that will encourage communication and will not exclude the child with the stuttering or articulation problem or the child who is hearing impaired. A teacher who shows kindness and understanding toward the child with a disability is not only assisting that child but also is showing other children in the classroom how to treat individuals who are disabled. Sometimes it takes more time and patience to deal with handicapped children, but the rewards in terms of the child's performance are many. The teacher in the classroom takes the lead in establishing the emotional climate in that setting, and the children learn by example.

The classroom teacher is also a teacher of speech and language by example. If you doubt this, watch a group of children "playing school" sometime. Teachers provide the models for communication and children imitate the teachers. Teachers must have an awareness of their use of language, the quality of speech, the rate and volume of speech, and the use of slang or dialect.

The SLP can expect the teacher to help identify children in the classroom with speech, language, or hearing problems. Some children with communication

260

**Chapter 9:
Working with
Others:
Collaboration
and
Consultation**

problems are not spotted during a routine screening, and teachers who see children on a day-to-day basis will have more opportunity to identify the children and refer them to the SLP.

The clinician can expect the classroom teacher to send the children to therapy at the time scheduled. The SLP will need to supply the teacher with a schedule, and both teacher and clinician should stick to it. The SLP can also expect the teacher to inform him or her of any changes in schedules that would necessitate a child being absent from therapy.

One of the most important areas of cooperation between the SLP and the classroom teacher is the carryover, or generalization stage—when speech and language behavior learned in therapy is brought into the classroom. For this to be accomplished it will be necessary for the SLP to keep the teacher well informed about the child's goals in therapy, progress in therapy, and steps in development of new patterns. This must be done not in general terms but in very specific ones. The teacher needs precise information on the child's problem and what is being done in therapy before there can be a carryover into classroom activities. The teacher can provide the SLP with information concerning how well the child is able to utilize the new speech or language patterns in the classroom.

When confronted with the idea of helping the child with a communication impairment in the classroom, the teacher's reaction is apt to be "I don't have time to work with Billy on his speech when I have 25 other children in the room." The SLP's role in this situation is to give the teacher specific suggestions on how this can be accomplished as a part of the curriculum. This of course means that the clinician will have to be well acquainted with classroom procedures, practices, and activities. It also means the SLP will have to know what can be expected of children of that age and on that grade level.

To integrate fully the speech, language, and hearing program into the school, there must be a continuous pattern of sharing ideas and information between the SLP and the classroom teacher.

We have considered what the SLP can expect of the classroom teacher. Now let us look at the other side of the coin—what the teacher can expect of the clinician.

If you are new in the school, starting off on the right foot is important. Being friendly and open with teachers, showing an interest in what they are doing in their classrooms, and showing a willingness to give them information are all things that can be done to help build trust and understanding. There are many ways in which this can be accomplished. One way is to plan to eat lunch with the teachers in the teachers' lunchroom. Another is to participate in some of their social activities. Because clinicians deal with many teachers in different schools it is not wise to become identified with little cliques and associate only with a very small group. Outside the school you will have your own circle of friends, but inside the school be friendly with everyone.

If you have a schedule, keep to it, and if you make changes in it, as you surely will, be sure to tell the classroom teachers who are affected. If you send a child back to the classroom late, you will have no basis for complaint if the teacher fails to send a child to you on time.

Share information with teachers through informal conferences, arranged conferences held periodically, invitations to observe therapy sessions, and observation in classrooms. Always make arrangements in advance for conferences and observations. The principal can often help make arrangements for any of these activities. In one school where I worked, the principal volunteered to take over each classroom for a half-hour so that each teacher in the school could observe in the therapy room.

Information can also be transmitted in written form. *Short* descriptions or definitions of the various speech, language, or hearing problems or any aspects of the program will help teachers understand the program better. *Short* is emphasized because realistically teachers are not going to take the time to read long treatises.

In working with classroom teachers the school SLP is a partner in effecting the best possible services for the child who has a communication disability. The more help that is given to the teacher, the more opportunity there will be for integrating the speech, language, and hearing program into the schools.

Due to mainstreaming, teachers are faced with the task of integrating children with special needs into regular classrooms. Providing in-service programs or short courses for credit are excellent ways of supplying teachers with information about children with communication disorders.

What are some of the things that classroom teachers will need to know about communication and communication disorders? Following is a list of topics that might be included in an in-service program:

1. The speech, language, and hearing program in the school, including the preventive, diagnostic, and remediation aspects. Describe policies and procedures for case identification, selection, enrollment, and dismissal.

2. Normal speech, language, and hearing development.

3. A brief description of the major types of communication impairments to be expected in the school-age population (i.e., articulation, delayed language development and language/learning disorders, fluency, voice disorders) and impairments associated with specific disability conditions including autism, developmental disabilities, emotional disturbances, traumatic brain injury, organic disorders, and the like. Briefly describe the characteristics, range of severity, possible causes and related factors, diagnosis and assessment procedures, criteria for selection, intervention strategies, impact on school performance, and the role of the classroom teacher for each disorder category.

4. The importance of hearing for learning and information related to hearing problems including the anatomy of the ear, nature of sound, types of hearing loss, causes of hearing loss, identification and measurement of hearing loss, role of the classroom teacher, rehabilitation and habilitation of hearing deficiencies, hearing aids and assistive listening devices.

5. The relationship of speech, language, and hearing to the educational/learning process.

262

Chapter 9:
Working with
Others:
Collaboration
and
Consultation

6. Medical and dental intervention where applicable for specific disorders such as cleft palate.

7. The roles of other professionals in treatment such as physicians, physical therapists, occupational therapist, psychologists, and counselors.

8. Therapy techniques and intervention strategies that can be successfully implemented in the classroom.

9. Areas of the curriculum where focus can be placed on improving students' communication skills and where communication goals can be integrated.

10. Assistive devices and augmentative communication systems used to facilitate communication in students with severe impairments.

Figure 9-1 shows an observation form developed to facilitate teachers' awareness and understanding of their own classroom communication style. It can be given to teachers (or others) for self evaluation or used as an observation tool. Analyzing the results jointly with the teacher can lead to meaningful discussion about how to modify communication style in order to meet a particular child's needs. For example, if Johnny cannot process language at a fast rate and the math teacher, Mr. Butler speaks very quickly, Johnny will be at a disadvantage for learning math. Therefore, a reasonable and do-able modification for Mr. Butler would be to slow his rate of speech when presenting important information or new concepts to his class. Figure 9-2 outlines numerous communicative strategies which can be recommended to teachers who are interested in modifying their communication styles in order to accommodate a child in their classroom who has a communication impairment.

FIGURE 9.1. Communication Style Observation Form

Instructions

During communication interactions with (student's name), pay close attention to your own communication manner and style. As completely as possible, describe the characteristics of your communication manner and style in the categories listed below. In consultation with a speech-language pathologist, determine those characteristics which can potentially pose difficulty for the student. Place a minus (−) next to them. Place a plus (+) beside those behaviors which can be used to promote the use of good communication skills.

1. _____ Average rate of speech
2. _____ Typical length and complexity of sentences
3. _____ Use of sarcasm, humor, and puns
4. _____ Word choice (simple, difficult, technical)
5. _____ Attentitiveness to students during conversations
6. _____ Organization of conversations
7. _____ Use of hand and body gestures
8. _____ Use of objects to help make explanations
9. _____ Manner of responding to students' questions
10. _____ Manner of giving directions and instructions
11. _____ Patience while waiting for someone else to talk or answer
12. _____ Ability to understand students with communication impairments

FIGURE 9.2. Recommended Strategies for Modifying Communication Styles to Accommodate the Needs of Children with Communication Impairments

Following is a list of communication strategies which teachers and others can use while interacting with a child who demonstrates a communication impairment.

Based on the results of formal and informal assessment procedures, indicate those strategies which will facilitate development of communication skills or correct speech and language productions.

For example, when GIVING INSTRUCTIONS AND DIRECTIONS, it is recommended that the communication partner make attempts to modify his or her communication style by reducing the length of complexity of the utterance, reducing the rate of utterance, repeating the instructions, altering the mode of instruction delivery, or giving prompts and assistance.

Giving Instructions and Directions

_____ Reduce length of instructions
_____ Reduce complexity of instructions
_____ Reduce rate of delivery
_____ Repeat instructions more than once
_____ Alter mode of instruction delivery
_____ Give prompts and assistance
_____ Vary voice and intonation patterns to emphasize key words

Explaining New Concepts and Vocabulary

_____ Give definitions for terms
_____ Show visual representations of concepts and vocabulary
_____ Present only a limited number of new concepts at a given time
_____ Ask questions to verify comprehension

Reading to the Student

_____ Reduce rate
_____ Reduce complexity
_____ Reduce length
_____ Determine comprehension through questioning
_____ Redirect student's attention to important details and facts

Practicing Memory Skills

_____ Encourage the student to categorize information and make associations
_____ Provide opportunities for rehearsing information
_____ Encourage the student to visualize information

Practicing Higher Level Thinking and Communicating

_____ Provide opportunities for problem solving
_____ Provide opportunities for decision making
_____ Provide opportunities for making judgments
_____ Ask questions to elicit solutions, judgment, decisions

Announcing and Clarifying the Topic of Discussion

_____ Introduce the topic to be discussed
_____ Restate the topic frequently throughout the conversation

(continued)

264

Chapter 9:
Working with
Others:
Collaboration
and
Consultation

FIGURE 9.2. (Continued)

Attending to Student's Behaviors, Queries, Comments
_____ Reinforce queries and comments
_____ Inform the student if the message is not understandable
_____ Request repetition of utterances not understood
Relaying Important Information to Students
_____ Avoid sarcasm, idiomatic expressions, puns, humor
_____ Reduce rate, complexity, length of utterance
_____ Use or reduce gestures dependent on student's responses and needs
_____ Incorporate visual cues and imagery for clarification
_____ Permit ample time for student response
_____ Introduce alternative and/or augmentative communication systems if necessary
_____ Arrange the physical environment to reduce distractions, eliminate barriers, and invite communication
_____ Invite questions
_____ Present information in clusters and groups
_____ Introduce information with attention-getting words
_____ Select materials appropriate for skills, age, interest levels

Special Education Teachers

Speech-language pathologists and audiologists relate to all the providers of special instructional services in the schools. This includes teachers of children who present emotional disturbances, specific learning disabilities, cultural and linguistic diversity, developmental disabilities, physical impairments, visual impairments, and hearing impairments. Instructional services are available to children in all of these groups and more as mandated by Public Laws 94-142, 99-457, and 101-476. The collaborative team should be comprised of those educators who have the greatest expertise in the areas of need defined for each particular student.

Because the laws do not clearly define the areas of professional specialization which must be involved in the delivery of services to particular groups of children, confusion sometimes arises concerning the professional scopes of practices. This is especially evident between SLPs and learning disabilities specialists because many children with learning disabilities demonstrate problems processing and producing spoken or written language. Their deficits negatively effect learning and result in academic problems in subject areas such as reading, spelling, writing, mathematics, and other academic and social areas that require adequate language abilities.

At this writing the interacting roles of the learning disabilities specialist and the SLP are not yet clearly defined. The working relationship is dependent on the local school and the individual professional persons involved, including the principal and the classroom teacher. Some issues are clear: The SLP has the academic background, interest, and competence in language development and disorders. Also, the fields of speech-language pathology and audiology have a solid backing of research in language disorders.

The Committee on Language-Learning Disabilities of the American Speech-Language-Hearing Association (1982) supports the following activities:

It is the position of ASHA that speech-language pathologists be included as members of the multidisciplinary team involved in the management of individuals with learning disabilities. More specifically:

1. The speech-language pathologist must be included in the review of referral data. Regular classroom teachers, parents, and other specialists are not always aware of the importance of language skills to successful learning. Some prerequisite academic problems are manifestations of language process.

2. The speech-language pathologist must be included in the assessment process. PL 94-142 suggests that a speech-language pathologist be a member of the assessment team. However, many local educational agencies do not require a language assessment to identify children with specific learning disabilities.

3. As members of the multidisciplinary team, the responsibility of speech-language pathologists must be expanded to include educational planning. For children whose handicapping condition is primarily a communicative disorder or a language and learning disability, the speech-language pathologist must be a participant in the development and review of individual educational programs. For students with other handicapping conditions, the speech-language pathologist must be a participant when the child has an accompanying communicative disorder.

4. The speech-language pathologist must be able to provide both direct service and consultative functions by helping teachers with language programs for LD children in classrooms, analyzing the language of the curriculum, and conducting language therapy sessions for students where appropriate.

Despite the difficulties in defining areas of work, the learning disabilities specialist and the SLP on the local level have in many instances achieved satisfactory working relationships. This has been the result of each specialist recognizing and relying on the expertise of the other. The consequence has been more effective programming for children with language-learning disabilities.

Using the continuum of service delivery options, liaison with special educators may be provided under different plans. The service delivery options are not mutually exclusive. The SLP may function as a member of the diagnostic team during the initial evaluation procedures or on an ongoing staffing basis. Specific remediation may be provided to children placed in full-time special classes or transition classes. The SLP may function as the resource room professional or as a consultant to the other specialists in relation to general or specific problems. Obviously, different service delivery models would depend on each local school system's situation. The possibilities have not been fully exploited, and the creativity of the SLP may be utilized in determining innovative approaches to helping pupils with language-learning disabilities.

Crabtree and Peterson (1974), through a case study, described the role of the speech pathologist as a resource teacher for the child with a language-

266

**Chapter 9:
Working with
Others:
Collaboration
and
Consultation**

learning disability. They stressed the idea that the speech pathologist, to function successfully as a communication specialist, must have a theoretical background in language development; must be able to identify and develop prescriptive techniques for problems related to phonology, syntax, and semantics; and should be able to relate these aspects of linguistics to all levels of oral and written language. In addition, the speech pathologist must be a generalist as well as a specialist. In other words, the speech pathologist must know how academic learning is developed and the effect of sensory deprivation, from any cause, on learning.

Simon (1977) described a program in which the SLP worked closely with the learning disabilities teacher in a developmental program in expressive language. The essentials of the program involved cooperation, communication, and programming. Both professionals focused on how they could best combine their talents, expertise, and schedules to increase the linguistic sophistication of the children in the program.

The Educational Audiologist

The most evident interrelationship between specialists in education to children with hearing impairments and members of the speech-language profession is in audiology. Educational audiology, a comparatively new specialization in the field of communication disorders, was born out of a need for improved services for the children with hearing impairments in the school and the mainstreaming component of Public Law 94-142, which mandates that the child be placed in the least restrictive educational environment possible. An educational audiology program was pioneered at Utah State University in 1966 (Alpiner et al., 1970). Since that time some states have followed suit in providing training programs for educational audiologists, and several universities have established curricula. This specialization is still in its infancy, and there is still much to be done if children with hearing impairments in classrooms are to receive the kind of care that will enable them to perform at optimal levels in the school.

The adverse effects of hearing loss on schoolchildren has been well documented. The Ad Hoc Committee on Extension of Audiology Services in the Schools (1983) focused on three major issues:

1. It causes delay in the development of receptive and expressive communication skills (speech and language).
2. It causes learning problems that result in poor academic achievement.
3. It causes a reduced ability to understand the speech of others and to speak clearly which often results in social isolation and poor self-concept.

The educational audiologist plays a primary role in identifying children who are hearing-impaired through mass screening programs and/or teacher or parent referrals. The children who fail the screening are given a comprehensive audiological assessment. Air and bone conduction pure-tone tests are administered as well as speech-reception and speech-discrimination tests. Imittance or impedance testing evaluates the function of the middle ear and can provide valuable information about the presence or absence of middle-ear pathology (for example, otitis media).

Additional evaluative and/or therapeutic recommendations may be made by the audiologist if indicated by the tests. If audiological and medical evaluations reveal that amplification is necessary, the educational audiologist helps the parents to obtain the aid or assistive device and to continue to monitor the child's behavior and hearing ability to ensure their acceptance and proper use (Townsend, 1982).

In addition to parent counseling, it is necessary to provide classroom teachers with information to help them deal with students who are hearing impaired. The educational audiologist participates in multidisciplinary team meetings. The audiologist also monitors classroom acoustics, measures noise levels, makes recommendations for sound treatment, and calibrates audiological equipment.

Ideally, all these functions are performed by the educational audiologist. Unfortunately, they are in short supply and often must spread themselves very thin. There are only about 700 educational audiologists to serve the country's 16,000 school districts.

In a study by Wilson-Vlotman and Blair (1984) the roles and attitudes of professionals serving the child with a hearing impairment in the regular classroom revealed some areas of concern. According to the study there is no one dealing with case management for the child to ensure optimum coordination of services. The educational audiologist appears to be in the best position to be a case manager if the optimization of residual hearing is the starting point for learning. Moreover, the monitoring of hearing aids is typically done at present by the classroom teacher or an itinerant teacher of the hearing impaired, although the educational audiologist is the best-equipped person for this function.

Direct services provided for the child with a hearing impairment in the classroom are often termed *aural (re)habilitation* and are essential if the child is to develop skills that will enhance learning opportunities. The Wilson-Vlotman and Blair study found that 64 percent of educational audiologists did not engage in aural habilitation with any students, and a further 18 percent provided direct service for only one-half day per week.

Other areas of concern include the availability of counseling for parents and for the child as well as consultative services for teachers, administrators, and other resource personnel. According to Wilson-Vlotman and Blair, there must be a united effort and coordination of services among the professions serving the student with a hearing impairment.

Another factor that may hinder the delivery system of audiological services is that primarily, educational audiologists were trained as, were functioning as, and viewed themselves as clinical audiologists who were based in the school. They carried excessively large caseloads, which is in keeping with the medical model. In effect, educational audiologists had limited impact on the classroom and were not taking full responsibility for the total management of the hearing-impaired child.

In considering the role of the SLP in relation to the educational audiologist there are many possible areas of cooperation. The SLP is specifically prepared to provide a program of language and speech therapy and is the best qualified

268

Chapter 9:
**Working with
Others:
Collaboration
and
Consultation**

person to do so. As information is obtained from the audiologist concerning the child's need for auditory development, it can be incorporated into the speech and language program. Because most audiologists service a wide geographical area and are not in a specific building with the same regularity as the SLP, the latter is considered to be the critical link between the student in the classroom and comprehensive audiological services.

The SLP may work with the educational audiologist in the evaluation of the child with a hearing disability. Consultation with classroom teachers and visits to the classroom may be scheduled by both the SLP and the educational audiologist in an effort to better assess the needs of the student.

To summarize, it may be said that to provide the child with a hearing impairment with the best possible services, the SLP and the educational audiologist must work together in the evaluation, remediation, and psychosocial adjustment of the child.

School SLPs would do well to encourage the employment of educational audiologists who are either by training or experience familiar with schools and the process of education. Educational audiologists must utilize their clinical knowledge and awareness of the educational and communicative needs of the child with a hearing impairment in the classroom.

Although the number of educational audiologists employed in the schools is increasing, there are still many schools with partial or limited audiological services. The school SLP may be playing a larger role in the delivery of services in these situations. Without an educational audiologist in the school system the task of caring for the child with a hearing impairment falls to the SLP.

Northcott (1972) described the role of the speech clinician as an interdisciplinary team member in regard to the child with a hearing disability. The term *hearing impaired* was used to include every child with a hearing loss that was developmentally and educationally handicapping. The importance of early intervention was stressed. Northcott describes the school clinician's role as (1) providing appropriate components of supplemental services directly to hearing-impaired children; (2) serving as a hearing consultant to teachers, administrators, and resource specialists, helping them make reasonable accommodations to meet the special needs of the child in the integrated class setting; and (3) serving as a member of an interdisciplinary team developing new components of comprehensive hearing services within the school district.

The Psychologist

The school psychologist is a member of the team of professional persons helping the child with communication impairments. The psychologist can provide valuable information regarding the student's cognitive and academic abilities (Cummins, 1984). The school clinician may make referrals to the psychologist to obtain additional information about educational diagnosis, school adjustment, personality, learning ability, or achievement. The child's speech, language, or hearing problem may be closely related to any of these factors, either as a result, a cause, or an accompanying factor.

The school clinician and the psychologist will find that a close working

269

The Bilingual
Educator
and/or
English-as-
a-Second
Language
(ESL) Teacher

relationship is mutually beneficial. The school clinician will want to know the kinds of testing and diagnostic materials the psychologist uses. On the other hand, the clinician may be helpful to the psychologist in interpreting the child's communication problem so that the best possible tests may be used. In making a referral to the psychologist the clinician should ask specific questions in regard to the kind of information being sought. The school clinician can also furnish the psychologist with helpful information that would facilitate working with the child.

The school psychologist's role differs from one school system to another, so the clinician should make a note of that role and find out what additional kinds of psychological help are available in the community.

The Social Worker

A major role of the social worker is to facilitate referrals among tax-supported and voluntary agencies. This individual's thorough knowledge of social agencies in an area can be of considerable aid to the school clinician. The social worker is a key person in helping families find places where they may receive needed help. The social worker may do some counseling, both individually and in groups, may make home visits, and can be the liaison between the school and the family. When financial assistance is required for supplemental services, the social worker is the one who can be of assistance to the family in locating that aid.

Not all school systems are fortunate enough to have a social worker on the staff, but if there is one, the school clinician should explore ways in which they may work cooperatively.

The Bilingual Educator and/or English-as-a-Second Language (ESL) Teacher

America is truly a multi-cultural nation. Across the country there are children in our schools who do not speak the same language as their teachers and class-mates. They may speak a language other than English or a nonstandard dialect. They may be from families who have recently moved to the United States, have parents who do not speak English, or live in communities where a unique dialect is spoken. These children are classified as presenting cultural and linguistic diversity. Their traditions, values, attitudes, and beliefs may be different from their teachers and classmates. They often struggle in the school setting while trying to learn to communicate and participate in school activities.

Class placement and service to children in these groups varies widely. In communities where there are large numbers of children from different cultures, programs and protocols for meeting their needs may be established. The speech-language pathologist is often called upon to assist these children in developing communication skills which will permit them to learn and benefit from the education setting. In these cases, SLPs should work cooperatively with the bi-lingual educators or English-as-a-Second Language (ESL) teachers in the district to determine how to best assess and establish a plan for intervention.

270

Chapter 9:
Working with
Others:
Collaboration
and
Consultation

In a discussion of considerations when working with multi-cultural populations, Damico and Nye (1990) stressed the importance of selecting individuals who can act as informants or interpreters during interviewing, testing, planning, and intervention procedures. Inclusion of a person who speaks the child's native language and understands the child's culture will help ensure that the program developed is appropriate and relevant for the student's needs.

Chamberlain and Landurand (1990) indicated several competencies that are preferred when selecting informants. These include proficiency in both English and the child's language, an understanding of the importance of maintaining confidentiality, and other cognitive, personality, and experience factors which would facilitate cooperation during the time that the person is acting as an interpreter or informant. If using informants or interpreters in these functions, it will be important to provide training for them so they clearly understand their role and duties (Damico and Nye, 1990).

The Guidance Counselor and Vocational Rehabilitation Counselor

The guidance counselor works with students with adjustment or academic problems, helps students plan for future roles, and makes available to them information pertinent to their situation. This individual may also do individual counseling.

The guidance counselor is especially helpful in dealing with students in the junior high and high school. Students with communication problems are often known by the guidance counselor, so the school clinician may depend on this person for referrals, supplementary information, and cooperative intervention.

The vocational rehabilitation counselor is usually employed by a district or state agency. This individual assists students 16 years of age and older in overcoming handicaps that would prevent them from being employable at their highest potential. The vocational rehabilitation counselor, although not a member of the school staff, may work in conjunction with the school system.

The School Nurse

Depending on the size of the system, there may be a number of school nurses, only one, or one working part time. In some localities the school nurse may be part of the staff of the city, county, or district health department and work either part time or full time with the school. The new school clinician will want to know in which of these arrangements the school nurse functions.

The school nurse maintains the health and medical records of the children in the school. Children with hearing loss, cleft palate, cerebral palsy, and other physical problems are already known by the school nurse. The nurse is the one who arranges for medical intervention when it is needed, makes home visits, and knows the families. The school nurse is a storehouse of medical and health information. It goes without saying that the school nurse and the speech-language pathologist work closely together and need to share information on a continuing basis.

In some states, Ohio for example, the school nurse is legally responsible for conducting hearing screenings. The nurse, the school clinician, and the educational audiologist may work together in organizing and administering the hearing-conservation program of detection, referral, and follow-up. Medical referrals and follow-ups involving family doctors, otologists, and other medical specialists may be carried out by the school nurse. Medical problems in addition to those connected with hearing loss would be included.

The school nurse is one of the best sources of information for the school clinician and should be one of the clinician's closest working allies.

The Physical Therapist

By definition a trained physical therapist works in the general area of motor performance. The services may focus on correction, development, and/or prevention of motor-related problems. Physical therapists are more likely to be found in hospitals or home health care agencies than they are in public schools. They no longer work under a doctor's prescription but often under medical referral. Physical therapists usually develop a written treatment plan for each patient, which is countersigned by a physician.

Physical therapists work with persons with ambulatory problems, focusing on the improved use of the lower extremities in sitting, standing, walking, and movement with and without aids.

The school SLP and the physical therapist may work together in serving children with orthopedic and neurologic problems and on developmental programs for high-risk infants. Physical therapists may also provide information and assistance to SLPs in achieving good posture for optimal breath support and control and in the stabilization of extraneous movements for cerebral palsied children. In addition, physical therapists may evaluate motor abilities for students who are possible candidates for communication boards or augmentative communicative equipment.

The speech-language pathologist can provide the physical therapist with assistance in the establishment of methods of communication modes with their clients.

The Occupational Therapist

Because the work of the occupational therapist covers such a wide range it is difficult to define the scope of activities. The profession of occupational therapy is concerned with human lives that have been disrupted by physical injury, accident, birth defects, aging, or emotional or developmental problems. The programs in occupational therapy are designed to help persons regain their well-being and their "occupation." The word *occupation* does not necessarily refer to the individual's employment but rather to being occupied in meaningful day-to-day activities, including work, leisure, and play.

272

Chapter 9:
Working with
Others:
Collaboration
and
Consultation

Occupational therapists work in a variety of settings, and today an increasing number are employed in public school systems. The occupational therapist and the SLP will find many areas of cooperation that will enhance the disabled student's potential. These same areas, however, may also give rise to conflicts regarding professional responsibility as well as differences in therapeutic approaches. The answer to this problem seems to be the establishment of a truly cooperative working relationship. Each profession has unique skills, and the recognition and respect for each other's expertise will only serve to help the handicapped individual.

Occupational therapists may work with the severely disabled child, especially in the development of adaptive devices, such as conversation boards, that aid greater independence. They may work with children with visual-spatial perceptual problems or with children who are having trouble adjusting to handicaps. They may work with a child individually or with groups of students in such activities as role playing, games, work adjustment sessions, and discussion groups.

The Health and Physical Education Teacher

One staff member who may be in as close of contact with pupils as the classroom teacher is the health and physical education (HPE) teacher. This individual sees students in an environment where movement is stressed, where pupils are engaged in activities in which they may be more relaxed, and where talking may be more spontaneous. School SLPs may be able to work with the HPE teacher in generalized activities for the pupil with an articulation problem. The HPE teacher can also help with the pupil with a voice problem who yells too much. The HPE teacher is competent in teaching relaxation strategies and may help the mild cerebral palsied or dysfluent pupil. The HPE teacher on the elementary or secondary level can be a valuable resource person for the SLP.

Nonteaching Support Personnel

In every school building, there are many nonteaching support personnel with whom speech-language pathologists, audiologists, and students interact. This includes the clerical staff, cafeteria workers, bus drivers, gardeners, custodians, and volunteers who make the school function.

These individuals, who often know the students in different ways than the teacher, are important people without whom the school could not run smoothly. The SLP can rely on them for information on where to get things and where to find things as well as information on the school buildings, equipment, and classroom housekeeping. The custodian may be the only one who knows that in the back of a storage closet there are some textbooks, workbooks, chairs, or a portable chalkboard that the clinician could use.

All of these individuals can contribute something to the success of a school therapy program even if it is just a positive comment now and then. Their work and contributions to the operation of the school should be acknowledged. They will provide you with more efficient and effective services if you take the time to share information about your program with them. Oftentimes these individuals live in the school district community and will promote your program to their neighbors if they understand what it is that you do. In addition, they interact with children on a daily basis and can provide compliments and reinforcement to children on your caseload.

Working with Family

Throughout this book references are made regarding the importance of working with family. Public Law 94-142 and Public Law 99-457 have mandated the inclusion of parents and/or guardians in the planning and intervention process. This is not a new role for the SLP; most have always worked with the parents of children on their caseloads and the parents of children at risk. In this section the term family shall be used to include parents, guardians, and significant other family members who can contribute to the program designed for a child.

Involving families can facilitate development of meaningful intervention goals, better implementation of recommendations, and effective transfer of skills from the therapy room to daily life. Winton (1990) and Crais (in press) suggest observing several underlying principles when integrating families in the intervention process:

1. families are the constants in our client's lives, but service systems and individual professionals may be only sporadic;
2. families should be equal partners in the assessment and intervention process;
3. services should foster families' decision-making skills while protecting their rights and wishes;
4. professionals need to recognize the individuality of clients and families and modify their own services to meet those needs; and
5. services must be delivered within a coordinated and "normalized" approach.

There is no one set of rules on how the school SLP works with families, but for the beginning clinician it might be helpful to have some general ideas. As clinicians gain experience they develop their own "style" of working with family.

The first thing to remember is that parents are people, and the basic ingredients in working with people are understanding and respect. The inexperienced clinician sometimes approaches parents with a preconceived idea of how they are going to react and behave and, therefore, expects resistance. At the same time the parents may anticipate the clinician's role as that of the "expert" who has at hand all the information and know-how to "cure" their child's problem. Obviously, then, everyone gets off on the wrong foot. But if the clinician approaches the parents in a friendly open way and lets them see her or him as a person whose task is to apply the most appropriate principles of rehabilitation (or habilitation) to the situation, the clinician will set the stage for the next step in

274

**Chapter 9:
Working with
Others:
Collaboration
and
Consultation**

the process. It is the clinician's responsibility to establish the ground rules and create the climate. A knowledge of body language would be helpful to allow the clinician to "read" the parents more accurately. Many useful books are written on this topic.

Also important is the ambience of the parent conference. For example, is there a desk between the clinician and the parents? How are the chairs arranged and are they comfortable? (They can sometimes be too comfortable!) Are they all an equal height? Is the light from the window directly on the clinician's or the parents' faces?

In addition to discussing these questions in the university classrooms, it is helpful for prospective SLPs to use role playing as a vehicle for rehearsing situations commonly encountered by the school clinician. For example, here are a few role-playing situations involving parents:

1. Parents ask whether having their child's tonsils removed will help his speech problem.
2. Parents ask how long Johnny will be in therapy to cure his stuttering.
3. Parents ask how they can stop the neighborhood children from teasing their child because she "can't talk right."
4. A parent asks if her smoking during pregnancy caused her child to be hard of hearing.

Role playing allows the prospective clinician to act out situations in front of a critical but friendly audience. In this way future clinicians can share observations and feelings with their contemporaries and discuss various ways the comments and questions may be dealt with in real situations. Students shouldn't expect agreement on what may be considered the "right" answer, and it is not fair to use the evasive phrase, "It depends on the situation!"

Parent Groups

As the school clinician you will be working with parents on a group basis as well as in individual situations. Parent groups may be organized by the school clinician as support groups or by the parents themselves out of a felt need. The professional in this kind of relationship assumes the "helping" role in which parents can be encouraged to express both positive and negative feelings without being judged. Parents of handicapped children often have feelings of guilt, as if something they did or didn't do caused the child's handicap. Professionals need to understand this and to help parents use the group situation as an opportunity for change, growth, and personal development. The use of the words *ought* and *should* are best dropped from the SLP vocabulary when dealing with anxious parents.

Parents, especially mothers, can be the most reliable sources of information concerning the child's speech, language, and hearing behavior. For example, if a parent insists that her child stutters when playing with an older sibling, accept her word for it. Subsequent observation will often prove her correct.

Family patterns are changing in the modern world. There are many single-parent families, latchkey children, children who are cared for on a daily basis by someone other than a parent, and divorced and remarried parents in families in which the children are "his," "hers," and "ours." The effect of these family situations may often have negative effects on the child. The speech-language clinician needs to be sensitive to this possibility.

There are other family situations that the school clinician may have never encountered in his or her own experience but nevertheless should be prepared for. One is that of the child from the poverty-level or lower-income family. Unfortunately this condition is becoming more and more common. The school clinician should keep in mind that many of these children come to school hungry, malnourished, and inadequately clothed. The cutback in the school lunch programs by the federal government will cause even greater problems in the future. Children who are hungry have needs greater than the refinement of minor articulation problems. However, the school clinician should not assume that children from poverty-level families are children who are not cared for and loved. These children may have a rich and loving family life and may receive superior parenting.

Involving the Student

Too often, children with impairments are treated as inanimate objects. Other people talk about them and decide how to teach them or how to "fix" their communication problems. This eliminates them from the decision-making process and does not enable us to understand if the student feels the communication impairment is important or not. It also prohibits us from gaining insights about the student's interest or motivation for improving communication skills. Some students even have a perspective on how to structure therapy to benefit them most.

Whenever possible, the student should be included as a member of the collaborative team. Efforts should be made to provide the student with a clear understanding of the communication impairment and how it effects the performance academically and socially. When possible, the student should be asked to contribute ideas for developing a treatment program which can effectively meet his or her personal needs. Of course, the quality and quantity of a student's involvement as a member of the collaborative team will depend on how the involvement is sought and on the student's capability for understanding the problems and for providing information. The level of involvement should be commensurate with the student's cognitive and social maturity.

Working with Physicians in the Community

A good relationship with the physicians in the community enhances the speech, language, and hearing program. School clinicians should take every opportunity to establish such relationships by conducting their programs in a professional

276

Chapter 9:
Working with
Others:
Collaboration
and
Consultation

manner—following established local protocol in referral procedures, writing letters and reports that are professional in content and style, and giving talks to local medical groups if invited to do so.

A competent school clinician never oversteps professional bounds by giving medical advice or advice that could be construed as medical in nature. For example, the school clinician may think that a child's persistent husky voice may be the result of either vocal abuse or vocal nodules, or possibly a combination of both conditions. After collecting as much information as possible from parents and teachers and the child, the clinician then follows local referral policies established by the school system. These policies will differ from school system to school system. In some places all medical referrals are done through the school nurse, the school social worker, or some designated administrator. The school policy may allow the clinician to discuss the contemplated referral with the parents, who then follow through by taking the child to the family physician. The referral is accompanied by a letter from the clinician and includes results of diagnostic procedures, general impressions, and specific questions, as well as any other helpful information. The clinician should also include a request for the results of the physician's diagnosis and suggestions. It is best to request that the physician's results should be sent to the SLP, with a copy to the parents.

When parents ask the clinician to suggest a physician in the event they don't have a family doctor, the acceptable policy is to give the family the names of at least three doctors from which they can choose.

The question of who pays for the medical services has, at this writing, been addressed by Public Law 94-142. According to Dublinske and Healey (1978) the following interpretations of the law were made:

Must Medical Services Be Provided at no Cost to the Parents?

Yes and No. If the medical services are diagnostic in nature and necessary to determine if a child is handicapped, the cost of such services are to be provided at no cost to the parent. For example, medical diagnostic services could include assessments by laryngologists to determine that a child has a voice disorder or otologic assessments to diagnose hearing disorders if not available as part of the regular school program hearing conservation services. Medical services that are restorative or rehabilitative in nature cannot be funded under Public Law 94-142.

Nothing is more important than good health. The child who is ill or in need of medical attention cannot be expected to perform well in school. School clinicians should be alert to the child's physical condition. If there are any behaviors or symptoms that might be related to a health condition, the school clinician should discuss this with the school nurse and/or the principal, who would then take the proper referral steps.

Working with the Dentist

There are a number of areas of specialization within the dental profession, among them pedodontists, who are concerned with children's dental care; ortho-

277

**Maintaining
Ongoing
Communica-
tion with
Others**

dontists, who are concerned with dental occlusion; and prosthodontists, who are concerned with designing and fitting appliances to compensate for aberrations within the oral structure. SLPs may make referrals to, or may be the recipient of referrals from, these dental specialists as well as the dentist in general practice within a community. The referrals may be children whose articulation problems are related to dental or oral cavity problems, such as cleft palate or other craniofacial anomalies. Children with dysarthrias associated with cerebral palsy, as well as developmentally disabled children, may require special handling by dentists. Thus the professional relationship between the dentist and the SLP requires cooperation.

Maintaining Ongoing Communication with Others

How do SLPs bridge gaps in understanding? First, it must be emphasized that understanding is a two-sided coin and that although clinicians seek to be understood, they must also understand the roles and responsibilities of school administrators and personnel. Second, this is a continuous, ongoing process requiring a vigorous and assertive stance on the part of the SLP. Administrators and teachers are not about to invite us as SLPs to tell them who we are or what we can do. The pathologist must be like the Fuller Brush salesperson of the past and start by getting a foot in the door. Third, this responsibility should have the support and active participation of the American Speech-Language-Hearing Association, over 45% of whose members are employed in schools, as well as state and local professional organizations such as the Council for Exceptional Children.

Blosser and DePompei (1984) suggest that administrators are not likely to take steps independently to find out more about the SLP profession. They recommend that an assertive, proactive approach is needed to gain administrative support. To accomplish this, administrators must first be educated about the profession and be encouraged to work with the SLP to facilitate effective program changes. The SLP needs to establish a more visible position in the school so that administrative attention, understanding, and cooperation can be attained. Blosser and DePompei suggest that an Administrator Education Program be initiated in the following manner:

1. Conduct a quality program. No program change or growth can occur unless quality is already in operation.
2. Identify the key decision-makers within the school district. Determine who needs to be "educated." This may include principals, teachers, curriculum directors, central office administration, school board members and parents.
3. Continually supply key administrators at the building, central administration and top administration levels with facts and information that will challenge them to act on behalf of the speech-language therapy program when decisions are being made.

278

**Chapter 9:
Working with
Others:
Collaboration
and
Consultation**

4. Increase the visibility of the speech-language therapy program districtwide:

   a. Join school committees and attend building activities.

   b. Participate in prevention services and in-service activities.

   c. Host invitational days. ("Board of Education Day"; "Principal's Day"; "Administrator's Day"; "Teacher's Day.") Invite important people to observe therapy sessions.

   d. Establish an on-going mechanism for communication such as a monthly newsletter.

   e. Offer to speak at Board of Education meetings, local parent groups, church groups, etc.

   f. Serve as a source of information to other educators regarding communication skills. Forward informative clippings and articles about the importance of effective communication skills and/or therapy. An "FYI" ("For Your Information") approach could be effective.

5. Inform administrators of your aspirations and goals for your program. Arrange for a meeting with district leaders to share your ideas about the program's strengths, weaknesses, and potentials.

It is important to seize every opportunity possible to form working relationships with parents, students, and fellow professionals. Because there may be conflicting schedules and time is a precious commodity for all, it is essential for clinicians to be creative and use a wide range of mechanisms for exchanging information with others about communication disorders, program goals, and intervention strategies. These mechanisms can include face to face conferences, written communication (letters, reports, newsletters), audio and video tape recordings, discussion groups, inservice meetings, news articles, and observations.

Figure 9-3 shows a variety of mechanisms which can be used to form effective working relationships with specific constituency groups.

Community Information Program

Keeping the community informed about the speech, language, and hearing program in the schools has a number of advantages. First, it interprets the program of prevention, assessment, and remediation to the public at large and may remove any possible stigma attached to having a child enrolled in the program. It also builds a feeling of trust and confidence in the program and toward the school system in the community.

A community information program should not be a haphazard affair; it should be well planned and executed. It should not be a "one-shot" deal but rather continuous, consistent, and persistent. It should also be varied, informative, and interesting.

The school clinician may want to survey the types of media available within the community. The most commonly utilized are newspapers, radio, television, service clubs, lectures and presentations, and displays.

The clinician may wish to make arrangements with the local newspaper to run a series of articles on such topics as types of communication problems, how parents can help children learn to talk, the school therapy program, helpful

FIGURE 9.3. Methods for Communicating with Others

Listed below are several methods which can be used to form effective working relationships with others in order to develop awareness of the SLP program and cooperation for effective intervention.
Students
Visits to classrooms Interactions throughout the building Visual displays inside and outside the therapy room
Students' Parents
Discussion groups and training programs Written communication (newsletters, progress reports, homework notes) Conferences (face to face and telephone) Observation days and school visits
Teachers and Special Educators
Meetings and conferences to develop educational plans Written communication (notes, letters, reports, newsletters, summarizing relevant articles) Inservice meetings Audio and video tapes Discussion groups Informal interactions (lunch, school events, after school activities)
Administrators
Inservice meetings Meetings and conferences Written communication (budget requests, annual reports, summaries of relevant professional literature, service statistics, thank you notes, state association newsletters, reports describing conferences attended)
Community
Participation in school events Speaking and/or membership in community organizations
Local Professionals
Networking through professional organizations Inservice meetings Written communication (newsletters, letters, reports)

suggestions for families of children with fluency problems or hearing impairments, the importance of early referral, and the many other topics of interest to parents and community members.

In preparing articles for release in the local newspapers, it is best to inquire of the editor how long the article should be and then stick to the length suggested. If an article submitted is too long the editor is likely to trim it and may inadvertently cut out an important part. Most editors like to have articles submitted, but they should be well written and interesting. The school clinician can usually obtain from a member of the newspaper staff the pertinent facts on style and length. If pictures are used and they contain any children, it is an absolute *must* first to obtain written consent of the parents.

280

**Chapter 9:
Working with
Others:
Collaboration
and
Consultation**

Some school systems have a person in charge of community information or public relations, and this individual will often assist the clinician in preparing articles for publication.

Radio interviews or other types of radio programs are a good way of getting information across to the public. Local radio stations often welcome suggestions on programs of special interest. Clinicians can utilize such timely events as Better Speech and Hearing Month in May to focus attention on the needs of persons with speech, language and hearing disorders.

The same can be said of television programs. Often local television stations have programs during which various community figures are interviewed. Or the television station may cooperate in preparing a program on various aspects of the speech, language, and hearing program.

Talks to community service clubs, professional organizations, and other groups can yield innumerable benefits. Many of these groups sponsor special projects or programs as part of their community service activities. Another effective way of informing the community about the program is through displays at health fairs and similar events. Public libraries are often willing to add to their shelves books of interest to parents of handicapped children. The school clinician can make suggestions for specific books, which could then be made available to the public.

DISCUSSION QUESTIONS AND PROJECTS

1. Invite an elementary principal in to talk to the class on how he or she views the speech, language, and hearing program.

2. Interview a learning disabilities teacher on how he or she works with the school SLP.

3. Find out what your state requires in the certification of educational audiologists.

4. List ways the SLP in the school can work with the classroom teacher on the teaching of reading. How would you implement these strategies?

5. How would the SLP in the schools schedule time for collaboration?

6. Plan an in-service session or a group meeting for elementary-school principals to acquaint them with the speech, language, and hearing program.

7. Do a survey of the health and rehabilitation agencies in your community. What are their referral policies and their criteria for accepting clients?

8. Ask a practicing school pathologist what the policies are concerning medical referrals in that school system.

9. Write a brief article about a speech-language or hearing topic that could be submitted to a local newspaper or radio.

CHAPTER 10

A Sampling of Programs

Introduction

Students-in-training have often expressed interest in how school speech-language pathologists carry out their programs. To obtain information on the various programs, a questionnaire was sent to four individuals in various geographical areas of the United States. The purpose of the questionnaire was to obtain a sample of programs in different parts of the country. No attempt was made to query representative programs or to quantify the information received or even to draw any conclusions from the comments returned. Rather, it was felt that the information these individuals provided would be helpful to prospective speech-language pathologists in the schools.

All the respondents at the time the questionnaire was returned in 1991 were actively engaged in school programs, and all are holders of the Certificate of Clinical Competence in Speech-Language Pathology from the American Speech-Language-Hearing Association. Two of them represent one segment of their school's larger speech-language program. The other two sent questionnaires to various clinicians in their programs. Their answers represent a combination as well as a variety of roles. The school speech-language pathologists are: Deborah Kendall, Phoenix, Arizona, Elementary District Schools; Sally De-Witt Tippett, Peoria, Illinois, Elementary District Schools; Jane Frobose, Fulton County Schools, Atlanta, Georgia, and Lynne Coleman, Akron, Ohio, Summit County Public Schools.

The answers to the questions are not given in the order of the names as listed. However, the order given here is consistent throughout the series of answers. In other words, the number 1 answer throughout the series is always the same SLP each time.

The questionnaire asked the clinicians to provide the following information:

A. Describe the service delivery models you employ in your program.

B. Describe the process used for referral for speech-language hearing services (how and by whom?)

C. What diagnostic and assessment instruments do you use most frequently?

D. Do you conduct the screenings listed below?
   If someone other than you conducts these screenings (e.g., psychologist, nurse, etc.), indicate that person's discipline and the rationale for their involvement.

> Speech—
> Language—
> Hearing—

E. Do you conduct the follow-up assessments?
   If someone other than you conducts these assessments (e.g., psychologist, nurse, etc.), indicate that person's discipline and the rationale for their involvement.

> Speech—
> Language—
> Hearing—

F. Describe your procedure for caseload selection.

G. What are your program's strengths and areas in need of improvement?

A Sampling of Programs

A. Describe the service delivery models you employ in your program.

1. I have a self-contained preschool for three- and four-year olds with communication disorders. They must score at least one and one-half standard deviations below the mean and/or be unintelligible to the parent. This is the only self-contained program for communication disorders (for any age) in the district. School-age children receive services either in a pull-out setting (majority), in-class services with small groups or the entire class involvement, or consultation services.

2. I am currently assigned to one school only so I am able to provide two major types of service delivery models. First, traditional active therapy services through a "pull-out" model are provided in 25- or 30-minute sessions. Individual therapy sessions are minimal, but are offered if needed. Generally, students are seen in groups of three to four students. (The State of Georgia stipulates that an SLP can see no more than seven students per segment/hour.)
   Consultative services through an in-class intervention model are provided to students enrolled in a Modified Self-Contained Learning Disabilities class-

room. My current school houses three of these classrooms at this time. Students categorized as LD typically demonstrate developmental delays or gaps in their language abilities. The in-class model is designed to meet the communication needs of students exhibiting generalized delays as well as students exhibiting specific deficits.

3. The information below is based on the program designs of approximately 30 clinicians. These clinicians meet the needs of many different types of children (normally developing to multiply handicapped; preschool through high school) in ten local and small city school districts. Interestingly enough, although the situations in which the clinicians participate are different, their philosophies, concerns, delivery models and program designs are very similar.

The main service delivery model provided by our clinicians remains the individual, pull-out model for many of the children seen. The clinicians, however, are seeing the need for additional models due to the increased numbers and needs of the children being referred. At this point, many clinicians are using classroom-based collaborative and consultative models especially for younger and more handicapped children. More and more the clinicians are planning with teachers and other school professionals either using a consultative model (where the clinician still provides the service but consults with school personnel on content and logistics) or in collaboration with school personnel (where the clinician works with school personnel on program design and implementation). Parent programs are used by many clinicians, as well.

4. The delivery of services by each speech pathologist is somewhat dependent upon the type of program served. Most of the regular division speech pathologists serve paired primary and middle schools. They most frequently use the pull-out small group therapy model of service. This year, the Peoria Public Schools implemented two kindergarten programs—SKILLS and the classroom language program.

The parent program, SKILLS (Serving Kids in Language Learning Settings), is designed to provide parents with ideas and/or materials to teach language concepts to their children. Parents or guardians of *all* kindergarten children are invited to attend the SKILLS program presented by the speech pathologist at their child's school once a month.

The classroom language program has helped establish an active involvement between the speech pathologist and the kindergarten classroom teacher. A language lesson is presented in each kindergarten classroom twice a month by the speech pathologist. Both SKILLS and the classroom language program coordinate with the goals that are established in each unit of the reading program.

Special Education and Special Program speech pathologists currently have an opportunity to participate more actively in the classroom program. They can schedule more frequent classroom language lessons and, in some instances, deliver all or part of the therapy service in the classroom. The caseload may be somewhat smaller, which allows time for individual therapy for those with the most severe phonological and language disorders.

The high school speech pathologists each have two high schools and have an opportunity to do more individual therapy. One middle school speech pathologist has an elective class for speech improvement and another class where those in need of therapy meet daily during a regular class period for nine weeks. One speech pathologist services the speech-only and resource pre-school students. She is also involved in some teacher training with nursery school teachers.

B. Describe the process used for referral for speech-language-hearing services (how and by whom?).

1. For the preschool, we receive referrals from the local agencies that evaluate children, but do not provide services. Parents hear of the program and bring the child in for screening or hear of our "round-ups" we conduct in June every year.

2. Fulton County Schools do NOT implement a mass Speech-Language screening program. The Speech-Language Pathologist (SLP) presents an inservice to all schools at the beginning of each school year in order to educate the entire faculty as to the services provided by the Speech-Language Department along with its referral procedures.

Students may be referred to the SLP by any faculty member (i.e., administrator, classroom teacher, art/music/PE specialists, etc.). Parents may also refer their children.

The referring individual presents referral information and reports of attempted classroom interventions to the school's Educational Support Team (EST). The EST is composed of nonspecial education teachers, the school psychologist, a Student Support Teacher, and the SLP. The school's guidance counselor generally serves as the chairperson of this team.

The EST then determines if a referral for a Speech-Language Evaluation is warranted, or if additional classroom interventions are needed. The SLP then follows through with all Speech-Language Evaluations.

Mass hearing screenings are provided annually to all students in grades 1, 3, and 5. The initial screenings are completed by trained parent volunteers. All re-screenings must be completed by the school's SLP.

3. In regards to speech and language, most of our clinicians depend on teacher and other school professionals for referrals. The greatest number of referrals come from the teachers followed by the school psychologist, school nurse, counselors and parents. Screening also is used for speech and language referrals, but this is limited to preschool, kindergarten, new student, and special education classroom students only.

Referrals for hearing come, to a great extent, from screenings completed by the clinician or the clinician in conjunction with the school nurse and/or volunteers. In almost every school, the clinician completes some portion of the hearing screening or threshold/impedance testing and then does the follow-up. The teacher and/or school nurse is called in when the clinician, after repeated trials, is unable to contact the parents. Screenings for hearing, in most cases, follows the Ohio Department of Health guidelines for ages, grades and standards. In addition, almost all clinicians screen new students, their caseload, special education classroom students and kindergarten children on a yearly basis for hearing. The reason for completing screenings for each of these groups of children is due to the higher percentage of communication and/or hearing difficulties that may be found in these groups.

4. Many of our students are identified early through an extensive preschool screening program. Developmental screening is offered to every child ages three through five who resides within the boundaries of our school district. This is conducted by a trained SCREEN team and the areas of vision, hearing, speech, language, cognitive development, fine and gross motor, social and self-help skills are included in the screening process.

We also accept referrals from private agencies who may have identified and worked with the families and children from birth through age two. Some referrals may come from other qualified professionals, parents, or teachers who are asked to indicate students in their classes who might need speech/language services.

C. What diagnostic and assessment instruments do you use most frequently?

1. We use the *Brigance Preschool Screen for three- and four-year-olds* for the screening. We use the *Test of Auditory Comprehension of Language* and the *Expressive One-Word Picture Vocabulary Test* for the testing along with a language sample. The articulation assessment is with the *Alpha Test.* Spanish speaking children are given a translated version (locally translated—no norms) of both tests and the decision is predominantly based upon the language sample. School-age students are screened with a local screening instrument that includes parts of the Woodcock and TOLD. Assessment is each clinician's decision with a budget for ordering assessment instruments of their choice.

2. *Articulation:* Goldman-Fristoe Test of Articulation
Computer Analysis of Phonological Processes

Language:	PPVT-R	Language Processing Test
	EOWPVT-R	WORD Test
	TOLD-P	TOPS
	CELF-R	Preschool Language Scale
	TACL-R	SPELT-II

Fluency: Protocol for Differentiating the Incipient Stutterer (Rebekah Pindzola)

Stuttering Severity Instrument

Voice: Fulton County Voice Evaluation Form

3. *Articulation:*

1. Test of Minimal Articulation Competence (T-MAC),

2. Goldman Fristoe Test of Articulation and Phonological Process Analysis,

3. Photo Articulation Test

Language:

1. Test of Language Development (TOLD-P, TOLD-I)
2. CELF-R and CELF Screening-R
3. Test of Adolescent Language (TOAL)
4. Test of Written Language (TOWL)
5. PPVT-R
6. Language Processing Test and The Word Test
7. Test of Auditory Comprehension of Language (TACL-R)
8. SPELT (Pictographic Expressive Language Test for Syntax)

As well as tests for auditory comprehension (i.e., VADS, Token Test, TAPS), teacher checklists for educational verification, language and phonological process samples of spontaneous speech and clinician-made tests based on curriculum.

4. A survey of the speech pathologists in our district revealed a wide variety of tests used, particularly for language assessment. Those speech/language tests mentioned most frequently were:

Expressive One Word Picture Vocabulary Test

Peabody Picture Vocabulary Test

Hodson Phonological Test

Bankson Language Screening

Test of Language Development—Primary and 2

The Word Test

Goldman-Fristoe Articulation Test

Woodcock Language Proficiency Battery

Language Processing Test

Test of Auditory Perceptual Skills

Receptive One Word Picture Vocabulary Test

The Fullerton Language Test for Adolescents

Wilson's Voice Evaluation

In addition to the standardized tests, a developmental skills assessment is used in some of our special programs to test children who are functioning at or below the 72-month level. The speech pathologist tests the receptive and expressive language skills while the teacher, occupational therapist, and sometimes the psychologist, are involved in evaluating the cognitive, fine motor, and gross motor sections of the test. The Stuttering Severity Instrument is sometimes used with those who have fluency disorders; however many of our speech pathologists use this with some suggestions for evaluation not yet published that were recently presented in a class.

D. Do you conduct the screenings listed below?

If someone other than you conducts these screenings (e.g. psychologist, nurse etc), indicate that person's discipline and the rationale for their involvement.

    Speech—
    Language—
    Hearing—

1. We all do the speech and language screening and assessments. Hearing is accomplished as a team with the school nurses. The nurses are responsible for the follow-up so they are involved in the initial testing and screening. Pure tone and impedance testing is included.

2. SPEECH—YES
LANGUAGE—YES
HEARING—YES. The Student Support Teacher may complete initial hearing screenings for students that are in the referral process. The SLP must complete all re-screenings as needed, and then implement any necessary referrals to the Audiology Department.

3. Screening is completed in the areas of speech, language, and hearing to decide on the need for subsequent evaluation and/or services. Each kindergarten child is seen for communication and hearing screening as best practice for early intervention. Recently, H.B. 140 has mandated that each kindergarten child or first grade child new to the system (who has not previously received a screening) be screened by November of the school year in which the child first attends.

Our clinicians screen each child referred to the school psychologist for special education programming and at each three year re-evaluation for special education students.

The teacher is involved in the screening process as a second party to validate the need for services and to give information to the clinician on how the communication and/or hearing deficit affects the child educationally (verification of educational adverse affect). Information also is received from the child's parents, school nurse and other professional who is involved in service provision to the child.

4. Regular division students are screened by the City/County Health Department for hearing and vision. The Health Department can then make a medical referral for the child, if necessary.

Special education students are screened annually by the school health technicians. They also screen regular division students who are referred for a case study evaluation and children participating in the preschool screening program.

The speech pathologist screens the hearing each year of the children enrolled in therapy. He/she is also responsible for the speech/language screening of students newly enrolled in the district, and those enrolled for the first time in a public school setting. Those transferring from another district are rescreened and/or the screening results of the previous district are reviewed. The trained staff of Project SCREEN conducts the speech/language screening of preschool children during the developmental screening program.

E. Do you conduct the follow-up assessments?

If someone other than you conducts these assessments, (e.g., psychologist, nurse, etc.), indicated that person's discipline and the rationale for their involvement.

> *Speech—*
> *Language—*
> *Hearing—*

1. We do the follow-up of the speech and language testing. We do compare results of our testing with the psychological test results if the child is being totally evaluated at the time. The nurses follow up on the hearing, but are apt to ask some speech pathologists to help with the more difficult to test children or those with inconsistent test results.

2. Yes.

3. It is the responsibility of each clinician to complete follow-up assessments.

4. The speech/language pathologists do all of the evaluations for speech and language.

Audiological evaluations are done by the audiologist for regional programs who is located in a central facility in our school district. The audiologist also does re-evaluations for those who have hearing problems which require annual monitoring.

F. Describe your procedure for caseload selection.

1. For preschool, we select the children who fall within the moderate range. The severe children (below 2.5 SD below the mean) are sent to other programs shared by some districts for financial reasons. As we are now mandated to serve all qualifying children reaching the age of four, we fill up the program I have, and then will refer the "extras" to other programs in other districts. As mandating expands, we will establish more programs of this type.

2. The SLP completes the Speech/Language Evaluation and then writes an Eligibility Report. The SLP then reviews the Eligibility Report with her assigned Eligibility Team (comprised of 6–8 SLPs from within our county). Eligibility Teams are important to ensure continuity of student placement throughout the county, which employs 35–40 SLPs. The team can also offer a firmer guarantee that county guidelines for placements and dismissals are adhered to closely.

Specific guidelines for caseload eligibility have been formulated by the county and/or State of Georgia, and are found in the SLP Procedure Manual.

3. Each clinician considers a formula based on evaluation scores and team judgment of need as established by at least the clinician, teacher, parents and a

district representative in caseload selection. The greatest number of children selected show a standard deviation of 1. or more below the mean or at least one year of age below chronological age as seen in standardized testing for articulation and/or language. Team and parent judgment to show need and educational adverse affect also are considered in caseload selection.

Consistency of the problem and adverse affect are considered most often in fluency and voice caseload selection with the addition of medical clearance in the area of voice.

Written criteria for eligibility and dismissal has been established as a guideline in caseload selection in the Summit County Schools. This criterion is now being revised.

4. The caseload selection process varies with each speech pathologist and the population served. In the special education program I serve, most of the students are enrolled in speech/language and have that service as part of their IEP. Those who do not have speech/language as an immediate priority are part of the classroom language program once a week.

Regular division speech pathologists take into consideration developmental factors, age, test results in relation to school placement and achievement, and the severity of the child's speech/language disorder. The effect of the child's speech/language skills on academic performance, communication, and social functioning is also considered.

After considering these factors, the SLP makes a priority list of the most severe to the mild cases. Those in the very severe, severe, and moderate range are usually enrolled in therapy. Mild problems are re-screened later. Those with severe phonological disorders, poor intelligibility, severe language, voice, or fluency problems would be high priority cases. Those with both speech and language problems and those with multiple articulation errors would take precedence over those with single sound errors.

According to district criteria, a student is eligible who demonstrates any delay from the expected age of developmental acquisition of one or more separate phonemes in any word position as measured by standardized articulation assessments of sound in word production and sound in sentence or conversational sample, or demonstrates less than 75% intelligibility in conversational speech and errors in more than four separate phonemes in any word position.

Criteria for language include a kindergarten to fifth grade student who demonstrates a language age of at least 8 to 12 months below his/her chronological age or a sixth to twelfth grade student who demonstrates a language age of at least 18 months below his/her chronological age. Students may also be enrolled if language performance is at or below the tenth percentile or if the scaled scores fall more than one standard deviation below the mean of the test, as measured by two standardized language assessments. For the Educable, Trainable, or Profoundly Mentally Handicapped, the mental age rather than chronological age is utilized in determining eligibility.

Any student is eligible who evidences more than one stuttered word per minute during the stuttering evaluation and whose teacher and/or parent indicates the presence of stuttering behavior.

Any student is eligible who evidences voice characteristics which consistently deviate from normal, as measured by Wilson and whose teacher and/or parent indicates the presence of deviant voice characteristics.

G. What are your program's strengths and areas in need of improvement?

1. The major strength is the *early* intervention with the child and the family. By exposure to school setting, readiness skills and speech/language services, the children are brought much closer to being ready for kindergarten. Many do still need speech/language services in the early grades, but have gained other skills (e.g., readiness skills, small motor and gross motor coordination, social skills, self-discipline, etc.). The improvements that are needed include better assessment of Spanish-speaking children. A test that is written in the same Spanish spoken in the area (there is great variation between that spoken in Arizona, Texas, Mexico, Spain, etc.) is greatly needed. We teach the children in Spanish if they are Spanish dominant, so we need to evaluate (pre- and post-testing) properly. This is also true for the school-age children in the district. They need good evaluation instruments for the Spanish-speakers and we greatly need Spanish speaking SLPs.

2. *Strengths:*

1. The fact that I am assigned to one school full-time allows me to function as a true member of the faculty. It enables me to better "inservice" other teachers as I am always accessible to them. It also allows me that extra time required to provide the in-class service model to our Self-Contained LD students, (time which an itinerant SLP spends packing up and travelling to two or more schools.)

2. Another strength of my program/"county" is related to the materials that are available. I have an adequate selection of assessment and therapy materials. At my particular school, I also have an Apple IIGS computer in my room two days per week.

3. The Eligibility Teams are a strength of our county as they support the SLP's recommendations and provide evidence that those recommendations are agreed upon by several professionals. It also enables SLPs to have some time to associate with peers and have some time to "talk shop" or share ideas/concerns/gripes.

4. Students receiving active services are given Speech-Language folders (by this SLP) in which to keep all therapy activities and worksheets. This enables parents to see what is being done in therapy and to complete home practice assignments if they are given. The folder also serves as a vehicle for communication between the SLP and the parents.

Weaknesses:

The areas in need of improvement are time/funding related. I am in desperate need of planning time so that I can be more creative with my therapy activities. We are allowed 4 hours of "release" time per week for planning, assessment, etc. However, the referral lists are never-ending so this "release" time is always spent as diagnostic-time with no time left for planning or the completion of paperwork.

Paperwork is very demanding and is truly a "second" job. It seems as though the amount of paperwork time is the equivalent of student-contact time, most of which is handled after school hours.

As with all SLPs in the schools, the number of students on our caseloads is higher than we would like; Georgia's maximum caseload size is 55 students—this does NOT account for severity.

Finally, additional staff development time is needed to stimulate new ideas and to keep up with trends and developments in our field. Staff development sessions used to be held monthly by the Speech-Language Administration, but they have stopped due to lack of funding, increased caseload demands, and lack of "release" time due to state regulations.

3. The area of greatest strength in our program(s) is the professionalism of the speech-language pathologists who have been hired in each school district. Each of the clinicians with whom I work spend a great deal of time in not only screening, assessment, and intervention, but also in documentation of services provided, dissemination of information to parents and other professionals on the communication and hearing processes of specific children and communication in general, program development, staff development, certification and knowledge improvement, creativity of programming and working with other members of the school environment as a school professional (our clinicians do bulletin boards, schedule inservices, take bus and lunchroom duty, etc.).

Our speech-language professionals need more time. The need for intervention, testing, paperwork and professional involvement all take time. Now that school professionals know how much our clinicians can add to an educational program, their services are in demand. Most of our clinicians are most reactive to the needs of the children and professionals in the schools. This often leaves little time to be proactive or to try other service options.

Our speech-language professionals need more financial resources for purchase of equipment (i.e., FM units, impedance audiometers, augmentative communication devices, tests and protocols, etc.).

Our speech-language professionals need more resources. Though our speech-language professionals often provide information and help to teachers, administrators and parents, they find it difficult to depend on these people for their own support needs.

4. Strengths of our speech/language program are:

A. Emphasis on language development in the kindergarten through classroom language lessons by the speech pathologist, suggestions for language tables to coordinate with skills learned in the reading program, and identification of difficult vocabulary in each unit.

B. SKILLS program for helping parents teach language skills to their children.

C. Well qualified professional staff who work together and continue to take college classes and attend meetings and seminars to update their skills.

D. A sincere interest in meeting the special needs of the population we serve.

E. Computerized IEP program written by our staff to meet our needs and updated annually. This provides a consistency as students move from one school to another in the district.

F. Speech pathologists are hired for some of our special programs to allow more time for each population to be served.

G. An effective team approach with the active involvement of the psychologist, social worker, teacher, speech pathologist, and, in some cases, the occupational therapist working together to meet the needs of the children.

Areas in need of improvement are:

A. More parent involvement.

B. A smaller caseload mandated by the state to adequately service the severity of the population we serve.

C. Adequate and convenient space is sometimes difficult to obtain in the primary schools.

CHAPTER 11

Student Teaching

Introduction

Student teaching is sometimes regarded with trepidation by the prospective student teacher, probably because like all new experiences it contains the element of the unknown. The unknown is usually anticipated with a mixture of fear, curiosity, and excitement. The actual experience may bear out what was anticipated, and it may also contain some surprises.

The following comments from student teachers provide insights for contemplation, not only for prospective student teachers but for school and university supervisors as well:

> The thought that occupied my mind as I drove home after my first day of being a student teacher, was, "How will I ever make it?" I had come face to face with part of my "Sammy Snakes," "quiet sounds," "growling sounds," "frog sounds," and I foresaw ten weeks of writing lesson plans and thinking up activities. And now, here I am ten weeks later. I can look back to that first day and laugh when I think of how my ideas have changed. It doesn't seem possible that I could have experienced all that I did. My student teaching was in all aspects a total learning situation.

> Student teaching has been a great experience and has been more of a benefit, not only from the professional point of view, but also from the personal point of view, than I ever imagined it would be. It has been a lot of hard work and a lot of time invested, but the satisfaction, rewards, and learning that this has created has made it all worthwhile.

> Without having had the opportunity to student teach, the answers would have been a long time coming.

I suddenly realized that I didn't need to be unsure, for I could handle the situation that I feared, adequately and surprisingly well.

I have met with many new experiences as a member of a school system. I have met many teachers, talked with them and have gotten to know them as fellow educators. I feel much more confident being out in the schools since I am no longer regarded as a "student." When the teachers ask my professional opinion about various children, their confidence in me boosts my confidence in myself.

I feel the most important things I learned from my student teaching experience were through my own mistakes. I had a very intelligent school supervisor who allowed me to experiment and try new things on my own. When I failed, I learned a great deal. Instead of telling me my ideas were inappropriate, she allowed me to find out for myself through my own mistakes.

As a student teacher I have grown to understand the daily routine, unexpected problems and hassles a school clinician must go through and accept. I have also experienced the rewards a therapist obtains when a child achieves progress and success. Being able to take over many of the responsibilities has opened my eyes and allowed me to see how fulfilling it is to be able to help children improve in their speech communication.

One fact which cannot go without mentioning is that in this field we are all professionals and must uphold a certain dignity and respect for our position while complying with ethical standards. Through my student teaching experience I have had a taste of the professional dignity and hope in the future I will be able to combine the professional and personal components for a complementary balance.

My student teaching experience was the most rewarding one of my college career and I owe most of this to my school supervisor, who allowed me to experiment with my own ideas while watching me with a critical eye.

One mistake I feel that I made at the beginning of student teaching was in failure to ask questions about everything that was going on around me. I don't know if I was afraid to ask them or if I didn't know which questions to ask but either way it was a mistake. I think I went in with the attitude that I was "supposed" to know everything. This is, of course, the wrong attitude to take. The whole purpose of student teaching is to learn and what better way to learn than by asking questions?

The seminars during student teaching have been very helpful. The discussions were relaxed, free, and very relevant.

My supervising clinician was very helpful when I asked questions. She gave me her professional opinions and/or referred me to other professional sources. Although she informed me of reasons why some therapy sessions were less successful, she did not fail to commend the progress she saw and my success in therapy.

Student teaching has shown me how a school can function, how to deal with faculty, staff, and parents, and possible procedures to follow in making referrals and recommendations.

Another thing I've learned is that the activity is not terribly important. I've wasted a lot of time trying to be like Milton-Bradley or some of the other games and toy makers. What is important is getting the child to use his good speech and language as much as possible during the session.

The most valuable information I obtained was how to schedule clients and set up a therapy program.

Mrs. Harms maintained an atmosphere of organization, responsibility, cordiality and resourcefulness throughout the entire ten weeks. Because of such outstanding qualities in my supervising school clinician, I had a very fulfilling and rewarding student teaching experience.

I consider the practical experience that student teaching afforded me to be the most effective learning device in my college education. It was a positive and growing experience. Student teaching has started a growing in me, and a desire to grow more which I can continue for the rest of my life.

What is the purpose of student teaching in speech-language pathology and why is it a necessary and important part of the preparation of school SLPs? According to Anderson (1972),

The purpose of the school practicum as a part of the training program of the speech-language pathologist and audiologist is to provide certain learning experiences which the university or clinic setting cannot provide. If the practicum is to be meaningful there must be a careful delineation of those learning experiences which can and/or should be provided in each of those settings. It must be recognized that the student who begins his practicum in the schools is not a "finished" clinician but a student who needs certain types of experiences before he is ready to assume the responsibility of a job of his own.

The Student Teaching Triad

Basically, three persons are directly involved in the process of student teaching. The first is the student teacher who is doing his or her practicum in an off-campus school system; the second is the pathologist employed by the school system, who is directly responsible for the day-to-day supervision of the student intern; the third is the university supervisor.

Too often the roles and responsibilities of the various participants in the student teaching process are not clearly defined and these individuals are put in a situation of not knowing what is expected of them, what to do, or how to do it. Following is a list of the roles, qualifications, and responsibilities of the persons involved in the clinical practicum in the schools. This is by no means a complete list, and others may wish to add to it or delete from it (Neidecker, 1976).

I. *Qualifications of the University Supervisor:*

A. Shall have a master's degree in speech pathology and, or, audiology.

B. Shall have ASHA Certificate of Clinical Competence in speech-language pathology and, or, audiology.

C. Shall have had experience as a full-time public school pathologist for a minimum of three years.

D. Shall be a competent speech-language pathologist.

E. Shall have had experience in teaching on a university speech pathology and audiology staff.

F. Shall demonstrate ability in supervision techniques, evaluation methods, counseling, and in-service training.

G. Shall have knowledge of school administration; general and special education policies and laws; physical planning of speech-language and hearing facilities; the process of developing programs for children with speech, language, and hearing disabilities; available social and welfare agencies and services; and the practice and psychology of management techniques.

H. Shall be aware of the current issues facing educators and contemporary trends in education.

I. Shall have the following personal characteristics:

   1. Shall be an effective communicator.

   2. Shall be objective and flexible and able to adapt to change.

   3. Shall have the capacity for self-evaluation and the ability to profit from mistakes.

II. *Responsibilities of the University Supervisor:*

A. Shall be responsible for establishing criteria in regard to the time when a student is ready for practicum in the public schools.

B. Shall be responsible, in part, for selection of the cooperating pathologist.

C. Shall assume that the university still has the ultimate responsibility for the student's practicum experience.

D. Shall be responsible for conducting in-service training for cooperating pathologists.

E. Shall act as consultant to the cooperating pathologist.

   1. Shall provide time for conferences to keep the cooperating pathologist informed of the university program and policies.

   2. Shall provide written materials concerning the university policies and procedures.

   3. Shall provide information on the background of the student teacher, both general and specific.

   4. Shall be able to provide a wide variety of resource materials, approaches, and techniques which are based on sound theory, successful therapy, or documented research.

F. Shall establish goals with the student teacher which are realistic and easily understandable.

   1. Shall prepare informational material about the expectations of the

student teacher and policies of the university regarding the school practicum.

2. Shall observe the student teacher during the practicum.

3. Shall confer with the student teacher each time a visit is made to the school.

4. Shall provide opportunity for the students to give feedback on their practicum experiences both during and after the practicum experience, either in writing or through conferences.

G. Shall promote communication between the university and the public school setting.

H. Shall act as mediator between the student teacher and school administration.

I. Shall act as mediator between the cooperating pathologist and the student teacher.

J. Shall participate in conferences with the student teacher and the cooperating pathologist individually and collectively.

K. Shall establish that the responsibility for the student teacher's practicum is shared equally by the university supervisor and the cooperating clinician, but that the daily supervision of the student is the responsibility of the cooperating pathologist.

L. Shall be able to demonstrate therapy for both the student and the cooperating pathologist during the therapy session.

M. Shall share with the cooperating clinician in making the final evaluation of the student teacher.

III. *Qualifications of the Cooperating Clinician:*

A. Shall have had at least three years experience in the public schools as a speech, language, and hearing pathologist.

B. Shall have the appropriate credentials as a speech-language pathologist in the schools.

C. Shall be recognized by colleagues as a competent professional person.

D. Shall be willing to have a student teacher.

IV. *Responsibilities of the Cooperating Clinician to the Student Teacher:*

A. Shall be responsible for the day-to-day supervision of the student teacher.

B. Shall acquaint the student teacher with available materials and equipment for screening and diagnostic procedures.

C. Shall acquaint the student teacher with materials available for therapy.

D. Shall encourage the student teacher to create and develop his or her own materials.

E. Shall supplement the student teacher's background information through reading lists and other references.

F. Shall provide the student teacher with information regarding the school system in reference to school policy, location of schools, the community, dismissal and fire drill procedures, and other appropriate information.

G. Shall provide the student teacher with opportunities to:

1. Observe the cooperating pathologist doing therapy.

2. Assist in screening and diagnostic programs.

3. Plan for and evaluate therapy sessions.

4. Visit classrooms where children with speech, hearing, and language impairments are enrolled.

5. Meet other school personnel informally and also confer with them about specific children.

6. Write progress reports, case history reports, letters, therapy logs, and individual educational programs.

7. Become familiar with the reporting, recording, filing and retrieval systems used by the cooperating pathologist.

H. Shall provide feedback to the student teacher regarding strengths and weaknesses. The feedback shall be done on a regular basis and may take the form of verbal communication, written communication, tape recordings, video taping and, or, demonstration therapy.

I. Shall encourage the student to develop behavioral objectives regarding himself and the children with whom he works.

J. Shall encourage and assist the student to utilize supportive personnel and aids when available.

K. Shall encourage the student to become increasingly independent in thinking and problem solving.

V. *Responsibilities of the Cooperating Clinician to the University Supervisor:*

A. Shall inform the university supervisor immediately of any problems that arise.

B. Shall be aware of and assist the student in fulfilling university requirements.

C. Shall provide the university supervisor with feedback concerning the student's progress.

Qualifications of the Student Teacher:

A. Shall, after completion of practicum, be no more than one quarter or semester away from completing the degree program in speech-language pathology and, or, audiology at an accredited university.

B. Shall have completed the required clinical practicum.

C. Shall have had observation experience in a school setting prior to school practicum.

D. Shall demonstrate physical, mental, and emotional stability.

E. Shall possess acceptable speech and language patterns and adequate hearing.

VII. *Responsibilities of the Student Teacher:*

A. Shall be aware of and adhere to the Code of Ethics of the American Speech-Language-Hearing Association.

B. Shall be aware of and carry out the university requirements during school practicum.

C. Shall adhere to the policies and practices of the school to which assigned.

D. Shall comply with the directives of the cooperating pathologist as to working in the school therapy program.

E. Shall expect to be treated as a professional person and act accordingly.

F. Shall demonstrate ability to be dependable and assume responsibility while realizing that the cooperating clinician is legally responsible for the children being treated.

G. Shall contribute to the fullest extent to the school therapy program based on academic background and university clinical practice.

H. Shall demonstrate ability to establish and maintain appropriate interpersonal relationships with school personnel.

I. Shall demonstrate ability to establish and maintain appropriate rapport with children.

J. Shall demonstrate ability to evaluate self in therapy and a willingness to accept and utilize constructive criticism.

K. Shall be aware of the criteria for evaluating the practicum experience.

L. Shall recognize status as a learner and regard the practicum as a learning situation from which much is to be gained.

M. Shall expect the practicum experience to assist in the development of skills enabling one to function as an independent professional person.

N. Shall demonstrate interest in continued professional growth by making use of resource centers, attending in-service meetings, workshops, and professional meetings.

The Student Teaching Program

Universities have many ways of carrying out the student teaching program in speech, language, and hearing. Obviously, there are many different patterns that are followed successfully depending on conditions and factors present in local areas and on the philosophy of the university concerned. There are, however, some commonalities that we will consider.

Schedules. It is important that the student teacher submit a day-by-day schedule to the university supervisor. Because many school therapy programs are on intermittent program schedules, several centers may be involved in the student teacher's assignment. Important also is the obligation of the student teacher to keep the university supervisor informed of the hours he or she will be at the

schools, as well as times when therapy may not be going on as a result of interruptions to the school's daily schedule.

Log of Clinical Clock Hours. In addition to fulfilling the university's requirements
for daily attendance, the student clinician must also consider the future possibility of verification of clinical clock hours for certification by the American
Speech-Language-Hearing Association, licensing in various states, and certification by state departments of education. Most universities use a weekly reporting
system, and the forms used to record this information vary. Besides the identifying information, the forms should include places to record the age range of the
children; the various types of communication problems; and the amount of time
actually spent in diagnosis, audiometric testing, screening, and group and individual therapy sessions. The student teacher and the cooperating pathologist
should sign the completed form. A summary form may be filled out at the
conclusion of student teaching.

Lesson Plans. A daily written plan of intervention for each child with whom the
student teacher works is a necessary tool of therapy. The plan should include
both long- and short-range goals for each child, procedures, materials used, and
evaluation of the therapy session. The evaluation is done by both the cooperating pathologist and the student teacher and may include the progress of each
child, the effectiveness of the procedures and the materials used, and the effectiveness of the approach used by the student teacher. There is no one universally
accepted form for a lesson plan, but most forms include the same basic elements.

Seminars. It is common practice to hold seminars for the student teachers on a
periodic basis. These seminars may be held weekly or less often, depending on
the philosophy of the university. Frequently, the seminar time may be used for
discussions and sharing of information and problems; speakers may be invited to
discuss pertinent issues, panels may be utilized to familiarize student teachers
with current information, demonstration therapy or diagnosis may be carried
out, visits may be made to agencies or centers, and one seminar may be devoted
to an explanation of school policies and practices. It is valuable for student
teachers in speech, language, and hearing pathology to attend at least several
seminars that include all student teachers in a school system.

Evaluations. Assuming that self-evaluation and evaluation by supervisors is an
ongoing procedure, it also may be useful to have a more formal type of written
evaluation at the midpoint and at the conclusion of student teaching. The form
used for these evaluative procedures should be in the hands of the student
teachers during the first week of student teaching, or even prior to it, so that they
know exactly what will be expected of them.

The midpoint evaluation should let the student teacher know his or her
weak points, strengths, areas needing improvement, and how these improvements may occur. The student teacher then has the responsibility to act on the
suggestions.

The final evaluation may be an evaluation of the student teacher during
that experience, and it may also contain the perceived professional potential of
that individual. It is important to differentiate between these two items. No

student teacher emerges from the experience a "finished product," and this should be conveyed in the final evaluation report.

ASHA Certification Requirements

The American Speech-Language-Hearing Association has set standards in regard to the supervision of student clinicians on both the graduate and undergraduate levels. They have specified that in states where credential requirements and/or state licensure requirements differ from ASHA certification standards, the supervised clinical experiences, including student teaching, must be supervised by ASHA certified personnel (CCC) in order to satisfy ASHA requirements.

At this writing, in some states, there are discrepencies among state requirements, state licensure requirements, and ASHA certification requirements. Student teachers seeking ASHA certification should be aware of these discrepencies. The university supervisor with ASHA certification (CCC) is ethically bound to inform the student in student teaching and other clinical practice that the experience obtained under non-ASHA-certified personnel cannot be applied to ASHA certification (ASHA, 1991).

Additional Guidelines for Student Teachers

Student clinicians should know something about the community in which they are doing their teaching. Knowing the socioeconomic backgrounds of the families in the school districts helps student teachers to understand better the children with whom they will be working. This may be especially important for student teachers whose own backgrounds are different from those of their prospective clients.

There are additional requirements for student teaching that many university training centers have found productive and valuable in assisting student teachers to become full-fledged, competent professional persons. One is a checklist of experiences the prospective student teacher has had before the teaching experience. Such a checklist submitted to the cooperating pathologist is helpful in acquainting that person with the student teacher's capabilities. It might include information on any experience in child care such as baby-sitting or teaching church school; observational experience; clinical practicum experience; diagnostic experience; academic experience; and experience with tape recorders, audiometers, assistive listening devices, video tape machines, duplicating machines, and computers and augmentative devices.

Each university training center has developed its own requirements and often includes policies regarding the behavior of student teachers. The following partial list was adapted from the Student Teaching Handbook at Bowling Green State University (Weinberger, 1991).

A. Student teachers should not be used as substitute therapists nor should they be used to perform such activities as playground, cafeteria, or recess duties.

B. Dress and grooming of student teachers should be consistent with the standards of the schools to which they have been assigned.

C. Many school speech-language pathologists visit several schools during the course of their work week. Policies on transportation for student teachers among schools and to and from the school system should be clearly understood and adhered to prior to starting the student teaching assignment. Most student teachers provide their own transportation.

D. Outside activities such as jobs or coursework are discouraged during the student teaching experience. Student teaching is a full-time job and the stakes are high for a successful performance.

E. Under no circumstances should a student teacher administer corporal punishment to a child or serve as a witness.

F. Student teachers should not become involved in strikes, boycotts, work stoppages, or riots. In fact, it is not advisable for a student teacher to report for work should any of these things occur (Weinberger, 1991).

It goes without saying that student teachers should be well versed on the university's policies and keep in mind that during the student teaching or field experience they are guests of the school system.

Competency-Based Evaluation of the Student Teacher

Competency-based evaluation systems can be used to evaluate the student teaching experience. Johnson et al. (1982) developed a form comprised of 89 competencies which was field-tested on 34 student teachers and 30 supervising clinicians for two semesters (see Figure 11-1). The results indicated that the two groups favored the competency-based form to that of the traditional numerical form to evaluate knowledge, skill, and value objectives.

According to Johnson et al., the procedures are as follows:

At the beginning of the semester, the university supervisor distributes the competency-based forms to both the supervising clinician (the public school speech-language pathologist to which the student is assigned in the schools) and the student teachers. The university supervisor meets with the supervising clinician and student teachers to discuss the use of the form. At this time, several aspects of the competency-based form are explained:

1. An explanation of a minimal competency is given. This is the minimal requirement that the student must meet by the end of the student teaching experience.

2. For each competency a choice of "yes", "no", or "not applicable" is given. A review of competency-based systems throughout the education field utilizes a yes/no format. According to a strict competency-based format, the student either demonstrates the competency (by meeting the criteria) or does not. The N/A category was included to cover the skills and cases the student does not experience (e.g., type of caseload).

3. A competency is achieved if the student demonstrates a skill with 85% accuracy by the end of the semester.

4. At mid-term the supervising clinician is to review the form with the student teacher and discuss the student's strengths and weaknesses in various areas.

5. At the end of the semester the supervising clinician is to complete the competency-based objectives form and discuss these results with the student teacher. (At Miami University student teaching is graded on a pass/fail basis.)

In conjunction with the competency-based objectives form, a traditional numerical rating form was used at both mid-term and at the end of the semester. The numerical form, which utilized a scale from 1 to 7, rates the same skills evaluated on the competency-based form with the exception of those skills that could not be rated on a 1-7 basis, that is, the entire laws and standard section.

Guidelines for the Cooperating Clinician

In a chapter dealing with student teaching it is appropriate to include information useful to the person who plans and directs the student internship. That person is the cooperating clinician in the schools.

An article by Hess (1976) contains many excellent suggestions. According to Hess,

It is vital for the cooperating clinician working with a student clinician to realize the importance of student teaching. The student deserves the chance to be involved in a worthwhile program, and it will be worthwhile if he is met with leadership, an opportunity for growth, and a well-planned program.

Hess discusses the responsibilities of the cooperating clinician in the first week of student teaching. They are

1. Communicate with the student clinician before the first week, by telephone call or letter, or an invitation to visit the school ahead of time.

2. On the first day provide orientation for the student by having him meet with the program director and other school pathologists and student teachers to discuss school policies, complete necessary forms, map out routes to the schools, and generally to minimize anxieties. He could also be informed of time schedules of the various schools, as well as the school calendar.

3. During the first week the student teacher should be given a tour of the school buildings and should be introduced to the principal and secretary of each building to which he has been assigned, as well as the teachers, school counselor, nurse, and psychologist.

(*Continued on page 309*)

FIGURE 11.1. Competency-Based Objectives for Student Teaching in Speech and Hearing

By the end of the student teaching experience, the student teacher will be able to:

Laws and Standards—Demonstrate knowledge of laws and standards. He or she will demonstrate the competency by:

YES NO N/A

1. Explaining the mandates of PL 94-142 (HB 455)

2. Outlining the procedures for due process safeguards as determined by the school district.

3. Preparing Individualized Educational Plans (IEP) for at least five children.

4. Participating in a placement team conference.

5. Explaining the state standards for speech therapy services in the school.

COMMENTS:

Screening—Plan and implement an efficient and effective speech-language and hearing screening program. He or she will demonstrate the competency 85% of the time by:

YES NO N/A

1. Explaining the procedures of screening and referral.

2. Select and utilize appropriate screening materials.

3. Screening the speech, language, and hearing of pupils with 85% agreement with the supervising clinician:

   a. Articulation disorders

   b. Language disorders

   c. Voice disorders

   d. Fluency disorders

   e. Hearing disorders

4. Recording results accurately on school records.

5. Interpreting and communicating screening results.

COMMENTS:

Diagnosis—Diagnose speech, language and/or hearing problems. He or she will demonstrate this competency 85% of the time by:

YES NO N/A

1. Selecting appropriate diagnostic instruments and procedures.

2. Administering effectively:

   a. An oral peripheral examination

   b. 2 diagnostic tests for articulation

   c. 2 diagnostic tests for language

(*continued*)

FIGURE 11.1. (*Continued*)

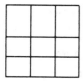

d. A diagnostic assessment for voice

e. A diagnostic assessment for fluency

f. Diagnostic test for auditory perceptual skills.

g. Hearing thresholds

3. Recording diagnostic results accurately on school records.

4. Interpreting and communicating diagnostic results to speech pathologists and key persons/other professionals.

COMMENTS:

Scheduling—Effectively schedule public school therapy programs. He or she will demonstrate this competency 85% of the time by:

YES NO N/A

1. Selecting case load based upon eligibility criteria established by school district.

2. Scheduling program in relation to the needs of the children to be served.

3. Communicating with school personnel about schedule.

COMMENTS:

Planning Procedures—Write effective and appropriate objectives and therapy plans. He or she will demonstrate this competence 85% of the time by:

YES NO N/A

1. Utilizing diagnostic information to determine long-term objectives.

2. Utilizing diagnostic information to determine short-term objectives.

3. Planning a service strategy to meet long-term objectives.

4. Planning a service strategy to meet short-term objectives.

5. Using information and evaluations from previous therapy sessions.

6. Preparing lesson plans in advance.

COMMENTS:

Materials—Demonstrate the ability to select, produce, and utilize a variety of appropriate materials. He or she will demonstrate the competency 85% of the time by:

YES NO N/A

1. Selecting a variety of commercial materials.

2. Making new materials.

(*continued*)

FIGURE 11.1. *(Continued)*

3. Utilizing materials appropriate to client's interests, abilities, and age level.

4. Learning how to manipulate equipment and materials before therapy sessions.

COMMENTS:

Therapy—Conduct effective therapy sessions. He or she will demonstrate this competency 85% of the time by:

YES NO N/A

1. Providing the rational for selection of specific therapy techniques.

2. Using therapy procedures appropriate to child's age level.

3. Establishing and maintaining good rapport with client.

4. Giving directions clearly.

5. Handling child's behavior effectively.

6. Demonstrating creativity in materials and techniques.

7. Beginning and ending therapy on time.

8. Providing for carry-over to classroom and home.

9. Communicating goals and techniques to parents.

10. Communicating goals and techniques to teacher.

COMMENTS:

Articulation Therapy—Conduct effective articulation therapy sessions. He or she will demonstrate this competency 85% of the time by:

YES NO N/A

1. Explaining the theories and demonstrating ability to conduct two types of articulation therapy techniques:

   a. List name of technique: _____

   b. List name of technique: _____

2. Conducting therapy consistent with goals.

3. Discriminating correct/incorrect sound production with 85% agreement with supervising clinician for 85% of the articulation caseload.

4. Obtaining maximum number of responses per therapy session.

5. Providing appropriate and consistent reinforcement.

6. Demonstrating flexibility in therapy situations.

7. Evaluating the pupil's performance with respect to moving on to the next therapy step.

COMMENTS:

(continued)

Language Therapy—Conduct effective language therapy session. He or she will demonstrate this competency 85% of the time by:

YES NO N/A

1. Eliciting a spontaneous language sample.

2. Analyzing a spontaneous language sample.

3. Demonstrating ability to conduct 2 types of language therapy techniques:

   a. List name of technique: _____

   b. List name of technique: _____

4. Conducting therapy consistent with goals.

5. Recognizing correct/incorrect language productions with 85% agreement with the supervising clinician.

6. Obtaining appropriate number of responses per therapy session.

7. Utilizing a variety of appropriate activities.

8. Providing appropriate reinforcement.

9. Demonstrating flexibility in therapy situations.

10. Evaluating the pupil's performance with respect to moving on to the next session.

COMMENTS:

Stuttering Therapy—Conduct effective stuttering therapy session. He or she will demonstrate this competency 85% of the time by:

YES NO N/A

1. Conducting therapy consistent with goals.

2. Explaining the procedures of one therapy program.

3. Teaching fluency techniques.

4. Demonstrating flexibility in therapy situations.

COMMENTS:

Voice Therapy—Conduct effective voice therapy sessions. He or she will demonstrate this competency 85% of the time by:

YES NO N/A

1. Conducting therapy consistent with goals.

2. Counseling pupils about causes of vocal abuse.

3. Discriminating correct/incorrect voice production with 85% agreement with the supervising clinician for 85% of the voice cases.

4. Explaining the procedures of one therapy program.

(continued)

FIGURE 11.1. (*Continued*)

5. Demonstrating flexibility in therapy situation.

6. Explaining the steps of making a medical referral.

COMMENTS:

Other Disorders—Conduct effective therapy sessions. He or she will demonstrate this competency by:

YES NO N/A

1. Explaining the procedures of one aural rehabilitation technique.

2. Explaining the procedure of a program for improving auditory perception skills.

COMMENTS:

Observation and Self Evaluation—Observe and evaluate him- or herself. He or she will demonstrate this competency by:

YES NO N/A

1. Evaluating therapy through audio or video tapes.

2. Compiling data on child's performance in order to plan future session.

3. Following through on suggestions from the supervising clinician.

4. Setting personal objectives for change as a result of self evaluation.

COMMENTS:

Professionalism—Demonstrate a professional attitude. He or she will demonstrate this competency by:

YES NO N/A

1. Attending professional meetings.

2. Exhibiting interest and enthusiasm about his/her work.

3. Interacting with parents.

4. Interacting with school personnel.

5. Dealing appropriately with supervising clinician.

6. Arriving at school on time.

7. Demonstrating regular attendance.

8. Demonstrating initiative.

9. Demonstrating dependability.

10. Dressing appropriately.

11. Demonstrating correct articulatory skills.

12. Utilizing appropriate vocal quality, rate, and intonation.

COMMENTS:

4. The cooperating pathologist should prepare the children enrolled in therapy for the arrival of the student teacher in such a way that they understand his role in relation to them.

5. The cooperating pathologist and the student teacher should discuss the university's materials, requirements, and suggestions so they are mutually understood.

6. The major goals for the student teaching program, as well as assignments and weekly goals, should be discussed. The cooperating pathologist should discuss his expectations of the student teacher and encourage the student to express his own expectations.

7. The student teacher should be made aware of rules, regulations and policies of individual schools, the school system as a whole, and of the speech-language and hearing program in the state.

8. The first week of student teaching should include the opportunity to observe therapy sessions and to become acquainted with the children. During the first week the student teacher may assist with segments of the therapy sessions.

9. If the student teacher is assigned at the beginning of the school year he may assist in the screening programs.

According to Hess, the assigned weeks of student teaching should be utilized effectively and efficiently, but the student teacher should not be overloaded.

There are numerous school activities the student clinician can take part in during the weeks of student teaching. It is important for the cooperating clinician to have a list of priorities or activities that seem most valuable for the student. The list can be compiled from various sources: university information, other clinicians, published articles, and discussions with the student clinician. The student should have the opportunity to take part in as many phases as possible of the school therapy program. Besides learning to organize and carry out a therapy program, the student clinician will want to become familiar with related activities. For instance, it is helpful for the student to attend meetings of the clinicians as well as those meetings held in the individual schools.

The cooperating clinician should discuss with the student clinician how to begin and how to terminate the school year. The clinician will want to include the student in obtaining referrals for therapy and in conferences with teachers and parents. Furthermore, the cooperating clinician can discuss with the student clinician bulletin board ideas, newsletters for parents, parent conferences, and special therapy ideas that have proven successful. The student should learn to use the copy machine and any other office equipment that is applicable to the therapy program. Also the student clinician will want to have information about the many sources of therapy materials.

A Word of Advice to Student Teachers

Are you ready to start your student teaching? Here are some suggestions that might be helpful:

1. Work in harmony with your cooperating pathologist and university supervisor. Their job is to help you become a better speech-language pathologist and/or audiologist.

2. Be enthusiastic about your work and sincerely interested in the children with whom you will be working.

3. Keep healthy; get plenty of rest and eat the right foods.

4. Take advantage of every opportunity to become involved in the unique experiences a school has to offer.

5. Ask questions when you aren't sure, and ask questions even if you *are* sure.

6. Know what you can expect of children at various age and ability levels.

7. Be firm, fair, consistent, and compassionate in all your dealings with children. Every human being deserves respect.

8. Know the ground rules of the various schools and adhere to them.

9. When making professional decisions always ask yourself, "Is this in the best interests of the child?"

10. Enjoy your student teaching experience!

DISCUSSION QUESTIONS AND PROJECTS

1. Interview a current student teacher on his or her suggestions to beginning student teachers.

2. Invite a principal to talk to your class on what he or she expects of the student teacher.

3. What is the student teacher's role when a child must be punished for misbehavior?

4. What is the student teacher's role in relation to children in therapy? Defend your choice.
   a. A buddy
   b. Mother or father figure
   c. "One of the gang"
   d. Authority figure
   e. Permissive big brother or big sister
   f. Teacher
   g. Counselor
   h. One who "lays down the law"
   i. Referee

5. What do you hope to learn from student teaching?

6. Interview a school SLP on what he or she expects from a student teacher.

7. Ask a first-, second-, or third-grade child what he or she likes best about a favorite teacher. Ask a junior high and high-school student the same question. Did you find any differences or similarities in their answers?

CHAPTER 12

Life After College

Introduction

Changes in the field of speech-language pathology and audiology are occurring rapidly. As Heraclitus once said, one may not step in the same river twice, not only because the river flows and changes, but also because the one who steps into it changes, too, and is never at any two moments identical.

What does this mean to you as a beginning SLP? And more specifically, what does it mean to those of you who will be employed in education? First, it means that this is an incredibly interesting time to be alive and in the field of communications. This era has been called the "age of communication," and the SLP or audiologist will be in the thick of it. You will need to be knowledgeable and involved in the world, not only the world of the therapy room and the classroom, but also the community beyond.

In this chapter we will look at some of the ways you will be able to keep abreast of current information through professional journals and continuing education programs. Your role as a researcher will also be examined. Collective bargaining and the school SLP is an issue of importance to you. We will also look at ways you may provide interviewers and prospective employers with information about your skills, knowledge and attitudes, in order to enhance your employment opportunities.

The importance of being familiar with state and federal laws is discussed. Due process procedures in the light of malpractice claims are described, as well as liability insurance.

There IS life after college. Welcome to a very interesting, challenging, and important profession. Be your best self and do your very best.

Professional Publications and Resources

As the roles of the school SLP and audiologist expand, there is a need to keep abreast of current information. This is particularly crucial for school clinicians working in remote areas or in areas where there is no access to academic libraries, medical libraries, or even public libraries. School libraries usually do not have publications pertinent to a school pathologist's needs.

Throughout the United States regional resource centers have established a statewide network system with regional centers that have among their services the collecting and distributing of special education materials as well as providing information about the materials. They also help school personnel create new materials when commercially produced products are not available. Information is provided by newsletters concerning the services and materials available.

The American Speech-Language-Hearing Association publishes the *Journal of Speech and Hearing Research; Language, Speech, and Hearing Services in Schools; The American Journal of Speech-Language Pathology: A Journal of Clinical Practice; The American Journal of Audiology: A Journal of Clinical Practice; ASHA Monographs; ASHA Reports;* and *Asha.* The National Student Speech-Language-Hearing Association publishes *The NSSLHA Journal.*

Public libraries in almost all communities have an interlibrary loan service whereby library materials are made available by one library to another for use by an individual. In addition to books, materials may include audiotape, videotape, film, and microfilm. The community public library can be of great assistance to the school clinician, and librarians are always helpful in obtaining materials. The school clinician may want to visit the library and find out what kinds of services are available.

Language and Language Behavior Abstracts is published quarterly and examines the contents of approximately 1,000 publications for articles to be summarized. The subject categories are speech and language pathology, special education, verbal learning, and psycholinguistics. Subscriptions can be obtained by writing to P.O. Box 22206, San Diego, California 92122.

The Council for Exceptional Children publishes *Exceptional Child Education Resources (ECER)*, a quarterly journal that contains abstracts of books, articles, research, and conference proceedings. It also offers reprints of selected computer searches from *ECER* and ERIC (Educational Resources Information Center). *Resources in Education* is published monthly and contains abstracts of research reports and materials, with the exception of journal articles.

Continuing Education

Another way in which the SLP keeps up to date on professional matters is through continuing education, in the form of workshops, short courses, seminars, miniseminars, in-service training courses, professional meetings highlighted by competent speakers, university courses, extension courses, teleconferences, televised courses, and presentations by film and videotape. Continuing education can be carried on by a structured program or on a more informal basis. It is a lifelong process for an individual expecting to remain accountable and qualified. It is a process by which one keeps one's skills and knowledge up to date.

Continuing education is not only necessary to the individual currently practicing but also helps those persons who interrupt their professional lives and wish to reenter at a later date.

Continuing education is not the responsibility of any one institution or agency but should represent the coordinated efforts of a number of groups. Universities cannot offer extension courses in a geographical area unless there is an expressed need concerning the content area of such a course. For the university to plan for such courses, the need should be expressed to the university staff by the school clinicians. By the same token, universities should be willing to offer courses at a time that would be convenient to the school clinicians and in a location that would be accessible to them.

Members and nonmembers of the American Speech-Language-Hearing Association who are holders of the Certificate of Clinical Competence may apply for an award called the ACE (Award for Continuing Education). Credits are earned through continuing education activities under ASHA-approved sponsors. A specific number of CE units are awarded to the participant for each instructional activity, and a national CE registry is maintained; on the completion of the required number of units the ACE is awarded.

Research

It is doubtful that anyone would argue against the need for research about public school speech, language, and hearing programs. Neither is there any question that the public school is a fertile field for research in communication disorders. To add further emphasis, PL 94-142 has created pressure to find answers to questions about prevalence of speech, language, and hearing problems; comparison of delivery systems; efficacy of therapeutic methods; and other important issues.

Unquestionably a fertile field for possible research, the school programs have produced little in the past. There are a number of possible reasons given by school clinicians. Among them are lack of time, lack of funding, lack of support by school boards, lack of cooperation by university staff members, and lack of interest by journals. The fear of performing statistical analyses, the lack of training in research methods on the university level, and the lack of rewards have also been suggested as reasons for the lack of research in the schools. Another reason may be that SLPs may simply be more interested in being clinicians than researchers. This is understandable in light of their employment setting. On the other hand, school clinicians are always eagerly reading journals and attending professional meetings in the hope of finding answers to questions.

A profession must be based on a body of knowledge, and this body of knowledge is accumulated by research. There must be interested individuals to pose questions and interested individuals to seek answers and solutions. Collaboration by researchers in universities, specialists in departments of education and special education on both the state and federal levels, and school SLPs is one of the methods for generating research on the public school level.

The publications *Language, Speech & Hearing Services in Schools* and the *Journal of Childhood Communicative Disorders* contain reports of collaborative research between school SLPs and university faculty members. Public schools provide a good base for research projects, and university personnel are a good source of information for consultation on research design. It should be kept in mind by school-based SLPs, however, that university faculty members are also busy people; the SLP can't just call the local university for help with research and expect an immediate response.

Other sources of collaboration are state and local departments of education and special education and area speech, language, and hearing professional organizations.

Single-subject studies are especially amenable to research projects by the school SLP. The clinician can carry out this type of research without disruption of schedule and without ethical constraints on using school-age clients for research. Parents and school administrators need only to be advised. Single-subject studies can yield information on therapy methods and case management options. The two previously mentioned publications contain numerous examples of single-subject studies by school SLPs.

Longitudinal studies, in which a single subject or a group of subjects are followed for months or even years, are ideally suited for public school researchers in speech-language pathology. An example of this type of study involved a 15-year follow-up of 50 children initially diagnosed as communicatively impaired (King et al., 1982). Although the study was not conducted by school-based investigators, it has implications for the school SLP in terms of methodology and research. According to King et al.,

> The kind of results collected in this study suggest that some alteration in the expected outcome of academic, social, and emotional difficulties seen along with speech and language problems can be observed. This alteration may be related to early and long-term speech-language services. What appears to be critical is a need for careful records from standardized and documented nonstandardized evaluation procedures, progress toward stated therapy goals, progress and/or lack of progress in the classroom setting, results of standardized academic achievement tests, and results of teacher rating scales ranking the child's social and emotional development. It is hoped that the clinic will work diligently with school personnel to collect these data. Although the task requires some additional time on the part of all concerned, the information is desperately needed.

The school clinician of the future will undoubtedly be involved in research on the local level, the state level, or as part of a national research project. The questions are everywhere, and the need to find answers is urgent. The questions of the school clinician in Mississippi may be the same ones asked by the clinician in Montana. Not only is the search for answers important, but equally important is the need to exchange professional information. By recording data on standardized forms they can then be computerized and related to data collected and recorded in other geographical areas. The use of computers has already proven to be effective in speech, language, and hearing, and will continue to grow as a valuable method of storing, retrieving, and displaying data.

Collective Bargaining and the School
Speech-Language Pathologist

The unmistakable trend toward collective bargaining in the public sector clearly indicates that school speech-language pathologists and audiologists need to develop procedures for negotiations. Collective bargaining has a long history in the private sector and since 1962 when New York City teachers negotiated a collective bargaining agreement it has become a significant factor in American education. Collective bargaining is an outgrowth of the desire to have a say in such issues as salary, fringe benefits and working conditions.

Whether the American Federation of Teachers and the National Education Association call themselves labor unions or professional organizations is a moot point. If they bargain collectively with management they are functionally labor unions. The American Speech-Language-Hearing Association and the various state speech, language and hearing associations are professional organizations because they do not negotiate salaries, contracts, and fringe benefits.

Many, but not all, states have collective bargaining laws and the laws differ from state to state. Your state's labor relations board can give you information on your state's collective bargaining law. Whether you, as a speech-language pathologist or audiologist, are considered management or labor will depend on your state's collective bargaining law. If your state classifies you as management, during a strike you may be called on to staff a classroom. If you are classified as labor, it is important to become involved in and work with the union or unit at the local level to make sure the issues and concerns important to you are brought to the bargaining table.

The decision of whether or not to affiliate with a local collective bargaining unit depends on the local situation. If you belong to the local unit of either AFT or NEA you must also belong to the state and national organization. If you do not join the locally designated unit it is required by law that the unit must bargain for you regardless.

School speech-language pathologists and audiologists are at a disadvantage primarily because they comprise a very small percentage of persons covered by the bargaining unit. During negotiations when concessions are made it would be easier for a unit to give up a demand affecting the few speech-language pathologists in favor of a demand affecting all the classroom teachers.

According to Dublinske (1986): "It appears that speech-language pathologists can have the most impact in the collective bargaining process if:

1. ASHA works with the NEA and AFT at the national level to make them aware of the general needs related to the working conditions of speech-language pathologists and audiologists employed in the schools;

2. state speech-language-hearing associations work with the NEA and AFT affil-

iates at the state level to make them aware of specific state needs and to work on state legislation that will improve working conditions; and if

3. individual speech-language pathologists and audiologists get involved in the collective bargaining process at the local level. If speech-language pathologists and audiologists are going to be able to use the collective bargaining process to improve their working conditions it is important to become knowledgeable about their state's collective bargaining law and how negotiations are handled locally."

According to Johns (1974):

A strong local teachers' organization can offer representation before the school board, county board, or state legislature; communications including action reports, news releases, and media coverage for educational problems; professional services and developments such as negotiations with the school board (concerning salary), arbitration of grievances, attainment of better employment conditions, and greater voice in curriculum matters; and such advantages as tax-sheltered annuities, notary service, legal service or legal defense, housing placement, civic representation, and discounts with local merchants.

You and the Law

Free and appropriate education for all children with handicaps was mandated by Public Laws 94-142, 99-457, 101-476 and Section 504 of the Civil Rights Act of 1978. These laws also described procedures for parents and other parties to appeal when they believe it is not being provided. The 1986 Public Law 99-372 provided for the recovery of attorney's fees when the parents prevailed. This legislation has opened the door for the possible increase in the number of appeals generated. Due process hearings are the proceedings between the school and the family, presided over by a presumably impartial hearing officer. Often, prior to the due process hearing, the school district attempts to amicably resolve the misunderstandings.

How can the school SLP prepare for a due process hearing? A checklist of activities was compiled by staff members of the Montgomery County Public Schools, Rockville, Maryland (Clausen, Gould, Corley-Keith, Lebowitz, 1988). These activities include the following:

1. *Case Background:* Review student school files; review speech/language file, note reason for referral; consult with pertinent staff (teachers, therapist, etc.); compile a chronology of significant dates and events.

2. *Individual Education Program (IEP):* Check inclusion of and be familiar with: disability code; model of service recommended, and intensity of program; evaluative instruments, including validity and norms; data reported, both formal and informal; strengths and needs; goals and objectives related to needs; mas-

tery criteria; committee members, parent's presence; other special education services.

3. *Program Implementation:* Review therapy logs and note: attendance, group size/composition, techniques and materials, and progress; review observations of student in educational program; note parent contacts, frequency and content.

4. *Testimony:* Be prepared to: summarize your credentials, educational background and experience; discuss your knowledge of the case; discuss evaluative finds and the basis for recommendations; describe test characteristics, validity and normative data; discuss the program in relation to student needs; describe progress and how measured.

Some behavioral do's and don'ts were also recommended. They suggested maintaining professionalism and formality at all times, taking notes on any points you hear that may help your case presenter, and stop testifying and wait until the question is resolved if there is an objection from either side. They also advise not to panic if you are placed under oath and not to talk except when testifying. Conversing with the hearing officer and discussing hearing issues with the opposing side during breaks should not occur (Clausen et al.).

Further information on the ethical and legal considerations of the speech, language and hearing profession and due process issues may be found in the following documents and publications:

Downey, M., "Due Process Hearings and PL 94-142," *Asha,* 22 (1980), pp. 255–57.

Downey, M., "Conduct of the Due Process Hearings," *Asha,* 22 (1980), pp. 332–34.

Dublinske, S., "PL 94-142 Due Process Decisions," *Asha,* 22 (1980), pp. 335–38.

Dublinske, S., Healey, W., "PL 94-142: Questions and Answers for the Speech-Language Pathologist and Audiologist," *Asha,* 20 (1978), pp. 188–205.

Edminister, P., Ekstrand, R., "Lessening the Trauma of Due Process," *Teaching Exceptional Children,* 19, (1987), pp. 6–10.

Flower, R. M., "Legal and Ethical Considerations," *The Delivery of Speech-Language and Audiology Services.* (Baltimore/London: Williams and Wilkins, 1984), pp. 252–90.

Malpractice claims are a continuing risk for speech, language, and hearing professionals. There are preventive measures such as maintaining good client relationships, careful documentation of therapy procedures, and knowledge of current state and federal regulations. But the best guide to avoiding malpractice claims is strict adherence to the American Speech-Language-Hearing Association's Code of Ethics. (See Chapter Two.) The Code of Ethics not only serves as a model of behavior for you, as a professional person, but it also protects the consumer (in this case, the student) against dangerous practices of inexpert and injudicious individuals.

As a school speech-language pathologist, you may be the subject of a claim in a malpractice suit but you are much more likely to be called as an "expert witness" in a trial. An expert witness does not have direct knowledge of the case at hand but by virtue of education, research, or experience is qualified to testify.

Professional Liability Insurance

As the school speech-language clinician's caseload and role expands to include a wide variety of communication disorders and intervention tasks, the possiblity of situations occurring for which the clinician may be held liable is increased. Though this may be a sad commentary on the state of our world today, it is nevertheless a reality. Thus, it may be important to maintain professional liability insurance in case such an event should occur.

The decision to be covered by liability insurance as a protective measure is a purely personal one. It is also dependent upon the kind of working situation you are in. Check with your local school system to see if there is coverage through an educational agency. Another source of information is ASHA or your state speech-language-hearing association. Liability insurance for speech-language pathologists and audiologists would cover all professional activities but may not cover corporal punishment, transportation by private auto, and travel by aircraft or watercraft.

Your personal insurance agent is also a source of information; you may already be covered under your own insurance plan.

Insurance for student teachers is usually offered by universities at a nominal sum. It is incumbent upon the student to find out what is specifically covered. Student teachers may also be covered under their parent's insurance plans.

Getting Your First Job

In this section of the chapter, we are indebted to Bowling Green State University, Bowling Green, Ohio, and JoAnn Kroll, director of Placement Services. The information herein is based on and has been adapted from the university's publication *Job Search: A Guide for Success in the Job Market.*

Where to Start

The job search for you, as a beginning SLP, may start any time during the last year of college. The best place to start is your university placement office. The service is available at most universities and is usually free to students and alumni. The first step in your job search will be to visit your university placement office to find out what specific services are available. Generally speaking, this is what they have to offer:

1. Individual counseling
2. Vacancy listings
3. Credential services
4. On-campus interviews
5. Placement seminars and guest speakers
6. Library with information concerning employment strategies, career opportunities, alumni placement services, videotapes, and slide/sound presentations

7. Mock interview training and critique sessions

8. Staff referrals of qualified candidates

After you find out what services are available, which ones are applicable to you, and which ones you want to utilize, it is time to plan your strategy. Timing is important here. You will want to visit the placement office after you have completed most of your academic work and clinical practice but before you start your student teaching.

The Credential File and Portfolio

School personnel administrators expect to see well-organized and up-to-date credential files on prospective SLPs. The credential file you accumulate must document your past achievements and support your candidacy for a position. It is important to begin early to complete the necessary forms required by your university's placement office and gather the appropriate letters of recommendation from faculty members and past employers.

A complete credential file should include the following:

1. *Letters of recommendation.* Most university placement services have a reference form on which the student writes his or her name, address, social security number, and so on. There is a place on the form for the reference writer to make statements regarding your professional or personal relationship and how long the writer has known you. There should be a description of your academic or career growth and potential, a review of your principal achievements, an estimate of future promise at this point, a paragraph on your personal qualities, and a final summary paragraph.

2. *Student teaching evaluation.* An evaluation is made by the student teaching supervisors during the experience. This may also include the perceived professional potential of the student teacher in the final evaluation report.

3. *Transcript of grades.* This is obtained from the registrar of the university.

If you intend to use someone's name as a reference it is always necessary to request that person's permission in advance. The reference letter may be sent directly to the university placement office or to you. If it is sent to the placement office it is desirable to request a copy for yourself. Always enclose self-addressed stamped envelopes.

Regardless of immediate or long-range plans, establishing a credential file at the university placement office is strongly advised for all students and alumni. Be sure you keep it up to date by informing the office of current professional addresses and positions and by periodically including letters of reference from employers.

One of the most successful "marketing tools" is the use of the student teaching portfolio. Your résumé, samples of lesson plans, photographs of displays or bulletin boards, and statements verifying your participation in educational projects both before and during the student teaching should be placed in the portfolio. Your student teaching supervisor can offer excellent recommendations concerning the content and layout of the portfolio.

One of the keys to successful interviewing is preparation. It is also one of the best ways to combat nervousness during the interview. The beginning point of your preparation is to know yourself. Review your personal inventory and background thoroughly and always in light of the position you are seeking. Be prepared to answer questions regarding your education, grades, courses, jobs, extracurricular activities, goals, strengths, weaknesses, and other information. Keep in mind that the interviewer is asking himself or herself the question, "Why should I hire you?" In answering this question be prepared to give examples and illustrations of your abilities, skills, leadership, effectiveness, and potential.

Successful preparation for the interview also entails knowing the school system. Your placement office may be able to assist you. Other sources for general information include newspaper articles, school board minutes, parent-teacher organizations, or your university education department. However, you would also be interested in learning about the speech, language, and hearing programs, information you would be able to obtain by asking the interviewer questions. Pertinent questions would include the following: How many SLPs are presently on the school staff? How long has the program been in existence? What is the school population? How many buildings and grade levels are being serviced by the speech-language program? To whom is the speech-language clinician directly responsible?

Another important way to prepare for the interview is to practice. With a friend, relative, another candidate, or a placement staff counselor, role-play a mock interview. Pay especially close attention to questions that may deal with some weaknesses or problem areas in your background. Don't wait until you reach the interview to think about responding to a question concerning a weakness.

Another facet of interview preparation is appropriate dress. First impressions are often lasting impressions, and you must look as if you fit the role before an employer will let you act the role. How you dress is a statement about how you feel about the significance of the interview and who you will be meeting. Careful attention to dress and grooming is a way of putting your best foot forward. When in doubt it is best to be conservative in your dress.

What can you expect the interviewer to be like? Because you really don't know in advance you will need to take your cues from the content of the interview. If the interviewer wants you to do most of the talking and wants to assess your ability to communicate and reason, this individual's style will be nondirective. If the interviewer is concerned with eliciting specific and precise responses, the style will be more formal and structured. Sometimes interviewers will create some stress to ascertain how the candidate will react.

How you handle the interview is important. Avoid short responses, as they tell the interviewer little or nothing or perhaps the wrong things, about you. Use this opportunity to capitalize on your assets. Use anecdotal information to demonstrate your strong points, for example, "During my spring vacation I helped the school clinician in my hometown with the preschool screening program. We screened over 500 children for speech, language, and hearing problems. She was pleased with my work and wrote a letter describing my contribution. The letter is in my portfolio and I would like to have you read it." This tells the interviewer not only that you were able to function well in a professional situation and that you have gained some experience but that you were also interested in improving your skills by spending your spring vacation doing so.

Be prepared for questions like these: What is your philosophy of education? How would you plan to work with the learning disabilities teacher? What do you think a speech, language, and hearing program can add to a school system?

Inappropriate behaviors elicit negative impressions during an interview. They include candidates who show up late, chew gum, smoke without permission, bring uninvited guests, have poor hygiene, are braggarts and liars, are overly aggressive or too shy, lack confidence and poise, fail to look the interviewer in the eye, show lack of interest and enthusiasm, and ask no questions or poor questions.

Follow-up on the interview is important. Write a thank-you letter, noting anything that was said that you want to reemphasize; thank the interviewer for the opportunity to discuss your mutual interests and clarify any questions or ambiguities from the meeting. If you are interested in this position restate your desire to work for this particular school system. If you are undecided write a thank-you letter anyhow.

The Résumé

Another important tool is the résumé, a written document that introduces your education, background, skills, and experience to the prospective employer. It is a document that is used not only for the first job but also for subsequent employment searches throughout your professional life. The résumé, whether we like it or not, has become a cornerstone of the job-hunting process. Its worth is seldom questioned; its necessity is simply assumed. However, despite its importance as a marketing tool, many people express anxiety and frustration about preparing it.

A résumé is neither an autobiography nor merely a listing of your employment history. When properly done, it is an advertisement which excites an employer's interest in a particular product—*namely, you.* Because there are no absolutes in résumé writing, you will ultimately decide how it looks and what it says. Its style, format, and length should be determined by your employment interests or target markets and your background and qualifications.

An effective résumé can be prepared in different styles or formats and contain widely diverse information. Making the strongest presentation of your unique and individual qualifications will contribute to the kind of distinction that will set your résumé apart from others. So although there are no absolute rules on what "all" resumes should contain—except who you are and how you can be contacted—the following general rules address issues of honesty, accuracy, neatness, grammar, layout, and content that should be carefully observed:

Do not exaggerate your accomplishments to give the impression that you did more than you did. Employers know the difference between a restaurant hostess and an executive vice president for customer relations.

Be reasonably brief. You are writing a résumé, not an autobiography. Tailor your information to fit the employer's needs.

Be careful with your grammar and the design and layout of your résumé. There is no excuse for sloppy writing and poor grammar.

Do not include information that will work to your disadvantage. Negative or harmful information is best handled in a personal interview.

Use strong action verbs to make your résumé as impressive as possible. This is essential since employers will most often see your résumé before they see you.

Always present accurate information. Honesty really is the best policy.

The résumé on page 329 is designed to help you produce a document that strongly reflects your interests, qualifications, and potential. By itself, a résumé cannot get you the job you want; yet without it, you most likely will not even get started.

A Final Word

Not all interviews result in a job offer. Sometimes the supply of SLPs exceeds the demand, especially if you are interested in obtaining a position in a particular geographic area. The individual who is willing to locate anywhere has a much better chance of finding a job.

The classified section of *ASHA* lists open positions. And don't neglect the classified pages of the newspapers although these are unlikely to yield a great amount of information about positions in school systems.

The newsletters of state speech, language, and hearing associations often list job openings in schools, and the state consultants in speech, language, and hearing know of job openings within that state. The names and addresses of the state consultants can be obtained by writing to the state departments of public instruction, division of special education. They are located in or near the state capital cities. Information can be found in educational directories.

Begin now to build a network of persons who may be able to provide you with information concerning job possibilities. This will be valuable not only for your first job but also for subsequent job searches.

DISCUSSION QUESTIONS AND PROJECTS

1. Check a school library and a public library against the lists of publications in this chapter. How many did you find from the list in each facility?

2. Which universities, organizations or other facilities in your state are ASHA approved sponsors of continuing education programs leading toward the ACE? Do you think continuing education should be mandatory?

3. Do you think it is feasible for school SLPs to conduct research studies? What is the rationale for your answer?

4. Using the résumé form in this chapter write your résumé.

(*Discussion questions continued on page 324*)

Marrisa Cheney

Current Address: Permanent Address:
302 Jackson Hall   179 Elm Street
Bowling Green State Univ.   Hudson, Ohio 44100
Bowling Green, Ohio 43403   (000) 000-0000
(000) 000-0000

PROFESSIONAL OBJECTIVE

This is usually the most difficult section to write. Many people believe that listing a job objective on a résumé is too limiting. However, if you have a clear objective that applies to many organizations, it is to your advantage to include it. You may also state your professional objective in your cover letter rather than on the résumé. Include the job function desired and the type of organization. For example: Position as a speech-language pathologist in an inner city, medium size school system that will allow me to work with bicultural, speech, and language handicapped adolescents. Or: Position as a speech-language pathologist in a rural school system that will allow me to do diagnostic and remediation work with K-12 students, as well as consultative and preventive work with preschoolers and their parents.

EDUCATION

List highest or most recent degree first. Include name of college(s), major(s) (minor optional), date(s) of graduation. Add any special emphasis in your studies, such as relevant courses or research projects. If your grade point average is noteworthy include it. College expenses earned also can be included here.

EXPERIENCE AND WORK HISTORY

This is a summary of your work experience, highlighting your most recent or most relevant employment first. Include descriptions of your responsibilities, titles of positions held, names of companies or organizations, and dates you were employed. Summer employment, volunteer work, student teaching, and internships may be included. If you are a recent college graduate without experience, do not be concerned; you are in the majority. Stress the level of responsibility, achievement, and motivation you demonstrated in previous jobs. This section should be an active statement of what you <u>can</u> do. How you describe the experience is the key.

ACTIVITIES/ INTERESTS

Extracurricular involvement hightlights your leadership skills, sociability, and energy level. Thoose activities that support your professional objective by demonstrating your leadership or organizational skills. If you have many activities, select the ones in which you were most involved and describe your degree of responsibility. If you have limited activities, point out that you worked and include hours worked per week as well as the percentage of school expenses earned.

REFERENCES

It is not necessary to include names and addresses of references. If requested, these can be provided on a separate sheet or included on an application form. State either "Available upon request" or "Available upon request from (<u>your university placement service address</u>).''

OPTIONAL INFORMATION

This includes honors and awards, publications, professional association, research projects, study abroad, and personnal information. It is illegal for an employer to solicit personal data (age, weight, height, marital status, number of children, or disability) unless a genuine occupational requirement. Include this information only if pertinent to the job you are seeking.

5. Interview a school SLP or audiologist working in the schools to find out what they do on a typical day.

6. If the school SLP is paid more than classroom teachers will the collective bargaining union argue the SLP's cause with zeal even if they accept the SLP for membership?

7. In the case of a strike should the SLP man a classroom even though he or she is not a member of the teacher's union?

8. If the school SLPs align themselves with the classroom teachers, cannot the school administrators realistically expect them to have playground or lunchroom duties?

9. Should the state speech-language and hearing association provide assistance to SLPs whose local school district is on strike?

10. Caseload size could conceivably be a negotiable issue. What other issues of interest to the school SLP might be negotiable?

11. Contact ASHA or your state speech-language and hearing association to find out about professional liability insurance policies offered through their organization.

APPENDIX A

Classification of Procedures and Communication Disorders

Speech-Language Pathology and Audiology Diagnoses

The disorders section is designed to provide codes for communication diagnoses established by speech-language pathologists and audiologists. These codes are consistent with ASHA definitions approved in 1981 (*Asha,* November 1982, p. 949). Whenever more than one disorder is ascribed to a communicatively impaired individual, all disorders should be reflected in a listing of codes for that individual. The auditory disorders classification does include the traditional "mixed" classification as well as a more specific combination disorders such as middle ear plus cochlear disorders.

The coding system permits entry of time of onset at the second integer to the right of the decimal: __1 unknown time of onset; __2 prelingual time of onset; __3 postlingual time of onset; or __4 not applicable (noting time of onset is not appropriate or necessary).

For example, a motor speech disorder-dysarthria (131.1) is coded as 131.11 for unknown time of onset, 131.12 for prelingual onset 131.13 for postlingual onset and 131.14 if time of onset if time of onset is not applicable. A conductive hearing loss, right ear (230.1) is coded 230.11 for unknown time of onset, 230.12 for prelingual onset, 230.12 for prelingual onset, 230.13 for postlingual onset, and 230.14 if time of onset is not applicable.

Speech-Language Pathology and Audiology Procedures

01.0   **HEARING SCREENING:** A pass-fail procedure to identify individuals who require further hearing evaluation.

326

**Appendix A:
Classification
of Procedures
and Commu-
nication
Disorders**

02.0   **SPEECH SCREENING:** A procedure to identify individuals who require further speech evaluation.

03.0   **LANGUAGE SCREENING:** A procedure to identify individuals who require further language evaluation.

04.0   **DYSPHAGIA SCREENING:** A procedure to identify individuals who require specific assessment to determine the presence or absence of a swallowing disorder.

05.0   **FOLLOW-UP PROCEDURE:** A procedure needed to complete an assessment. May refer to repetition of a test, continuation of a previous evaluation, or procedure to establish validity of a previous test.

06.0   **CONSULTATION:** A procedure to provide professional expertise which may include, but is not limited to: conferring with other professionals during case staffings and team conferences, or in individual communication, providing information to business and industry and public and private agencies; and engaging in program development or supervision activities. Expert testimony is also a form of consultation.

07.0   **COUNSELING:** A procedure to facilitate the client's recovery from or adjustment to a communication impairment. Specific purposes of counseling may be to provide the client and his/her family or significant others with information and support, make appropriate referrals to other professionals, and to help the client to develop problem-solving strategies to enhance the rehabilitation process.

08.0   **AURAL REHABILITATION ASSESSMENT:** A procedure to assess the impact of hearing loss on communication which may include but is not limited to, speech reading, auditory training, and counseling.

09.0   **AURAL REHABILITATION:** A procedure to improve the communicative abilities of a hearing impaired individual. This procedure may include but is not limited to, speech reading, auditory training, and counseling.

10.0   **PRODUCT DISPENSING:** A procedure by which a prosthetic device (e.g., hearing aid, assistive listening device, and/or augmentative communication device) is prepared and dispensed.

11.0   **PRODUCT REPAIR/MODIFICATION:** A procedure to restore or adjust a product used to facilitate an individual's communication abilities.

Audiologic Procedures

20.0   **BASIC AUDIOLOGIC ASSESSMENT:** A procedure to determine the status of the peripheral auditory system. This procedure may include, but is not limited to, the following: case history, developmentally appropriate behavior tests, acoustic immittance tests, communication handicap inventories, speech-language screening, interpretation of audiometric test results, written report preparation, and counseling.

21.0   **COMPREHENSIVE AUDIOLOGIC ASSESSMENT:** A procedure to determine the status of the auditory system that cannot be determined by basic audiologic assessment (20.0) and/or to establish the site of the auditory disorder. This procedure may include items contained in the basic assessment in addition to electrophysiologic measurements (e.g., auditory evoked potentials, electronystagmography, tests of auditory adaptation, specialized speech tests, tests for non-organic hearing etiology, written report preparation, and counseling).

22.0   **ELECTROPHYSIOLOGIC ASSESSMENT:** A procedure to determine or monitor the status of a physiologic system(s), e.g., auditory evoked potentials, electronystagmography, electrocochleography.

23.0   **HEARING AID ASSESSMENT:** A procedure to determine the appropriateness and design of individual amplification systems. This procedure may include, but is not limited to, assessment of an individual's performance with different hearing aids, assistive listening devices, and/or tinnitus management devices, cochlear implant management, and counseling.

24.0   **HEARING AID FITTING/ORIENTATION:** A procedure to assist an individual in achieving maximum understanding of, and performance with, their individualized amplification system. This procedure may include electracoustic performance evaluation of the system.

25.0   **OCCUPATIONAL HEARING CONVERSATION SERVICE**

       25.1   **ENVIRONMENTAL ACOUSTICAL SURVEY:** A procedure to determine sound levels in settings where noise levels may be injurious to hearing or interfere with communication.

       25.2   **OCCUPATIONAL AUDIOMETRIC THRESHOLD TEST:** A pure-tone air conduction threshold procedure to identify the presence or absence of a hearing loss.

       25.3   **AUDIOGRAM REVIEW:** A procedure to determine change in hearing status and need for monitoring, follow-up, and/or referral.

26.0   **UNLISTED AUDIOLOGIC PROCEDURE:** Any audiologic procedure which is not listed above. Describe by report.

Speech-Language Pathology Procedures

30.0   **SPECIFIC ASSESSMENT:** A procedure to assess a specific aspect of speech, voice, language systems, and/or oral and pharyngeal sensorimotor competencies. Includes case history, assessment, written report preparation, and patient/family conference. Specific assessment is appropriate when the patient has a preliminary diagnoses. The assessment is usually completed for purposes of consultation reevaluation.

       30.1   **LANGUAGE**

       30.2   **SPEECH ARTICULATION**

       30.3   **SPEECH RATE, RHYTHM, FLUENCY**

       30.4   **VOICE**

328

Appendix A:
Classification
of Procedures
and Commu-
nication
Disorders

30.5 **RESONANCE**

30.6 **ORAL/PHARYNGEAL DYSFUNCTION**

30.7 **COGNITIVE/COMMUNICATION**

31.0 **COMPREHENSIVE ASSESSMENT:** A procedure for detailed analysis of speech, voice, language systems and/or oral and pharyngeal sensorimotor competencies; may include evaluation of comprehension and expression, structure and function, behavioral relationships, and adaptation. Includes initial interview and patient history, diagnostic procedure, patient/family conference, and written report preparation.

32.0 **PROSTHETIC/ADAPTIVE DEVICE ASSESSMENT:** A procedure to determine the appropriateness of augmentative communication systems and devices, oral or laryngeal prostheses, and artificial larynges.

33.0 **TREATMENT:** A procedure to apply intervention strategies that improve, alter, augment or compensate for comprehension, speech, voice, language, and pharyngeal sensorimotor competencies.

34.0 **SPEECH-LANGUAGE INSTRUCTION:** A procedure to teach various communication strategies with the primary goal of providing assistance in academic subject areas.

35.0 **COMMUNICATION INSTRUCTION** (Speech Enhancement): A procedure designed to improve the communication abilities of an individual who does not exhibit a disorder. Includes instruction in public speaking and elimination of foreign dialect.

36.0 **UNLISTED SPEECH-LANGUAGE PROCEDURE:** Any speech-language pathology procedure which is not listed above. Describe by report.

Speech, Language, and Related Diagnoses

100.0 **SPEECH AND LANGUAGE WITHIN NORMAL LIMITS**

101.0 **COMMUNICATION VARIATION**

    101.1 **LANGUAGE**

    101.2 **SPEECH**

    101.3 **VOICE**

    101.4 **RATE, RHYTHM, FLUENCY**

111.0 **LANGUAGE DISORDER**

    111.1 **SPOKEN LANGUAGE COMPREHENSION DISORDER**

        111.1 **PHONOLOGIC**

        111.2 **MORPHOLOGIC**

        111.3 **SYNTACTIC**

        111.4 **SEMANTIC**

	111.5	PRAGMATIC
	111.6	MIXED OR UNDIFFERENTIATED

112.0 SPOKEN LANGUAGE PRODUCTION DISORDER

    112.1   PHONOLOGIC

    112.2   MORPHOLOGIC

    112.3   SYNTACTIC

    112.4   SEMANTIC

    112.5   PRAGMATIC

    112.6   MIXED OR UNDIFFERENTIATED

113.0 WRITTEN LANGUAGE COMPREHENSION DISORDER (READING)

114.0 WRITTEN LANGUAGE PRODUCTION DISORDER (WRITING)

115.0 ARITHMETIC-CALCULATION DISORDER (DYSCALCULIA)

116.0 NON-SPOKEN COMMUNICATION RECOGNITION DISORDER

117.0 NON-SPOKEN COMMUNICATION PRODUCTION DISORDER

120.0 COGNITIVE/COMMUNICATIVE DISORDER

130.0 SPEECH ARTICULATION DISORDER

131.0 MOTOR SPEECH DISORDER

    131.1   DYSARTHRIA

    131.2   DYSPRAXIA

    131.3   DYSARTHRIA AND DYSPRAXIA

132.0 STRUCTURALLY BASED SPEECH DISORDER

    132.1   FACIAL

    132.2   LABIAL

    132.3   DENTAL

    132.4   MANDIBULAR

    132.5   LINGUAL

    132.6   PALATAL

    132.7   PHARYNGEAL

    132.8   MIXED

133.0 DEVELOPMENTAL ARTICULATION DISORDER

134.0 OTHER SPEECH DISORDER

140.0 SPEECH RATE, RHYTHM, OR FLUENCY DISORDER

    140.1   STUTTERING

    140.2   CLUTTERING

    140.3   DYSPROSODY

150.0 VOICE DISORDER

    150.1   MOTOR-VOCAL

330

Appendix A:
Classification
of Procedures
and Commu-
nication
Disorders

	150.2	STRUCTURAL (E.G., LARYNGECTOMY)
	150.3	FUNCTIONAL
	150.4	MIXED
160.0		RESONANCE DISORDER
	160.1	MOTOR-VOCAL
	160.2	STRUCTURAL
	160.3	FUNCTIONAL
	160.4	MIXED
170.0		ORAL/PHARYNGEAL DYSFUNCTION
171.0		DYSPHAGIA
	171.1	ORAL PREPATORY PHASE (CHEWING, BITING, FEEDING)
	171.2	ORAL PHASE (SUCKING, BOLUS MANIPULATION, SWALLOWING)
	171.3	PHARYNGEAL PHASE (AERODIGESTIVE DYSFUNCTION)
172.0		TONGUE THRUST
173.0		ORAL TICS
180.0		UNLISTED CATEGORY
190.0		RESULTS NOT CONCLUSIVE
	190.1	COULD NOT TEST
	190.2	COULD NOT DETERMINE

Auditory and Other Diagnoses

	200.0		HEARING WITHIN NORMAL LIMITS
		200.1	UNDIFFERENTIATED
		200.2	RIGHT
		200.3	LEFT
		200.4	BILATERAL
	210.0		MIDDLE EAR DYSFUNCTION, HEARING WITHIN NORMAL LIMITS
		210.1	RIGHT
		210.2	LEFT
		210.3	BILATERAL
	220.0		HEARING LOSS, TYPE UNDETERMINED
		220.1	UNDIFFERENTIATED
		220.2	RIGHT
		220.3	LEFT
		220.4	BILATERAL

230.0	**CONDUCTIVE HEARING LOSS**	
	230.1	**RIGHT**
	230.2	**LEFT**
	230.3	**BILATERAL**
240.0	**SENSORINEURAL HEARING LOSS**	
	240.1	**RIGHT**
	240.2	**LEFT**
	240.3	**BILATERAL**
241.0	**SENSORINEURAL HEARING LOSS, COCHLEAR**	
	241.1	**RIGHT**
	241.2	**LEFT**
	241.3	**BILATERAL**
242.0	**SENSORINEURAL HEARING LOSS, RETROCOCHLEAR**	
	242.1	**RIGHT**
	242.2	**LEFT**
	242.3	**BILATERAL**
243.0	**SENSORINEURAL HEARING LOSS, COMBINED COCHLEAR AND RETROCOCHLEAR**	
	243.1	**RIGHT**
	243.2	**LEFT**
	243.3	**BILATERAL**
250.0	**MIXED HEARING LOSS**	
	250.1	**RIGHT**
	250.2	**LEFT**
	250.3	**BILATERAL**
251.0	**MIXED HEARING LOSS, CONDUCTIVE AND COCHLEAR**	
	251.1	**RIGHT**
	251.2	**LEFT**
	251.3	**BILATERAL**
260.0	**CENTRAL AUDITORY DISORDER**	
270.0	**PSEUDOHYPACUSIS**	
	270.1	**RIGHT**
	270.2	**LEFT**
	270.3	**BILATERAL**
280.0	**VESTIBULAR FUNCTION**	
	280.1	**WITHIN NORMAL LIMITS**
	280.2	**PERIPHERAL DISORDER**
	280.3	**CENTRAL DISORDER**
	280.4	**NON-LOCALIZED DISORDER**

332

Appendix A:
Classification
of Procedures
and Commu-
nication
Disorders

290.0   SEVENTH NERVE DISORDER

   290.1   RIGHT

   290.2   LEFT

   290.3   BILATERAL

300.0   OTHER DISORDER

301.0   TINNITUS

   301.1   RIGHT

   301.2   LEFT

   301.3   BILATERAL

302.0   VERTIGO

310.0   UNLISTED CATEGORY

320.0   RESULTS NOT CONCLUSIVE

   320.1   COULD NOT TEST

   320.2   COULD NOT DETERMINE

American Speech-Language-Hearing Association. "Classification of Speech-Language Pathology and Auditory Procedures and Communication Disorders," *Asha* 29 (12) (1987): 49–53.

Data Bank of IEP Goals and Objectives

Goals

1.

2. The student will be seen on a consultation basis by the Speech/Language Pathologist.

3. The student will be seen on a consultation basis along with direct services by the Speech/Language Pathologist.

4. The student will improve intelligibility of the following sound(s):

   _____

5. The student will improve intelligibility on a whole word accuracy measurement, using a multiphonemic approach to therapy.

6. The student will improve intelligibility through remediation of phonological rules.

7. The student will improve receptive language skills.

8. The student will improve expressive language skills.

9. The student will improve receptive/expressive language skills.

10. The student will improve pragmatic (social) language skills.

11. The student will improve verbal/nonverbal communicative abilities through augmentative/alternative systems.

12. The student will improve auditory skills (listening, processing, recall, etc.).

13. The student will improve speech fluency.

14. The student will improve vocal pitch.

334

**Appendix B:
Data Bank of
IEP Goals
and Objec-
tives**

15. The student will improve control of vocal duration.
16. The student will increase/decrease loudness.
17. The student will improve vocal quality.
18. The Audiologist will periodically monitor the student's hearing status.
19. The Audiologist will provide an annual audiological evaluation.
20. The student will be seen a minimum of one 20 minute session per week.
21. Other

Objectives

1.
2. To discriminate between the target sound and other sounds, and between the target sound and the error sound.
3. To demonstrate correct tongue, lip and teeth positioning for the target sound.
4. To produce the target sound(s) in _____.
5. To produce the target sound(s) in conversational speech in the speech therapy setting.
6. To produce the target sound(s) in situations outside the speech therapy setting such as, the classroom, at recess and at home.
7. To self-monitor and self-correct his/her sound errors at each of the various stages of therapy.
8. To improve sequencing of unfamiliar multisyllabic words.
9. To demonstrate ability to imitate oral movement sequences.
10. To practice oral motor exercises and/or improve tongue mobility.
11. To maintain lip closure.
12. To practice management of drooling.
13. To maintain proper positioning for communication.
14. To increase rate and ease of production of the target words.
15. To improve auditory discrimination of sounds in all word positions.
16. To improve word analysis and sound blending skills.
17. To produce correct closure of final sounds in syllables and words.
18.
19. To imitate clinician's production of consonant sounds in isolation.
20. To improve intelligibility of frequently used significant words.
21.
22. To include syllables in multisyllabic words where the syllables are omitted.
23. To include consonant clusters where the sounds are omitted.
24. To include initial/final consonants where the consonants are omitted.

25. To produce the correct backing sounds (k, g, ng) to replace their frontal substitutions (t, d).

26. To produce the correct frontal sounds (t, d) to replace their backing (k, g, ng) substitutions.

27. To include the stridency feature (f, v, s, z, sh, ch, j) where it is deleted and/or substituted with stops (t, d, p, b, k, g).

28. To produce the stop consonants (t, d, p, b) to replace the continuant (f, v, s, z, sh, th, m, n) substitutions.

29. To add or delete the voicing feature as appropriate to consonants.

30. To produce the correct vowels in isolation/words etc.

31. To speak slowly and clearly to be more easily understood by others.

32.

33. To identify the type and frequency of his/her disfluencies in various settings.

34. To identify/modify/eliminate secondary characteristics of disfluencies.

35. To increase/maintain eye contact.

36. To demonstrate ability to use easy onset of speech.

37. To demonstrate ability to use continuous phonation, without and then with vocal inflection.

38. To use appropriate phrasing in and/or outside the speech therapy setting.

39. To reduce the speaking rate to achieve increased fluency.

40. To maintain fluent speech in structured settings.

41. To maintain fluency in conversational speech in the speech therapy settings.

42. To maintain fluency in situations outside of the speech therapy settings.

43. To gain confidence in his/her ability to speak fluently.

44. To self-monitor and self-evaluate his/her fluency.

45. To reduce the use of filler/starters (. . . uh . . . um . . . like).

46. To produce the appropriate prosody.

47.

48. To respond to/identify common environmental sounds.

49. To imitate gross body movements such as clapping.

50. To engage in functional play through meaningful exploration and manipulation of objects.

51. To get attention of others through vocalization or performative action.

52. To increase vocal play.

53. To attend during one-on-one and/or group situations.

54. To respond to pleasurable stimuli and/or own name.

55. To attempt to imitate sounds/words.

56. To vocalize differential vowel sounds.

336

**Appendix B:
Data Bank of
IEP Goals
and Objec-
tives**

57. To vocalize two or more identifiable consonants.

58. To improve vocalization of survival information such as, name, address and phone number.

59. To identify familiar body parts.

60. To localize/attend to auditory stimuli.

61. To recall in sequence, significant facts in a short paragraph presented aloud.

62. To initiate at least one communicative interaction.

63. To ask for and tell wants and needs.

64. To reduce echolalia.

65. To reduce repetitive comments/questions.

66. To attend to/comply with basic commands (stop, no, look at me, etc.).

67. To selectively attend to interactions/conversations.

68. To demonstrate ability to use strategies such as rehearsing, grouping, visualizing, linking and chunking to improve auditory memory.

69. To improve word recall and confrontation naming.

70.

71. To use appropriate gestures/facial gestures.

72. To demonstrate correct behavior to promote good listening and communication skills, such as, sitting in seat, keeping hands away from face, keeping hands to self, and eyes on speaker.

73. To express and respond to expressions of approval, support, congratulations and/or compliments.

74. To appropriately express emotions verbally, in writing and/or pointing to pictures.

75. To use language effectively for social interchange with peers and adults.

76. To maintain appropriate eye contact with listener, speaker and/or task.

77. To maintain appropriate distance from listener or speaker.

78. To make choices when asked.

79. To respond within an appropriate length of time.

80. To take turns appropriately in various activities.

81. To use appropriate conversational turn-taking.

82. To indicate old-new information.

83. To initiate, maintain and/or change a topic appropriately in conversation.

84. To respond to and initiate telephone calls.

85. To take and relay a message.

86. To respond to and formulate greetings and introductions and farewells.

87. To address people with appropriate titles. e.g. Mr., Mrs., etc.

88. To use appropriately polite tone when addressing and responding to others.

89. To give and respond to warnings and reminders.
90. To reduce inappropriate interrupting.
91. To protest and respond to protests.
92. To ask for and offer favors, help, assistance and/or directions.
93. To ask for and give directions.
94. To demonstrate the ability to form contractions (do not/don't, he is/he's).
95. To use the correct word order in sentences.
96. To use infinitive verb forms correctly.
97. To use compound phrases and sentences with conjunctions (and, or, but).
98. To ask questions with correct syntax and word order.
99. To use prepositions appropriately.
100. To use adverbs and adjectives appropriately.
101. To use comparative and superlative adjectives appropriately (big, bigger, biggest).
102. To repeat monosyllabic words in progressively longer sequences when presented aloud.
102. To demonstrate understanding and appropriate use of negation (no, not, never).
104. To demonstrate understanding of common nouns, verbs, adjectives and adverbs.
105. To self-monitor and revise messages to aid listener understanding.
106. To increase attention span without and with distraction.
107. To repeat verbatim ___ word(s) and sentence(s) presented aloud.
108. To demonstrate and describe functions of basic objects.
109. To name, describe and categorize objects and picture by likeness and difference.
110. To expand functional vocabulary.
111. To demonstrate understanding of specialized vocabulary required in academic coursework.
112. To improve word finding abilities.
113. To use grammatical, complex sentences with embedding and subordinate markers (as, although, etc.).
114. To give and follow directions using various basic concepts such as, size, location, quantity.
115. To produce the sentence-paragraph-story in correct grammatical form.
116. To demonstrate understanding of the following concepts:

    _____.

117. To arrange and tell or retell pictured sequence stories.
118. To follow ___ level commands of increasing linguistic complexity.
119. To answer yes/no questions correctly.

338

Appendix B:
Data Bank of
IEP Goals
and Objec-
tives

120. To answer 'Wh' questions such as, Who, What, How, Why, Where and When.

121. To recall basic content of orally presented material.

122. To relate and retell stories and experiences in correct sequential order.

123. To demonstrate reasoning ability and knowledge of cause and effect relationships appropriate for age and ability level.

124. To demonstrate understanding of conditional statements (if . . . . then).

125. To improve logical thinking skills such as, making inferences and predicting outcomes.

126. To demonstrate the ability to complete analogies.

127. To demonstrate understanding of common idioms and proverbs.

128. To identify verbal absurdities.

129. To expand utterences to _____.

130. To use present progressive verb forms (is/are ___ing).

131. To use the past tense of regular verbs (___ed).

132. To use the past tense of irregular verbs (came, ran).

133. To use the future tense of verbs (will ___).

134. To use the copula verbs correctly (the boy(s) is/are here).

135. To use the auxilliary verb ___ correctly.

136. To use 's' and 'z' language markers for plurals, possessives and present tense verbs (3rd person singular).

137. To use the irregular plural form of nouns (men, children).

138. To demonstrate subject-verb agreement (the boy walks/the boys walk).

139. To use subjectives pronouns correctly (I, he, she, we, they).

140. To use objective pronouns correctly (me, him, her, us, them).

141. To use possessive pronouns correctly (my, his, her, our, your, their).

142. To demonstrate correct use of articles (a, an, the).

143. To use modals correctly (can, would, should etc.).

144.

145.

146. To demonstrate the ability to access the system.

147. To identify vocabulary symbols used in the system.

148. To increase the number of vocabulary symbols used in the system.

149. To increase the rate of response utilizing the system.

150. To increase the length of response utilizing the system.

151. To initiate communication utilizing the system.

152. To ask and answer questions utilizing the system.

153. To utilize the communication aid in the classroom.

154. To expand utilization of the communication aid to situations outside of the classroom.

155. To independently program the electronic aid.

156.

157. The Audiologist will provide monthly hearing aid and/or FM checks.

158. The Audiologist will monitor the student's hearing status

_____.

159. To receive preferential seating.

160. To maximize use of auditory/visual cues to supplement hearing.

161. To use his/her amplification unit within the therapy setting.

162. To learn to use voice to communicate.

163. To develop different duration patterns.

164. To develop loud and quiet intensity patterns.

165. To develop a whisper.

166. To vary intensity patterns (loud, quiet, whisper) in a series.

167. To develop high and low pitch on separate breaths.

168. To develop high-low-high pitch on a single breath.

169. To develop 3 points on pitch range using separate breaths and/or single breaths.

170. To use voice in conjunction with pointing, gesturing, fingerspelling, signing, etc. when communication.

171. To attend to the visible aspects of speech by watching the speaker.

172. To improve basic speech reading skills.

173. To demonstrate understanding of body language and nonverbal cues.

174. To maximize use of auditory/visual cues to supplement hearing.

175.

176. To discriminate between normal and abnormal samples of voice production.

177. To identify the anatomy of the vocal mechanism.

178. To identify types and frequency of vocal abuse.

179. To monitor his/her own vocal abuses.

180. To decrease the incidence of vocal abuse in the therapy setting.

181. To decrease the incidence of vocal abuse outside the therapy setting such as, in the classroom, at recess and at home.

182. To reduce hard glottal attacks.

183. To improve vocal resonance by decreasing hypernasality/hyponasality.

184. To develop an oral openness to improve resonance.

185. To produce words/phrases/sentences with appropriate oral resonance.

340

**Appendix B:
Data Bank of
IEP Goals
and Objec-
tives**

186. To maintain oral resonance in a variety of situations.
187. To discriminate between oral and nasal sounds.
188. To maintain appropriate vocal quality.
189. To be able to identify optimum vocal pitch and use appropriate pitch.
190. To use appropriate vocal range.
191. To increase/decrease vocal loudness to be easily heard by others.
192. To maintain an appropriate loudness level.
193. To improve breath control for speech.
194. To achieve adequate velopharyngeal closure for oral phoneme production.
195. To do exercises to stimulate movement of the velum.
196. To reduce nasal emission.
197. To practice tension reduction and relaxation exercises.
198. To reduce vocal tension.
199. To maintain optimum speaking posture (head up, sitting up straight, etc.).

Criteria

1.
2. Informal assessment: __% accuracy.
3. Informal assessment: 50% accuracy.
4. Informal assessment: 75% accuracy.
5. Informal assessment: 90% accuracy.
6. Formal assessment: Improved score on standardized test.
7. Formal assessment: Within normal limits for age/ability on standardized test.
8. Teacher-made tests: __% accuracy.
9. Teacher-made tests: 50% accuracy.
10. Teacher-made tests: 75% accuracy.
11. Teacher-made tests: 90% accuracy.
12. Spontaneous speech sample: __% accuracy.
13. Spontaneous speech sample: 50% accuracy.
14. Spontaneous speech sample: 75% accuracy.
15. Spontaneous speech sample: 90% accuracy.
16. Spontaneous speech sample: Evidence of carryover of learned language structure outside the therapy setting.
17. Pathologist observation: __% accuracy.
18. Pathologist observation: 50% accuracy.

19. Pathologist observation: 75% accuracy.

20. Pathologist observation: 90% accuracy.

21. Pathologist observation: ___ minutes per session.

22. Pathologist observation: ___ out of ___ times.

23. Informal observation by the Pathologist/Classroom Teacher(s)/Others.

24. Informal observations by the Pathologist and Classroom Teacher(s): Adequate speech and language skills.

25. Hearing and/or hearing aid evaluations completed at the Goodwill Rehabilitation Center.

26. Annual hearing evaluation completed at the student's school of attendance.

27. Hearing aid(s) and/or FM units checked biologically and with the Fonix Hearing Aid Analyser at the student's school of attendance.

28. Periodic hearing evaluations completed at the student's school of attendance.

*This data bank was developed by speech-language clinicians in Canton, Stark County, and Cincinnati, Ohio (1992). Reprinted with permission.

Sample Language Arts Curriculum

Below are several excerpts representing examples of the major areas of focus and objectives of key portions of a Language Arts curriculum for the elementary grades. Examples are provided for six skill areas including listening, speaking, oral and dramatic interpretation, oral reading, grammar, and written composition. Due to space limitations, only one representative grade level is presented for each skill area. Classroom learning activities and teaching materials are developed to support these objectives.

These examples help illustrate the communication demands placed upon children as they progress through school as well as the types of learning activities that can be incorporated into the speech-language program.

Listening Skills
(Kindergarten)

Major Focus

- Direction following.
- Sound identification.
- Stories.
- Poems.

Sample Objectives

- Follow oral directions for drawing pictures.
- Follow directions for playing games.

- Follow directions for marking worksheets.
- Demonstrate body awareness of spatial words such as over, under, beside, in front, left, right, etc.
- Name a word that rhymes with a dictated word.
- Arrange in the proper sequence, four or five pictures related to the story.
- Answer questions using facts from the story.
- Recognize the main idea in an oral presentation or story.
- Name and describe the main characters in the story.
- Repeat short nursery rhymes, poems, finger plays, songs.

Speaking Skills
(Level 1)

Major Focus

- Story sequencing.
- Sharing experiences.
- Rhymes.
- Poems.

Sample Objectives

- Speak thoughts in complete sentences.
- Supply names for concrete items and pictures.
- Classification of familiar objects or pictures, (fruit—apple, orange; furniture—chair, table; clothing—dress, suit).
- Retell a story in the proper sequence.
- Relate a personal experience in front of a group.
- Express verbally human needs and emotions.
- Describe how two objects are alike or different.
- Take part in an informal exchange of ideas with others.
- Present facts and ideas in an organized manner.
- Recite familiar rhymes and poems.

Oral and Dramatic Interpretation
(Level 2)

Major Focus

- Pantomime.
- Role playing.

344

**Appendix C:
Sample
Language
Arts
Curriculum**

• Story characters.
• Human emotions.

Sample Objectives

• Take part in pantomiming activities; pretend to be the animal or character.
  —Animals or real people.
  —Non-living things.
  —Action or series of actions.
  —Emotion or series of emotions.
  —Story characters.
• Act out a situation in the classroom.
• Participate in role playing of real-life or storybook characters.
• Improvise familiar stories.
• Memorize written parts.
• Participate in a formal play.
• Dramatize a chosen role from a favorite book or play.

Oral Reading
(Level 3)

Major Focus

• Expression.
• Comprehension.
• Clear and distinct pronunciation.
• Punctuation.

Sample Objectives

• Read fluently in thought units.
• Use clear and distinct pronunciation when reading.
• Use expression to show the mood and emotion in the story.
• Re-read to locate information.
• Recall the sequence of the story.
• Recall details of the story.
• Identify the main idea of the story.
• Read orally for the enjoyment of others.
• Read a part in a play along with other readers.

Grammar Skills
(Level 4)

Major Focus

- Punctuation.
- Capitalization.
- Abbreviations.
- Irregular verbs.
- Prepositional phrases.
- Pronouns.
- Usage.
- Contractions.
- Possessives.
- Verb tense.

Sample Objectives

- Write and punctuate sentence types correctly.
- Use punctuation correctly in sentences.
- Use capital letters.
- Use correct plurals.
- Identify verbs in sentences.
- Identify the pronouns in sentences by underlining.
- Identify the two parts of a sentence by underlining the subject and the predicate.
- Identify the adjectives in sentences.
- Recognize that English sentences have definite word-order patterns.
- Show how changing the word-order of most English sentences will change their meaning.
- Make a list of words that show ownership by adding 's to singular nouns.
- Develop skill in proofreading.

Written Composition
(Level 5)

Major Focus

- Different points of view.
- Advertisements.

346

**Appendix C:
Sample
Language
Arts
Curriculum**

• Magazine articles, news stories.
• Poetry; limericks.
• Scripts; dialogues.
• Stories—surprise endings, interesting beginnings, science fiction.
• Letters.
• Note taking.
• Organization of ideas.

Sample Objectives

• Write from the point of view of animals or other people.
• Experiment with writing interesting book cards for a file as a means of pooling information about books.
• Develop skill in taking notes.
• Write an imaginary news story using notes.
• Use information from multiple sources when writing travel ads.
• Write a story about the future.
• Use correct form for a friendly letter.
• Combine concepts, principles and generalizations in written compositions.

Developed by Jean Blosser after reviewing curricula from numerous school programs.

References

Adler, S. "Data Gathering: The Reliability and Validity of Test Data Obtained from Culturally Different Children." *Journal of Learning Disabilities* 6 (1973): 429–34.

Ainsworth, S. *Speech Correction Methods, A Manual of Speech Therapy and Public School Procedures,* First Edition. 70 Fifth Ave., New York: Prentice-Hall Inc., 1948.

Ainsworth, S. "The Speech Clinician in Public Schools: Participant or Separatist?" *Asha* 7 (December 1965): 495–503.

Alpiner, J., Ogden, J.A., and Wiggens, J. "The Utilization of Supportive Personnel in Speech Correction in the Public Schools: A Pilot Project." *Asha* 12 (December 1970): 599–604.

American Speech-Language-Hearing Association. Ad Hoc Committee on Extension of Audiological Services in the Schools. "Audiology Services in the Schools Position Statement." *Asha* 25 (5) (1983): 53–60.

American Speech-Language-Hearing Association. "Asha Interviews Ann L. Carey, 1992 President." *Asha* 34 (1) (January 1992): 29.

American Speech-Language-Hearing Association. "Classification of Speech-Language Pathology and Audiology Procedures and Communication Disorders." *Asha* 29 (12) (1987): 49–53.

American Speech-Language-Hearing Association. "Clinical Management of Communicatively Handicapped Minority Language Populations." *Asha* 27 (6) (1985).

American Speech-Language-Hearing Association. "Code of Ethics." *Asha* 34 (March Supplement 9) (1992): 1–2.

American Speech-Language-Hearing Association. Committee on Audiologic Evaluation. "Guidelines for Identification Audiometry." *Asha* 27 (5) (1985): 49–52.

American Speech-Language-Hearing Association Committee on Definitions of Public School Speech and Hearing Services. "Services and Functions of Speech and Hearing Specialists in Public Schools." *Asha* 4 (4) (1962): 99–100.

American Speech-Language-Hearing Association. Committee on Language-Learning

Disabilities. "Position Statement on Language-Learning Disorders." *Asha* 24 (11) (1982): 937–44.

American Speech-Language-Hearing Association. Committee on Language, Speech, and Hearing Services in the Schools. "Definitions of Communicative Disorders and Variations." *Asha* 24 (11) (1982): 949–50.

American Speech-Language-Hearing Association. Committee on Language, Speech and Hearing Services in the Schools. "Guidelines for Caseload Size for Speech-Language Services in the Schools." *Asha* 26 (4) (1984): 53–58.

American Speech-Language-Hearing Association. Committee on Legislation. "The Need for Adequately Trained Speech Pathologists and Audiologists." *Asha* 1 (4) (1959): 138.

American Speech-Language-Hearing Association. Committee on the Status of Racial Minorities. "Clinical Management of Communicatively Handicapped Minority Language Populations." *Asha* 27 (6) (1985): 29–32.

American Speech-Language-Hearing Association. Committee on Supportive Personnel. "Draft Addendum to the Guidelines for the Employment and Utilization of Supportive Personnel." *Asha* 29 (12): 45–48.

American Speech-Language-Hearing Association. Committee on Supportive Personnel. "Utilization and Employment of Speech-Language Pathology Supportive Personnel with Underserved Populations." *Asha* 30 (11) (1988): 55–56.

American Speech-Language-Hearing Association. Council on Professional Standards. "Proposed Change in Scope of ESB Accreditation (Revised)." *Asha* 33 (11) (1991): 63.

American Speech-Language-Hearing Association. Educational Standards Board. "Supervision of Student Clinicians." *Asha* 33 (6/7) (1991): 53.

American Speech-Language-Hearing Association. "Guidelines for Screening for Hearing Impairment and Middle Ear Disorders." *Asha* 32 (Supplement 2) (1990): 17–24.

American Speech-Language-Hearing Association. *Professional Services Board Accreditation Manual.* Rockville, MD: American Speech-Language-Hearing Association (1984).

American Speech-Language-Hearing Association. "Starting in September: Referral Model Makes More Time for Services." *Asha* 31(1) (1989): 41.

American Speech-Language-Hearing Association. "Task Force Report on Traditional Scheduling Procedures in School." *Language, Speech, and Hearing Services in Schools,* 4(3) (1973): 100–109.

American Speech-Language-Hearing Association. Task Force on Clinical Standards. *Preferred Practice Patterns for the Professions of Speech-Language Pathology and Audiology.* Draft for Review. Rockville, MD: American Speech-Language-Hearing Association (1992).

American Speech-Language-Hearing Association. 33rd Annual Convention Proceedings. Netherland Hilton Hotel. Cincinnati, OH (1987).

American Speech-Language-Hearing Association. "Utilization and Employment of Speech-Language Pathology Supportive Personnel with Underserved Populations." *Asha* 30 (11) (November 1988): 55–56.

Anderson, J.L. *Handbook for Supervisors of School Practicum in Speech, Hearing and Language.* Bloomington, IN: Indiana University Publications (1972).

Anderson, K.L. Hearing conservation in the public schools revisited. In C. Flexer (Ed.). "Current Audiological Issues in the Educational Management of Children with Hearing Loss." *Seminars in Hearing* 12 (4) (1991): 340–64.

Autism Society of Ohio. "Information Brochure." (1992).

Backus, O. "The Use of Group Structure in Speech Therapy." *Journal of Speech and Hearing Disorders.* 17 (June 1952): 116–22.

Bankson, N.W. *Bankson Language Screening Test.* Baltimore: University Park Press (1978).

Bankson, N.W., and Bernthal, J.E. *Quick Screen of Phonology.* San Antonio, Texas: Special Press, Inc. (1990).

Barrett, M.D., & Welsh, J.W. Predictive articulation screening. *Language, Speech and Hearing Services in Schools,* 6 (1975): 91–95.

Beasley, J. Development of social skills as an instrument in speech therapy. *Journal of Speech and Hearing Disorders,* 16 (1951): 241–245.

Beitchman, J.H., Nair, R., Clegg, M., Patel, P.G. "Prevalence of Speech and Language Disorders in 5-Year Old Kindergarten Children in the Ottawa-Carleton Region." *Journal of Speech and Hearing Disorders* 51 (May 1986): 98–110.

Bender, R.E. *"The Conquest of Deafness."* Cleveland, Ohio: The Press of Western Reserve University (1960).

Berg, F.S. *Facilitating Classroom Listening: A Handbook for Teachers of Normal and Hard of Hearing Students.* Boston: College-Hill Press (1987).

Berg, F.S. "Classroom Acoustics and Signal Transmission." In F.S. Berg, J.C. Blair, J.H. Viehweg and A. Wilson-Vlotman (Eds.), *Educational Audiology for the Hard of Hearing Child.* New York: Grune & Stratton (1986).

Berg, F.S. *Educational Audiology: Hearing and Speech Management.* New York: Grune and Stratton (1976).

Berg, F. and Fletcher, S. *The Hard of Hearing Child.* New York: Grune and Stratton (1970).

Bergman, M. "Screening the Hearing of Preschool Children." *Maico Audiological Library Series, III,* Report 4, Maico Electronics, Inc. (1964).

Biklen, D. "Typing to Talk: Facilitated Communication." *American Journal of Speech-Language Pathology* 1 (2) (1992): 15–17.

Blake, A. and Shewan, C.M. "An Update on PL 94-142." *Asha* 52 (1992).

Blosser, J. and DePompei, R. "Proactive Response: A Model for Treating the Cognitive-Communicative Impairments in Students with Traumatic Brain Injury." In D. Eger and S. Chabon. *Clinics in Communication Disorders.* Andover Press (1992).

Blosser, J. and DePompei, R. *How to Encourage School Administrators to Support our Changing Roles.* Presentation at the American Speech-Language-Hearing Association Convention, San Francisco (1984).

Blosser, J. and Tomi, V. *Building Interdisciplinary Bridges.* Chicago, IL: Presentation at the National Coalition of Child Centers Annual Conference (1985).

Braunstein, M.S. "Communication Aide: A Pilot Project." *Language, Speech and Hearing Services in Schools* 3 (July 1972): 32–35.

Bryngelson, B. and Glaspey, E. *Speech Improvement Cards,* Scott, Foresman & Company (1941).

Byrne-Saricks, M.C. "School Services and Communication Disorders." *Asha* 31 (6/7) (June/July 1989): 79–80.

Caccamo, J.M. "Accountability—A Matter of Ethics?" *Asha* 15 (1973): 411–12.

Carrow, E. *Screening Test for Auditory Comprehension of Language; Test Manual.* Austin, TX: Urban Research Group (1973).

Chamberlain, P. and Landurand, P. "Practical Considerations—In the Assessment of Bilingual Students." In E.V. Hamayan and J.S. Damico (Eds.), *Limiting Bias in the Assessment of Bilingual Students.* Austin, TX: Pro-Ed (1990).

Chomsky, N. *Syntactic Structures.* The Hague: Mouton (1957).

Clark, J.G. "Central Auditory Dysfunction in School Children: Compilation Suggestions." *Language, Speech, and Hearing Services in Schools* (1980)a.

Clark, J.G. *Audiology for the School Speech-Language Clinician.* Springfield, IL: Charles C. Thomas, Publisher (1980)b.

Clausen, R., Corley-Keith, M., Gould, N.C., and Lebowitz, S. *Preparing for a Due Process Hearing.* Montgomery County Schools, Rockville, Maryland. Presentation at the American Speech-Language-Hearing Association Convention, Boston, MA (1988).

Connell, P.J., Spradlin, J.E., and McReynolds, L.V. "Some Suggested Critical Evaluation of Language Programs." *Journal of Speech and Hearing Disorders* 42 (1977): 563–67.

Costello, J., and Schoen, J. "The Effectiveness of Paraprofessionals and a Speech Clinician as Agents of Articulation Intervention Using Programmed Instruction." *Language, Speech, and Hearing Services in Schools* 9 (1978): 118–28.

Costello, M.R. and Curtis, R. "The Early Years: History of the Michigan Speech, Language and Hearing Association." *MSHA Journal* 23 (1989): 20.

Coventry, W.F., and Burstiner, I. *Management: A Basic Handbook.* Englewood Cliffs: NJ: Prentice-Hall, Inc. (1977).

Crabtree, M., and Peterson, E. "The Speech Pathologist as a Resource Teacher for Language/Learning Disabilities." *Language, Speech and Hearing Services in Schools* 5 (4) (October 1974): 194–97.

Crais, E.R. "Moving from "Parent Involvement" to Family-Centered Services." *American Journal of Speech-Language Pathology* 1 (1) (1991): 5–8.

Cummins, J.P. *Bilingualism and Special Education: Issues in Assessment and Pedagogy.* San Diego: College-Hill Press (1984).

Damico, J.S. and Nye, C. "Collaborative Issues in Multicultural Populations." In W.A. Secord and E.H. Wiig (Eds.), *Best Practices in School Speech-Language Pathology— Collaborative Programs in the Schools: Concepts, Models, and Procedures.* San Antonio, TX: The Psychological Corporation (1990).

Donnelly, C.A. *Changing Role of the Speech-Language Pathologist in the Public Schools.* Presentation at the American Speech-Language-Hearing Association Convention, San Francisco, CA (1984).

Downs, M., Mencher, G., Dahle, A., Gerber, S., Stein, L., Cherow, E., and Rubin, M. "Joint Committee on Infant Hearing: Position Statement." *Asha* 24 (1982): 1017–18.

Dublinske, S. "Children with Communication Disorders: Public Policy Issues." *Journal of Childhood Communication Disorders* 12 (2) (1989): 119–26. The Division for Children with Communication Disorders, The Council for Exceptional Children, Reston, VA.

Dublinske, S. "Preschool Programs for Children with Handicaps Ages 3–5." *Language, Speech, and Hearing Services in the Schools* 20 (2) (1989): 223.

Dublinske, S. "Collective Bargaining: What Can it Do for You?" *Asha* 28 (May 1986): 31–34.

Dublinske, S. "Special Reports: PL 94-142: Developing the Individualized Education Program (IEP)." *Asha* 20 (May 1978): 393–97.

Dublinske, S., and Healey, W.C. "PL 94-142: Questions and Answers for the Speech-Language Pathologist and Audiologist." *Asha* 20 (March 1978): 188–205.

Dublinske, S., Minor, B., Hofmeister, L., and Taliaferro, S. *School Issues: Effective Integration of Speech-Language Services into the Regular Classroom.* Asha Teleconference Seminar. Rockville, MD: The American Speech-Language-Hearing Association (1988).

Dunn, H.M. "A Speech and Hearing Program for Children in a Rural Area." *Journal of Speech and Hearing Disorders* 14 (June 1949): 166–70.

Dustrude, S.R. "Thoughts of a Speech-Language Pathologist: An Inside Perspective." *Computer Users in Speech and Hearing* 6 (1) (May 1990): 46–49.

Eger, D. *Indirect Services/Classroom Speeches and Language Programs.* ASHA Teleconference on Service Delivery in Schools. Rockville, MD: The American Speech-Language-Hearing Association (1988).

Eger, D.L., Chabon, S.S., Mient, M.G., Moreau, V.K. *The School Caseload Ain't What it Used to Be.* Presentation at the Annual Convention of The American Speech-Language-Hearing Association, Boston, MA (1985).

Eger, D., Adamczyk, D., Baker, A., Ekin, M.A., Hartman, K., Klein, D., Levy, M., Matta, C., Miller, R., Nalitz, N., Proto, J., Tempalski, D., Veraldi, J., Vukas, C., and Wood, M. "Planned Courses: Speech and Language Program." *Exceptional Children's Program*, Allegheny Intermediate Unit. Pittsburgh, PA (1990): ii.

Engnoth, G. "Public School Speech-Language-Hearing Administration." In Oyer, H. (Ed.), *Administration of Programs in Speech-Language Pathology and Audiology.* Englewood Cliffs, NJ: Prentice-Hall, Inc. (1987).

Erlbaum, S.J. "A Comprehensive PEL-IEP Speech Curriculum Overview and Related Carryover and Summary Forms Designed for Speech Therapy Services for the Hearing-Impaired." *Language, Speech, and Hearing Services in Schools* 21 (4) (1990): 196–204.

Finn, M.S., and Gardner, J.B. *Teacher Interview—A Better Speech-Language Screening Technique.* Area Education Agency AEA XI Ankeny, Iowa and Des Moines Public Schools. Presentation at the American Speech-Language-Hearing Association Convention, San Francisco, CA (1984).

Fisher, L.J. "An Open Letter to ASHA Members Employed in the Schools." *Language, Speech, and Hearing Services in Schools* 8 (April 1977): 72–75.

Flexer, C. *Facilitating Listening and Hearing in Infants and Young Children.* San Diego, CA: Singular Press (On Press).

Flexer, C. "Management of Hearing in an Educational Setting." In J.G. Alpiner and P.A. McCarthy, *Rehabilitation Audiology: Children and Adults (2nd ed.).* Baltimore, MD: Williams & Wilkins, Inc. (1992).

Flexer, C. "Access to Communication Environments through Assistive Listening Devices." *Hearsay: The Journal of the Ohio Speech and Hearing Association* 6 (1) (1991): 9–14.

Flexer, C. "Turn on Sound: An Odyssey of Sound Field Amplification." *Educational Audiology Association Newsletter* 5 (1989): 6–7.

Flexer, C. "Neglected Issues in Educational Audiology." *Journal of The Aural Rehabilitation Association* 22 (1989): 61–66.

Flexer, C., Baumgarner, H., and Wilcox, M.J. "Children with Sensory Impairment Series: Guidelines for Determining Functional Hearing in School-Based Settings." U.S. Department of Education, OSERS Deaf/Blind Communication Grant #G008730412 (1990).

Flexer, C., Millin, J.P., and Brown, L. "Children with Developmental Disabilities: The Effect of Sound Field Amplification on Word Identification." *Language, Speech, and Hearing Services in the Schools* 21 (1990): 177–82.

Flexer, C., Wray, D., Ireland, J. "Preferential Seating is NOT Enough: Issues in Classroom Management of Hearing-Impaired Students." *Language, Speech, and Hearing Services in Schools* 20 (1989): 11–21.

Flower, R.M. *Delivery of Speech-Language Pathology and Audiology Services.* Baltimore, MD: Williams and Wilkins (1984).

Fluharty, Nancy B. *Fluharty Speech-Language Screening Test.* Allen, Texas: DLM-Teaching Resources, 1978.

Frattali, C.M. "How to Establish a Quality Improvement Process: A Ten-Step Model." *Hearsay: The Journal of the Ohio Speech and Hearing Association* (On Press).

Frattali, C.M. "From Quality Assurance to Total Quality Management." *American Journal of Audiology* 1 (1) (1991): 41–47.

Frattali, C.M. "Quality Assurance Today: Learning the Basics." Adapted from Fratelli, C. "Are We Reaching Our Goals?: Developing Outcome Measures." In P. Larkins (Ed.), *In Search of Quality Assurance: What Lies Ahead?* Rockville, MD: American Speech-Language-Hearing Association (Workshop manual) (May 1986): *Asha* 32 (1) (1990): 39–40.

Freeman, G.C. "The Speech Clinician as a Consultant." *Clinician Speech in the Schools.* Roland J. Van Hattum (Ed.). Springfield IL: Charles C. Thomas, Pub. (1969).

Freeman, G.C. *Speech and Language Services and the Classroom Teacher.* Reston, VA: The Council for Exceptional Children (1969).

Fujiki, M., and Brinton, B. "Supplementing Language Therapy: Working with the Classroom Teacher." *Language Speech and Hearing Services in Schools* 15 (2) (April 1984): 98–109.

Galloway, H.F., and Blue, C.M. "Paraprofessionals in Articulation Therapy." *Language, Speech and Hearing Services in Schools* 6 (July 1975): 125–30.

Garrison, G. *et al.* "Speech Improvement." *Journal of Speech and Hearing Disorders,* Monograph supplement 8 (June 1961): 80.

Gillette, Y. and Robinson, J. "The Individualized Family Service Plan: A Systematic Approach." From *The CATCH Guide to Planning Services with Families: Coordinated Transition from the Hospital to the Community and Home* (1992).

Goldman, R. and Fristoe, M. *Goldman-Fristoe Test for Articulation.* Circle Pines, MN: American Guidance Service, Inc. (1971).

Gruenewald, L.J., and Pollak, S.A. "The Speech Clinician's Role in Auditory Learning and Reading Readiness." *Language, Speech and Hearing Services in Schools* 4 (July 1973): 120–26.

Haelsig, P. and Madison, C. "A Study of Phonoological Processes Exhibited by 3-, 4-, and 5-year-old Children." *Language, Speech and Hearing Services in Schools* 17 (2) (April 1986): 107–14.

Haines, H.H. "Trends in Public School Therapy." *Asha,* 7 (June 1965): 166–70.

Hammill, D.D., Brown, V.L., Larsen, S.C., and Wiederholt, J.L. *Test of Adolescent Language: A Multidimensional Approach to Assessment.* Austin, TX: Pro-Ed. (1982).

Hanson, M.J., Lynch, E.W., and Wayman, K.I. "Honoring the Cultural Diversity of Families When Gathering Data." *Topics in Early Childhood Special Education* 10 (1) (1990): 112–31.

Harris, G. "Considerations in Assessing English Language Performance of Native American Children." *Topics in Language Disorders* 5 (September 1985).

Healey, W.C. "Notes from the Associate Secretary for School Affairs, Task Force Report on Data Collection and Information Systems." *Language, Speech and Hearing Services in Schools,* 4 (2) (April 1973): 57–65.

Henoch, M.A., Scott, B.L., and Balentine, B. "Voice Interactive Computer-Assisted Therapy." *Texas Journal of Audiology and Speech Pathology* XII (2) (1986): 10–12.

Hess, R. "Guidelines for a Cooperating Clinician in Working with a Student Clinician in the Schools." *Ohio Journal of Speech and Hearing* 11 (Spring 1976): 83–89.

Hodson, B. and Paden, E. "Phonological Processes which Characterize Unintelligible and Intelligible Speech in Early Childhood." *Journal of Speech and Hearing Disorders* (1981): 369–73.

Hodson, B. *The Assessment of Phonological Processes.* Austin, TX: Pro-Ed., Inc. (1986).

Holzhauser-Peters, L. and Husemann, D.A. *Alternative Service Delivery Models for More Efficient and Effective Treatment Programs.* Alexandria, VA: The Clinical Connection (1988).

Hoskins, Barbara. "Collaborative Consultation: Designing the Role of the Speech-Language Pathologist in a New Educational Context." In W. Secord & E. Wiig (Eds.), *Best Practices in Speech-Language Pathology. Collaborative Programs in the Schools: Concepts, Models, Procedures.* San Antonio, TX: Psychological Corporation (1990).

Houle, G.R. "Computer Usage by Speech-Language Pathologists in Public Schools." *Language, Speech, and Hearing Services in Schools* 19 (3) (October 1988): 423–27.

Howerton, G.E. "What Can Be Done About Substandard Space for Speech Correction

Programs." *Language, Speech and Hearing Services in the Schools* 4 (April 1973): 95–96.

Hull, F.M., *et al. National Speech and Hearing Survey Interim Report.* Project No. 50978. Washington, D.C.: Department of Health, Education and Welfare, Office of Education, Bureau of Education for the Handicapped (1964).

Hyman, C.S. "Computer Usage in the Speech-Language-Hearing Profession." *Asha* 27 (November 1985): 25.

Hyman, C.S. "PL 94-142 in Review." *Asha* 8 (August 1985): 37.

Idol, L., Paolucci-Whitcomb, P., and Nevin, A. Collaborative Consultation. Rockville, MD (1986).

Iglesias, A. "The Different Elephant." *Asha* 27 (June 1985): 42–42.

Irwin, R.B. "Speech Therapy in the Public Schools: State Legislation and Certification." *Journal of Speech and Hearing Disorders* 24 (May 1959): 127.

Irwin, R.B. "Speech and Hearing Therapy in the Public Schools of Ohio." *Journal of Speech and Hearing Disorders* 14 (March 1949): 63–69.

Jackson, P. "Akron Public Schools Speech-Language Priority Rating and Eligibility Service Scale." *HEARSAY: The Journal of the Ohio Speech and Hearing Association* (1986): 55–58.

Jeffrey, R. and Freilinger, J.J. (Eds.). *Iowa's Severity Rating Scales for Speech and Language Impairments.* Austin, TX: Pro-Ed. (1986).

Jelinek, J.S. "A Pilot Program for Training and Utilization of Paraprofessionals in Pre-schools." *Language, Speech and Hearing Services in Schools* 7 (April 1976): 119–23.

Jerger, J. (Ed.) *Pediatric Audiology.* San Diego: College-Hill Press (1984).

Jimenez, B., and Iseyama, D. "A Model for Training and Using Communication Assistants." *Language, Speech, and Hearing Services in Schools* 18 (2) (April 1987): 168–71.

Johns, E.L. "Teacher Organization and the School Clinician." *Language, Speech and Hearing Services in Schools* 5 (July 1974): 73.

Johnson, A., Prudhomme, M., and Rogero, E. "Competency-based Objectives for the Student Teaching Experience." *Language, Speech and Hearing Services in Schools* 13 (July 1982): 187–96.

Jones, S.A., and Healey, W.C. *Essentials of Program Planning, Development, Management, Evaluation: A Manual for School Speech, Hearing and Language Problems.* Washington D.C.: American Speech and Hearing Association (1973).

Jones, S.A., and Healey, W.C. *Project UPGRADE: Guidelines for Evaluating State Education Laws and Regulations.* Washington D.C.: American Speech and Hearing Association (1975).

Khan, L.M.L. and Lewis, N.P. *The Khan-Lewis Phonological Analysis (KLFA),* Circle Pines, MN: American Guidance Services (1986).

King, R., Jones, C. and Lasky, E. "In Retrospect: A Fifteen-Year Follow-Up Report of Speech-Language-Disordered Children." *Language Speech and Hearing Services in Schools* 13 (January 1982): 24–32.

Kreb, R. *Third Party Payment for Funding Special Education and Related Services.* Horsham, PA: LRP Publications (1991).

Kroll, J. *Job Search: A Guide for Success in the Job Market.* Bowling Green, Ohio: Bowling Green State University (1985).

Krueger, B. "Computerized Reporting in a Public School Program." *Language Speech and Hearing Services in Schools* 16 (April 1985): 135–39.

Kulpa, J.I., Blackstone, S., Clarke, C.C., Collignon, M.M., Griffin, E.B., Hutchins, B.F., Jernigan, L.R., Mellott, K.E., Rao, P.R., Frattali, C.M. and Seymour, C.M. "Chronic Communicable Diseases and Risk Management in the Schools." *Language, Speech, and Hearing Services in the Schools* 22 (1991): 345–52.

Lass, N.J., Carlin, M.F., Woodford, C.M., Campanelli-Humphreys, A.L., Judy, J.M., and Hushion-Stemple, E.A. "A Survey of Classroom Teachers and Special Educators' Knowledge and Exposure to Hearing Loss." *Language, Speech, and Hearing Services in Schools* 16 (1985): 211–17.

Lastohkein, T., Glay-Moon, C., and Blosser, J. "Improving Collaborative Efforts Through the QI Process." *HEARSAY, The Journal of The Ohio Speech and Hearing Association* 7 (1) (1992): 19–22.

Lawrence, C., Katz, K., and Linville, J. "Ages of Phonological Process Suppression: A Clinical Assessment Tool." Poster session presented at The American Speech-Language-Hearing Association Annual Convention. Atlanta, GA (1991).

Leavitt, R.J. "Promoting the Use of Rehabilitation Technology." *Asha* 29 (4) (April 1987): 28–31.

Leith, W.R. *Handbook of Clinical Methods in Communication Disorders.* Austin, TX: Pro-Ed. (1984).

Lesner, S.A. "A Practical Update in Amplification for Speech-Language Pathologists." Miniseminar at the Annual Convention of the Ohio Speech and Hearing Association, Akron, OH (1991).

Listen Foundation. "Five Options for Teaching Deaf and Hearing-Impaired Children." *The Listener.* Englewood, CO: The Listen Foundation, Inc. (1991).

Luterman, D.M. *Counseling the Communicatively Disordered and Their Families.* Austin, TX: Pro-Ed. (1991).

Lynch, C. "1988 Policy Issues and Activities in the States." *Asha* 30 (12) (December 1988): 45–48.

Lynch, J. "Operation: Moving Ahead." *Language, Speech and Hearing Services in Schools* 3 (October 1972): 82–87.

Maclearie, E., and Gross, F.P. *Experimental Programs for Intensive Cycle Scheduling of Speech and Hearing Therapy Classes.* Columbus: Ohio Department of Education (1966).

Martin, E.W. "The Right to Education: Issues Facing the Speech and Hearing Profession." *Asha,* 17, no. 6 (June 1975): 384–87.

McCandless, G.A. "Screening for Middle Ear Disease on the Wind River Indian Reservation." *Hearing Instruments* (April 1975): 19–20.

McDonald, E. *A Deep Test of Articulation.* Pittsburg: Stanwix House (1964).

Marvin, C.A. Problems in school-based speech-language consultation and collaboration services: Defining the terms and improving the process. In W.A. Secord and E.H. Wiig (Eds.) *Best Practices in School Speech-Language Pathology. Collaborative Programs in the Schools: Concepts, Models, and Procedures,* San Antonio, TX: The Psychological Corporation (1990): 37–48.

Matkin, N. Educational Audiology Association. Membership application brochure (1992).

Matthews, E.C., Moore, K.A., and Harris, A. *Comparison of Screening Versus Teacher Referral in the Secondary Schools.* Phoenix High School District, Arizona presentation at the American Speech-Language-Hearing Association Convention, San Francisco, CA (1984).

Mechan, M., Jex, J.L., and Jones, J.D. *Utah Test of Language Development,* rev. ed. Salt Lake City, Utah: Communication Research Associates (1978).

Melnick, W., Eagles, E.L., and Levine, H.S. "Evaluation of a Recommended Program of Identification Audiometry with School-Age Children." *Journal of Speech and Hearing Disorders* 29 (February 1964): 3–13.

Moncur, J.P. *Institute on the Utilization of Supportive Personnel in School Speech and Hearing Programs.* Washington D.C.: American Speech and Hearing Association (1967).

Montgomery, J.K. "Building Administrative Support for Collaboration." In W.A. Secord and E.H. Wiig (Eds.), *Best Practices in School Speech-Language Pathology. Collaborative*

Programs in the Schools: Concepts, Models, and Procedures. San Antonio, TX: The Psychological Corporation (1990): 75–79.

Montgomery, J. *Handbook on Speech, Language, Services and Models.* Sacramento, CA: California State Department of Education (1988).

Moore, G.P. and Kester, D. "Historical Notes on Speech Correction in the Preassociation Era." *Journal of Speech and Hearing Disorders* 18 (March 1953): 48–53.

Moursund, J. *The Process of Counseling and Therapy.* (2nd ed.). Englewood Cliffs, NJ: Prentice-Hall, Inc. (1990).

National Joint Committee for the Communicative Needs of Persons with Severe Disabilities. "Guidelines for Meeting the Communication Needs of Persons with Severe Disabilities." *Asha* 34 (March, Supp. 7) (1992): 1–8.

Neal, W.R., Jr. "Speech Pathology Services in the Secondary Schools." *Language, Speech and Hearing Services in Schools* 7 (January 1976): 6–16.

Neidecker, E.A. "Supervision in the School Clinician Practicum Situation: Roles and Responsibilities." *Ohio Journal of Speech and Hearing* 10 (Spring 1976): 83–89.

Nelson, N.W. "Only Relevant Practices Can Be Best." In W.A. Secord and E.H. Wiig (Eds.) *Best Practices in School Speech-Language Pathology. Collaborative Programs in the Schools: Concepts, Models, and Procedures.* (1990): 15–28.

Northwest Ohio Special Education Regional Resource Center. *Operation and Management Plan for the NEOSERRC.* Bowling Green, OH (1983).

Northcott, W.H. "The Hearing-Impaired Child: A Speech Clinician as an Interdisciplinary Team Member." *Language, Speech and Hearing Services in Schools* 3 (April 1972): 7–19.

Northern, J.L. and Downs, M.P. *Hearing in Children* (4th ed.). Baltimore: Williams & Wilkins Company (1991).

Norris, J.A. and Damico, J.S. "Whole Language in Theory and Practice: Implications for Language Intervention." *Language, Speech, and Hearing Services in Schools* 21 (4) (1990): 212–20.

O'Brien, M. "Third Party Billing for School Services: The School's Perspective." *Asha* 33 (1991): 43–45

O'Connor, L. and Eldredge, P. *Communication Disorders in Adolescence.* Springfield, IL: Charles C. Thomas, Publisher (1981).

Ohio Department of Education, Division of Special Education, Statewide Language Task Force. *Ohio Handbook for the Identification, Evaluation, and Placement of Children with Language Problems.* Columbus, OH: Ohio Department of Education (1991).

Ohio Department of Health Hearing Advisory Committee. *Policies for Hearing Conservation Programs for Children: Requirements and Recommendations.* Columbus, OH: Ohio Department of Health (1990).

Ohio School Speech and Hearing Services. Worthington, Ohio: Ohio Division of Special Education (1972).

Operation and Management Plan for the Northwest Ohio Special Education Regional Resource Center, Revised. Northwest Ohio Special Education Regional Resource Center, 10142 Dowling Road, Route 2, Bowling Green, Ohio 43402 (August 1 1983).

O'Toole, T.J. "Accountability and the Clinician in the Schools." *Speech and Hearing Service in Schools* 3 (1971): 24–25.

O'Toole, T. and Zaslow, E. "Public School Speech and Hearing Programs: Things are Changing." *Asha* 11 (November 1969): 499–501.

Paden, E.P. *A History of the American Speech and Hearing Association 1925–1958.* Washington D.C.: American Speech and Hearing Association (1970).

Parker, B.L. "The Speech and Language Clincian on a Learning Center Team." *Language, Speech and Hearing Services in Schools,* 3 (3) (July 1972): 18–23.

Pascu-Godwin, V. *Lesson Plans for Communicative Disorders.* Unpublished. Akron, OH (1992).

Paul-Brown, D. *Communication Problems of Adolescents: Identification, Impact, Intervention.* Presentation to the New York Branch of the Orton Dyslexia Society Annual Conference (1991).

Paul, R. "Increasing Computer Literacy in Speech-Language Pathology Students." *Asha* 32 (4) (April 1990): 57–61.

Pendergast, K., Dickey, S., Selmar, J., and Soder, A. *Photo Articulation Test.* Danville, IL: The Interstate Printers and Publishers (1966).

Pennsylvania Speech-Language-Hearing Association Ad Hoc Committee on Issues in the Schools. (1989). Recommendations for speech-language services in the schools.

Peters-Johnson, C. "Medicaid and Third-party Reimbursement for Schools." *Language, Speech, and Hearing Services in the Schools* 21 (2) (1990): 121.

Peterson, H.A. and Marquardt, T.P. *Appraisal and Diagnosis of Speech and Language Disorders.* Englewood Cliffs, NJ: Prentice-Hall, Inc. (1990).

Phelps, R., Koenigsknect, R.A. "Attitudes of Classroom Teachers, Learning Disabilities Specialists and School Principles Toward Speech and Language Programs in Public Elementary Schools." *Language, Speech and Hearing Services in Schools* 8 (January 1977): 33–42.

Phillips, P. *Speech and Hearing Problems in the Classroom.* Lincoln, Nebraska: Cliff Notes, Inc. (1975).

Phillips, P. "Variables Affecting Classroom Teachers' Understanding of Speech Disorders." *Language, Speech and Hearing Services in the Schools* 8 (July 1976): 142–49.

Pickering, M. and Dopheide, W.F. "Training Aides to Screen Children for Speech and Language Problems." *Language, Speech, and Hearing Services in Schools* 7 (October 1976): 236–41.

Prather, E.M., Breneer, A. and Hughes, K. "A Mini-screening Test for Adolescents." *Language, Speech and Hearing Services in Schools* 12 (April 1981): 67–73.

Prentke-Romich. *How to Obtain Funding for Augmentative Communication Devices.* Wooster, Ohio: Prentke Romich Company (1989).

Ptacek, P. "Supportive Personnel as an Extension of the Professional Worker's Nervous System." *Asha* 9 (September 1967): 403–05.

Rap. "P.L. 99-457." *Monthly Resource.* Great Lakes Resource Access Project. Vol. 1, Issue 3 (1986).

Raph, J.B. "Determinants of Motivation in Speech Therapy." *Journal of Speech and Hearing Disorders,* 25 (1) (February 1960).

Rebore, R.W., SR. *A Handbook for School Board Members.* Englewood Cliffs, New Jersey: Prentice Hall, Inc. (1984).

Reed, V.A. and Miles, M.C. *Adolescent Language Disorders: A Video Inservice for Educators.* Eau Claire, WI: Thinking Publications (1989).

Reynolds, M.C. and Rosen, S.W. "Special Education: Past, Present, and Future." *The Educational Forum* 40 (May 1976): 551–62.

Rodgers, W.C. *Picture Articulation and Language Screening Test.* Salt Lake City, Utah: Word-Making Productions (1976).

Rollins, W.J. *The Psychology of Communication Disorders in Individuals and Their Families.* Englewood Cliffs, NJ: Prentice Hall, Inc. (1987).

Rules for the Education of Handicapped Children, Worthingon: Ohio Department of Education, Division of Special Education (1982).

Ross, M., Bracket, D., and Maxon, A. *Hard of Hearing Children in Regular Schools.* Englewood Cliffs, New Jersey: Prentice Hall, Inc. (1982).

Ross, M. and Giolas, T.G. (Eds). *Auditory Management of Hearing-Impaired Children.* Baltimore, MD: University Park Press (1978).

Savage, R. "Identification, Classification, and Placement Issues for Students with Traumatic Brain Injury." In J. Blosser and R. DePompei (Eds.) *Journal of Head Trauma Rehabilitation: School Reentry Following Head Injury*, 6 (1): 1–9.

Sarnecky, E. "Skills." *Asha* 2 (9) (September 1987): 35.

Scalero, A.M. and Eskenazi, C. "The Use of Supportive Personnel in a Public School Speech and Hearing Program." *Language, Speech and Hearing Services in Schools* 7 (July 1976): 150–58.

Scarvel, L.D. "Standardizing Criteria for Evaluating Physical Facilities and Organizational Patterns of Speech, Language and Hearing Programs." *The Journal of the Pennsylvania Speech and Hearing Association* 10 (June 1977): 17–19.

Schetz, K.F. "Computer Technology in Schools: Insights on the Future." *Computer Users in Speech and Hearing* 6 (1) (May 1990): 39–41.

Schoolfield, L. *Better Speech and Better Reading*. Magnolia, Massachusetts: The Expression Company (1937).

Seaton, W. *Managing Information in Communication Sciences and Disorders with Appleworks Software*. Hudson, Ohio: Seaton and Sibs (1991).

Sherr, R. Meeting to develop the individualized education program. *A Primer on Individualized Education Programs for Handicapped Children*. Ed. Scottie Torres. Reston, Virginia: The Foundation for Exceptional Children (1977).

Shewan, C.M. "ASHA Data: Speech-Language Pathologists in the Schools." *Asha* 31 (1) (1989): 56.

Shrewsbury, R.G., Lass, N.J. and Joseph, L.S. "A Survey of Special Educators' Awareness of, Experiences with, and Attitudes Toward Nonverbal Communication Aids in the Schools." *Language, Speech, and Hearing Services in the Schools* 16 (1985): 293–98.

Silverman, F.H. *Communication for the Speechless*. Englewood Cliffs, N.J.: Prentice Hall, Inc. (1989).

Simon, C.S. "A Profession in Transition: Thoughts on the Speech-Language Pathologist as a "School Language Specialist." *National Student Language Hearing Association Journal* 18 (1991): 26–33.

Simon, C.S. "Out of the Broom Closet and into the Classroom: The Emerging SLP." *Journal of Childhood Communication Disorders* 2 (1) (1987): 41–46.

Skinner, M.W. "The Hearing of Speech During Language Acquisition." *Otolaryngological Clinics North America* 11 (1978): 631–50.

Smith, J., Carter, M. and Gilder, G. "Trends in Time Allocations for the School Speech-Language Pathologist: A Need for Change." *HEARSAY: Journal of the Ohio Speech and Hearing Association* (Spring 1988): 45–48.

Sommers, R.K. Case finding, case selection, case load. *Clinical Speech in the Schools*. Ed. Rolland Van Hattum. Springfield, Illinois: Charles C. Thomas Publisher (1969).

Speech and Hearing Association of Alabama. School Affairs Committee. Recommended guidelines for physical facilities for the provision of speech-language services in the schools (1990).

Stark County and Cincinnati, Ohio Speech-Language Clinicians. *The IEP Generator Computer Program*. Canton, OH (1992).

Steer, M.D. and Drexler, H.G. "Predicting Later Articulation Abilities from Kindergarten Tests." *Journal of Speech and Hearing Disorders* 25 (November 1960): 391–97.

Steer, M.D. "Public School Speech and Hearing Services. A Special Report Prepared with Support of the United States Office of Education and Purdue University. *Journal of Speech and Hearing Disorders, Monograph Supplement 8* (July 1961): Washington, D.C.: U.S. Office of Education Cooperative Research Project No. 649 (8191).

Stephens, I. *The Stephens Oral Language Screening Test*. Peninsula, Ohio: Interim Publishers (1977).

Stimson, E. "Groping or Grouping: How to Reach the Individual." *Kappa Delta Pi Record* 16 (December 1979): 51–53.

Strong, B. "Public School Speech Technicians in Minnesota." *Language, Speech and Hearing Services in Schools,* 3 (1) (January 1972): 53–56.

Sudler, W.H. and Flexer, C. "Low Cost Assistive Listening Device." *Language, Speech, and Hearing Services in the Schools* 17 (October 1986): 342–43.

Swift, W.B. "How to Begin Speech Correction in the Public Schools." *Language, Speech and Hearing Services in Schools* 3 (April 1972): 51–56.

Templin, M. and Darley, F. *Templin-Darley Tests of Articulation, 2nd ed.* Iowa City, Iowa: Bureau of Educational Research and Services (1969).

Terrell, B.Y. and Hale, J.E. "Serving a Multicultural Population: Different Learning Styles." *American Journal of Speech-Language Pathology* 1 (2) (1992): 5–8.

Townsend, D. "Audiology in the Educational Setting." *Topics in Childhood Communication Disorders* 1 (December 1982): 12–14.

U.S. Department of Education. *Public Law 99-457. Education of the Handicapped Act Amendments of 1986, Title I, Handicapped Infants and Toddlers,* Washington, D.C., House Congressional Record (1986).

U.S. Department of Education. *Thirteenth Annual Report to Congress on the Implementation of The Individuals with Disabilities Education Act.* Washington, D.C.: U.S. Department of Education, Office of Special Education Programs (1991).

U.S. Department of Labor. *Dictionary of Occupational Titles.* Washington, D.C.: United States Government Printing Office (1979).

Vanderheiden, G.C. and Lloyd, L.L. "Communication Systems and Their Components." In S.W. Blackstone and D.M. Bruskin (Eds.), *Augmentative Communication: An Introduction* (1986): 49–161. Rockville, MD: The American Speech-Language-Hearing Association.

Vanderheiden, G.C. and Yoder, D.E. "Overview." In S.W. Blackstone and D.M. Bruskin (Eds.), *Augmentative Communication: An Introduction* (1986): 1–28. Rockville, MD: The American Speech-Language-Hearing Association.

Van Riper, C. and Erickson, R.L. *Predictive Screening Test of Articulation, 3rd ed.* Kalamazoo: Continuing Education Office, Western Michigan University (1973).

VanTasell, D.J., Mellinger, C.A. and Crump, E.S. "Functional Gain and Speech Recognition with Two Types of FM Amplification." *Language, Speech, and Hearing Services in Schools* 17 (1) (1986): 28–37.

Wall, L., Naples, G., Buhrer, K. and Capodanno, C. "A Survey of Audiological Services within the School System." *Asha* 27 (1985): 31–34.

Weinberger, H. (Ed.). *The BGSU University Supervisor.* Bowling Green, OH: Office of Field Experiences, College of Education and Allied Professions, Bowling Green State University (1990).

Weiner, F. and Wacker, R. "The Development of Phonology in Unintelligible Speakers." In N. Lass (Ed.), *Speech Advances in Basic Research and Practice* 8 (1982) 51–125. New York: Academic Press.

Westman, M.J. and Broen, P.A. "Preschool Screening for Predictive Articulation Errors." *Language, Speech, and Hearing Services in the Schools* 20 (1989): 139–48.

Wiig, K., Secord, W.A. and Wigg, E.H. "Deming Goes to School: Developing Total Quality Services in Speech-Language Pathology." In W.A. Secord and E.H. Wiig (Eds.), *Best Practices in School Speech-Language Pathology. Collaborative Programs in the Schools: Concepts, Models, and Procedures.* San Antonio, TX: The Psychological Corporation (1990).

Wilson, C.C., Lanza, J.R. and Evans, J.S. *The IEP Companion.* East Moline, IL: LinguiSystems, Inc. (1992).

Wilson-Vlotman, A.L. and Blair, J.C. *Educational Audiologists Working in Regular Schools:*

Practices, Problems and Directions. Utah State University, Logan, Utah. Presentation at the American Speech-Language-Hearing Association Convention, San Francisco, CA (1984).

Wing, D.M. "A Data Recording Form for Case Management and Accountability." *Language, Speech and Hearing Services in Schools* 6 (January 1975): 38–40.

Winton, P. "A Systematic Approach to Inservice Training Related to P.L. 99-457." *Infants and Young Children*, 3 (1990): 51–60.

Work, R.S. "Statewide Eligibility Criteria for Programs for the Speech and Language Impaired of Florida." *Tejas* XV (1989): 33–34.

Work, R.S. "The Therapy Program." *Speech-Language Programming in the Schools, 2nd ed.,* Ed. Van Hattum, R.J. Springfield, Illinois: Charles C. Thomas Publisher (1982).

Wray, D. and Watson-Florence, W. "Consultative Model: Implementing the Language-Reading Connection in the Classroom." University of Akron, Ohio. Presentation at the American Speech-Language-Hearing Association Convention, San Francisco (1984).

Yorkston, K.M. and Karlan, G. Assessment procedures. In S.W. Blackstone and D.M. Bruskin (Eds.), *Augmentative Communication: An Introduction* (1986): 163–96. Rockville, MD: The American Speech-Language-Hearing Association.

Zimmerman, J., Steiner, V. and Evatt, R. *Preschool Language Manual.* Columbus, Ohio: Charles E. Merrill Publishing Company (1969).

Index